T0314074

Democratizing Health

Consumer Groups in the Policy Process

Edited by

Hans Löfgren

Deakin University, Australia

Evelyne de Leeuw

Deakin University, Australia

Michael Leahy

Deakin University, Australia

Edward Elgar

Cheltenham, UK • Northampton, MA, USA

Published by
Edward Elgar Publishing Limited
The Lypiatts
15 Lansdown Road
Cheltenham
Glos GL50 2JA
UK

Edward Elgar Publishing, Inc.
William Pratt House
9 Dewey Court
Northampton
Massachusetts 01060
USA

A catalogue record for this book
is available from the British Library

Library of Congress Control Number: 2010939201

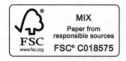

ISBN 978 1 84844 784 4

Typeset by Cambrian Typesetters, Camberley, Surrey
Printed and bound by MPG Books Group, UK

Contents

Figures, tables and boxes

FIGURES

TABLES

BOXES

Contributors

Karen Adams is Research Team Leader at the Victorian Aboriginal Community Controlled Health Organisation and Senior Research Fellow, Victoria University, Melbourne, VIC, Australia.

Wendy Armstrong has been affiliated with consumer organizations in Canada for more than twenty years.

Rob Baggott is Professor of Public Policy and Director of the Health Policy Research Unit, De Montfort University, Leicester, UK.

Roland Bal is Professor of Healthcare Governance in the Institute of Health Policy and Management, Erasmus University Rotterdam, the Netherlands.

Simon Barraclough teaches health policy and international health relations in the School of Public Health, La Trobe University, Melbourne, VIC, Australia.

Gudrun Braunegger-Kallinger is a researcher and doctoral student in the Department of Sociology, University of Vienna, Austria.

John Church is Associate Professor at the Centre for Health Promotion Studies and Department of Political Science, University of Alberta, Edmonton, AB, Canada.

Evelyne de Leeuw is Professor and Chair, Community Health Systems and Policy, Deakin University, Geelong, VIC, Australia.

Diana Delnoij is Professor at the Scientific Centre for Transformation in Care and Welfare, Tilburg University and director of the Dutch Centre for Consumer Experience in Health Care, Utrecht, the Netherlands.

Rebecca Edwards is Senior Administrative Officer in the School of Health and Social Development, Deakin University, Melbourne, VIC, Australia.

Rudolf Forster is Professor in the Department of Sociology, University of Vienna, and a researcher in the Ludwig Boltzmann Institute for Health Promotion Research, Vienna, Austria.

Michael H. Fox is Professor in the Department of Health Policy and Management in the University of Kansas Medical Center, Kansas City, KS, USA.

Bronwyn Fredericks is Senior Research Fellow in the Faculty of Health, Queensland University of Technology and at Monash University Melbourne, VIC, Australia.

Jens Geissler is Senior Consultant on Health Policy, Health Financing and Health Insurance at Sinopsis AG, Cologne, Germany.

Prem Chandran John is Co-Chair of the People's Health Movement, Cape Town, South Africa and Vice-Chair of Health Action International, Amsterdam, the Netherlands.

Kathryn Jones is Senior Research Fellow in the Health Policy Research Unit, De Montfort University, Leicester, UK.

Phua Kai Lit is Associate Professor at the Sunway (Malaysia) Campus of the School of Medicine and Health Sciences, Monash University, Melbourne, VIC, Australia.

Meri Koivusalo is Senior Researcher in the National Institute for Health and Welfare, Helsinki, Finland.

Karl Krajic is a researcher in the Ludwig Boltzmann Institute for Health Promotion Research in Vienna and Associate Professor in the Department of Sociology, University of Vienna, Austria.

Anna Lambertson is the Interim Director of the Kansas Health Consumer Coalition, Topeka, KS, USA.

Michael Leahy teaches in the School of International and Political Studies, Deakin University, Melbourne, VIC, Australia.

David G. Legge is Associate Professor in the School of Public Health at La Trobe University, Melbourne, VIC, Australia and Global Coordinator of the International People's Health University.

Hans Löfgren is Senior Lecturer in the School of International and Political Studies, Deakin University, Melbourne, VIC, Australia.

Timothy Milewa is Lecturer in the Department of Sociology and Communications, Brunel University, London, UK.

Christina Nuñez Daw is a research analyst at CPWR-Center for Construction Research and Training, Silver Spring, MD, USA.

Orla O'Donovan is Lecturer in the School of Applied Social Studies, University College Cork, Ireland.

Atie Schipaanboord is Director of the Dutch Nurses' Association and former Director of the Dutch Patient and Consumer Association (NPCF), Utrecht, the Netherlands.

Jonathan Tritter is Professorial Fellow in the Governance and Public Management Group in Warwick Business School, Coventry, UK.

Denise Truong holds a master's degree in public health from the University of Texas Health Science Center's School of Public Health in Houston, USA.

Pauline Vaillancourt Rosenau is Professor of Management, Policy, and Community Health in the School of Public Health, University of Texas at Houston, USA.

Agnes Vitry is Senior Research Fellow at the Quality Use of Medicines and Pharmacy Research Centre, Sansom Institute, University of South Australia, Adelaide, SA, Australia.

Abbreviations

ABPI	Association of British Pharmaceutical Industry
ABS	Australian Bureau of Statistics
ACCHO	Aboriginal Community Controlled Health Organisation
ACT UP	AIDS Coalition to Unleash Power
ADA	Americans with Disability Act
AFM	Association Française contre les Myopathies
AHMAC	Australian Health Ministers' Advisory Council
AIHW	Australian Institute of Health and Welfare
ALP	Australian Labor Party
AMA	Australian Medical Association
BAG Selbsthilfe	Bundesarbeitsgemeinschaft Selbsthilfe
CADTH	Canadian Agency for Drugs and Technologies in Health
CAP	Consumers' Association of Penang
CHF	Consumers Health Forum of Australia
CHI	Citizens' Health Initiative
CIL	Center for Independent Living
COAG	Council of Australian Governments
CRCAH	Cooperative Research Centre for Aboriginal Health
DDB	Deutscher Diabetiker Bund
DDU	Deutsche Diabetes Union
DPWV	Deutscher Paritätischer Wohlfahrtsverband
EAG	Expert Advisory Group
ECJ	European Court of Justice
EFPIA	European Federation of Pharmaceutical Industries and Associations
EMA	European Medicines Agency
EPHA	European Public Health Alliance
ESRC	Economic and Social Research Council
EURORDIS	European Organisation for Rare Disorders
FDA	Food and Drug Administration
FOMCA	Federation of Malaysian Consumers' Associations
FQHC	Federally Qualified Community Health Center
GP	general practitioner
Health GAP	Health Global Access Project
HSE	Health Services Executive

IAPO	International Alliance of Patients' Organizations
INCADDS	Irish National Council of AD/HD Support Groups
JSA	Jan Swasthya Abhiyan
KMS	Koori Maternity Services
MHA	Mental Health Association
MMA	Malaysian Medical Association
MSF	Médecins Sans Frontières
NACCHO	National Aboriginal Community Controlled Health Organisation
NAHS	National Aboriginal Health Strategy
NAM	Non-Aligned Movement
NAMI	National Alliance on Mental Illness
NATSIC	National Aboriginal and Torres Strait Islander Health Council
NCCC	National Consumer Complaints Centre
NHS	National Health Service
NICE	National Institute for Health and Clinical Excellence
NORD	National Organization for Rare Disorders
NPCF	National Patient and Consumer Federation
NPM	New Public Management
PBAC	Pharmaceutical Benefits Advisory Committee
PBPA	Pharmaceutical Benefits Pricing Authority
PBS	Pharmaceutical Benefits Scheme
PCT	Primary Care Trust
PHA	People's Health Assembly
PHM	People's Health Movement
PPI	patient and public involvement
QUM	quality use of medicines
SAPRIN	Structural Adjustment Participatory Review International Network
TABD	TransAtlantic Business Dialogue
TACD	Transatlantic Consumer Dialogue
TRIPS	Trade Related Intellectual Property Rights
UAEM	Universities Alliance for Essential Medicines
UMNO	United Malays National Organization
VACCHO	Victorian Aboriginal Community Controlled Health Organisation
VACKH	Victorian Aboriginal Council on Koori Health
VHA	Veterans Health Administration

1. Introduction – consumer groups and the democratization of health policy

Michael Leahy, Hans Löfgren and Evelyne de Leeuw

This book examines the extent to which consumer groups engage in the development of policy affecting their members' health and health *care*. Such engagement may be referred to as the 'democratization of health', but, as the contributions to this book show, there are considerable differences between national contexts as to what this means, both in theory and in practice. Before summarizing those differences, however, some account of the notion of democracy and the impetus to democratize human institutions is needed.

Democracy had its origins in ancient Greece, but its modern form stems from the French Revolution. In the name of the people the French Revolution cast off the shackles of the political and ecclesiastical hierarchies and proclaimed the 'liberty', 'equality' and 'fraternity' of all.[1] In the spirit of the Enlightenment the traditional authority of divine revelation was supplanted by the authority of scientific reason and the ideal of individual liberty, as in Immanuel Kant's notion of personal autonomy. This legacy subsequently developed in two streams. One of these emphasized individual liberty, which in the political sphere was conceived in negative terms as freedom from government, and in the economic sphere as market freedom. The other stream was the socialist/collectivist one, which placed the emphasis on 'fraternity' and thus a common good to be attained by collective action. Post-Enlightenment culture enjoins the exercise of the power of reason to bring both the physical world and the social world under human dominion.

In supporting the democratization of health policy and health care, contributors to this volume are not blind to the challenges to this culture. The tension between the liberal-individualist and the collectivist streams has already been acknowledged, and is reflected in some of the chapters that follow. But some authors also acknowledge the challenge to the status of reason – to the scientific paradigm of knowledge – found in the literature of both the philosophy and the sociology of science. The case for democracy, however, and thus for the democratization of all areas of human life, including health policy and health care, is not undermined by these challenges. If science cannot deliver the certainty claimed for it in modernist thought, it can at least deliver probability; moreover, to the extent that individuals have to rely on the judgements of their own reason as a result of science's shortcomings, space is created for democratic participation in decisions around such questions. The tension between the liberal-leaning and socialist-leaning streams of democratic culture can be cause as much for the fruitful development of the culture as for its erosion.

The collapse of the Soviet empire in 1989 led many on the liberal-individualist side of politics to proclaim it as definitively discrediting socialism as an alternative form of government. The global financial crisis of 2008 has prompted others to ask whether this crisis marks the demise of the liberal-capitalist paradigm (Wade 2008). Whether one leans towards the liberal or the social stream of democracy, it is fair to observe that the credit of democracy has been enhanced not primarily by its superior efficiency as a way of governing societies, but rather by its supposed moral superiority over its rivals: it is perceived rightly or wrongly as the only form of government capable of giving due recognition to human dignity. Globalization of democracy is thus thought to have a moral justification and perhaps even to be a moral imperative. In democratic polities the aspiration to democratize all areas of social life – to enable all those affected by particular policies and practices to have a significant role in determining them – is as much a moral as a political one. The realization of these democratizing aspirations is however conditioned by other factors in the relevant social contexts, particularly their economic systems. Since health is so central to human well-being, it is somewhat surprising that the progress of and obstacles to the democratization of health policy and health care have not been more fully researched. This volume tries to fill part of that research gap by presenting snapshots of the present status of the democratizing efforts of health consumer groups in the diverse social and political contexts of several nations.

The designation of such groups as 'consumer' groups immediately raises a problem. In capitalist economies the term 'consumer' has for many come to mean a purchaser of goods and services in markets, and thus to connote the rights attendant upon that role. But this term had an ordinary-language meaning before this market sense became so dominant, and it retains sufficient currency to permit its use today in a volume like this one. Thus while in some contexts in the following chapters the term 'consumer' is used in the market sense, in others it is used in its ordinary-language sense. 'Consumer groups' thus generally means groups who are actively working for the rights of citizens in health policy and care, though in some contexts they can be groups fulfilling the role assigned to them in market exchanges.

However, this distinction is not merely semantic. As the contributions to this volume show, underlying the semantic distinction is a real difference in the understanding of the role of consumer groups in health policy and care, particularly vis-à-vis other influential stakeholders in this arena. The role aspired to by some of the groups described in these chapters is that of activism in the struggle for human rights and the deepening of democracy, in this case in health. Their aim is to achieve emancipation from the structures which restrict those rights, and their general strategy is to enlist the power of the state in a process of reform to achieve those rights. The risk they run is that, having once contributed to the election of a reformist government, they become co-opted to its processes and policies and come under pressure to compromise their critical independence (Dryzek 2002). Groups that compromise that independence beyond a certain point become in some sense co-optees of the very state and private actors whose power they were founded to challenge. The success of democratizing efforts is limited, in other words, by the powers of the dominant actors in the field of health: the providers (both state and private), and the health professionals (Alford 1975).

In recent decades a major challenge has been levelled at the power of health professionals by the implementation of neo-liberal and New Public Management (NPM) approaches to health policy and care. Governmental and other service providers have enhanced their power vis-à-vis the medical profession through these approaches, and the theory underpinning these approaches accords a role to consumers. 'Consumers' in this context means consumers in the market sense. As purchasers of health services, consumers are entitled to such things as choice of services, quality of service and the lowest possible price. Since such entitlements are in part dependent upon provider policy, this theory concedes consumers some right to input into health policy as well as into service delivery. Some of the European contributions describe efforts to develop free markets in health and obstacles to that development. For some of these European authors, efforts to democratize health mean attempts to extend the operation of markets in the health domain. For other authors, such as those from Canada and Australia, the equation of marketization with democratization is a subversion of democracy because it reduces quality and affordable health care to a purchaser's entitlement rather than any citizen's right within an organic community. These differences could obviously be explained as leanings either to the liberal-individualist or to the socialist stream of the democratic tradition, but they also surely reflect conditions imposed by different social and political contexts.

Another title advanced here to consumer authority in health is that of 'experiential knowledge'. Structural reforms of the Irish health system purporting to enable consumer participation in shaping health policy and care have persisted in privileging professional knowledge. By doing so, according to the contribution on Irish health policymaking, they have ensured the failure of such reforms because they have systematically excluded that knowledge of health and illness which only patients and their close supporters possess. Democratization of health, on this argument, will require admission of experiential knowledge of health and illness to the discourse of policy and delivery.

But if, as several contributions to this volume argue, the claims of experiential knowledge are so strong, who has the strength to resist them and what is the source of that strength? According to one contributor, resistance to the admission of experiential knowledge to health discourse stems from 'the "scientization of decision-making", and the frequent medicalization of social problems as inevitable precursors to technical rather than social solutions, many of which directly remove power from consumers' (Brown and Zavestoski, in Fox and Lambertson in this volume). But as the term 'scientization' suggests, the privileging of scientific medical knowledge has deeper and stronger roots than the process of professionalization. Those roots lie in a particular paradigm of knowledge that has dominated the sciences generally and the human sciences in particular since the scientific revolution. According to that paradigm, the only valid forms of knowledge are those attained by the empirical methods of the natural sciences. Applied to medicine, this doctrine generates what might be called the 'pathogenic' paradigm[2] of health, which conceives health in terms of its opposite – disease – and defines the discipline of medicine as identification of the causes of and cures for diseases. Challenges to this paradigm, and to the account of the human sciences underpinning it, have long been common in the philosophy and sociology of science literature (see, for example, Kuhn 1970; Lakatos 1970; Mulkay 1979; Taylor 1985), but the upshot of this controversy for contributors to this volume is that the prevailing medical dominance is the result of a political rather than an epistemological contest.

Contests of power between interest groups or stakeholders, including consumer groups, would most likely result at best in realignments of power between conflicting groups. Such realignments would not be recognized by many as democratizations. As Timothy Milewa in this volume insists, 'autonomous health activist groups' need to develop 'new ideas of democratic practice and dialogue' if the discourse of democratization 'is to be anything more than an aspirational narrative'. Since the United Kingdom has been the location of pioneering research of efforts to democratize health policy and practice, this volume begins with chapters from these researchers.

According to Timothy Milewa (Chapter 2) the debate about the consumer role in health reflects a wider debate in sociology centred on the sociology of the body. Among the key features of that debate is the uncertainty of our knowledge of all things in life generally and of health in particular. This is the 'risk society' thesis of Ulrich Beck (1998) and Anthony Giddens (2000: 38–53). Debates about equity, justice and rights in the health area, and political mobilizations to promote views on them, are to be understood, according to Milewa, in the light of this wider debate about the amount of credit to be attributed to medical science, managerial expertise and lay/experiential knowledge. The focus on the body also draws into the political debate aspects of health that would previously have been excluded as belonging to the private realm, such as sexual health. This focus also exposes examples of 'ill health' being defined by social prejudice rather than physical condition, an egregious case of which is physical disability.

Milewa concurs with Goodin in noting the crumbling hierarchical structures of power in health policy and the consequent need for more democratic alternatives: 'health activist groups are in the business of attempting to produce (or co-produce) dialogic procedures and spaces of a particular "actionable form" that points to, but does not determine roles, norms and appropriate behaviours in connection with desired outcomes' (Goodin 1996: 31). The quest by consumer groups for 'procedures and spaces' for democratic dialogue among the three alternatives that Milewa identifies – managerial, asymmetrical co-option, and emancipatory – may, he concedes, seem fanciful. However, since it is driven by consumer dissatisfaction with existing structures, he believes the quest may not be in vain. The yearning for ever more democratic procedures and spaces can be deflected in various ways, but, if Milewa is correct, it cannot be entirely suppressed, especially in societies where hierarchies are breaking down because the knowledge which formerly authorized them has now been exposed as fallible. A case in point is the weakening of the classic pathogenic or biomedical model of health, which has been subjected to paradigmatic critiques by proponents of the social model of health and 'salutogenesis' (Antonovsky 1984).

Kathryn Jones and Rob Baggott (Chapter 3) draw on a pioneering study of the influence of health consumer groups on health policy and care in the United Kingdom (Baggott et al. 2005). These authors note Milewa's acclaim of new opportunities for activism in UK health policy but point to a continuing perception of a 'democratic deficit' in the National Health Service (NHS). Their 2005 study showed that the assumption that health consumer groups were powerless was facile and that these groups had contributed to the reduction of this deficit. However, the power of these groups in the NHS has not increased, they found, in the 20 years since the inception of the policy of patient and public involvement in health care. Changes in operating conditions have contributed to this stasis in the quest for greater influence: the shift to an emphasis on individualism, devolution within the United Kingdom and the influence of the European Union (EU). National Voices, a coalition of more than 200 health consumer groups in the United Kingdom, offers some hope of increasing consumer group influence, but the authors fear it may be too close to government to provide an independent perspective. They argue that more research is needed to assess the influence of health consumer groups in this changed environment, particularly at the local level. If Milewa has indicated the directions towards which consumer groups aspire in their efforts at democratization, Jones and Baggott have produced considerable empirical evidence from the English scene at least to show how far those aspirations have been realized.

Meri Koivusalo and Jonathan Tritter (Chapter 4) address the question of how EU structures and procedures affect citizen participation in policymaking in terms of representation and democratic participation in general. Who are the consumer representatives in the democratic sense, and who in the sense of front groups or stakeholders representing particular rather than common interests; and what access to the policy processes of the EU does each group have? Institutional context greatly influences groups' potential for democratization, and the EU, these authors argue, as did Jones and Baggott in the previous chapter, exemplifies the complexity such contexts can involve. To what extent is democratization of health policy doomed to reduction to a contest between stakeholders in this context, they ask, rather than a campaign for the emancipation of consumers from the dominance of the medical and managerial professions? They conclude that a critical watch is needed over EU regulations to ensure they enhance rather than limit consumer/democratic rights.

In Chapter 5, Prem Chandran John and David Legge locate the quest for democratization of health in the ideological and historical context of the post-Enlightenment struggle to bring human destiny under 'rational democratic control'. They see a '"modernist" confidence (perhaps faith in) the possibility of rational collective control over human destiny ... [as] integral to civil society/social movement activism'. The major challenges to this modernist faith, they claim, come from 'market and religious fundamentalisms'. Markets are the mechanisms that perpetuate the economic system and enrich the few at the expense of the many, and today markets are global forces. Religious fundamentalisms see a turning to God as necessarily involving a rejection of secular rationalism. Rational democratic control over health, the authors argue, is to be sought by disempowered people collectively confronting the obstacles to it at all levels: local, regional and global. While John and Legge do not address the challenge to this modernist faith posed by the exposure of the fallibility of scientific knowledge as Milewa does, they provide an important account of a collective effort they see as flowing from that faith: the international People's Health Movement.

In Chapter 6, Bronwyn Fredericks, Karen Adams and Rebecca Edwards present an Australian Aboriginal perspective on the democratization of health. That perspective is also cast in the terms of the post-Enlightenment quest for rational control over human destiny by disempowered people. The authors' argument is that Aboriginal peoples' problems in health, like their problems in other areas, are a direct result of their disempowerment, which was caused by colonization. The solution to their health problems therefore is essentially dependent upon their re-empowerment, interpreted by these authors as taking control of their own health policy and services. They see this re-empowerment exemplified in the establishment of Aboriginal Community Controlled Health Organisations, like that established in the Australian state of Victoria. Since the rise of Aboriginal Community Controlled Health Organisations is comparatively recent, however, virtually no research into the success or otherwise of their efforts to restore power to Aboriginal peoples has yet been carried out.

In Chapter 7, Orla O'Donovan criticizes the Irish state's claims to have redressed medical and managerial hegemony in its introduction of lay representation at the health policy table. She argues that such 'invited spaces' need not be entirely rejected as sources of gain for those striving for democratization; but, most importantly, they have not constrained the democratization of health in other contexts. She points to examples of groups in Ireland that have found spaces not dominated by 'credentialized experts', and indicates other spaces for democratizing efforts such as the media, the parliament and even the streets. Moreover, she contends that the tighter the regimes dominated by the privileged knowledge of experts the surer the weaknesses of that knowledge will be exposed – weaknesses that can be attacked by democratizers. It is the emancipation of the experiential knowledge of patients and their supporters from the hegemony of the expert knowledge of the medical and managerial professionals that must, in her view, produce 'epistemological justice'. Rendering judgement on recent experiments with new forms of lay involvement on expert committees, she attributes their failure to research why such experiments had failed in the past to blind faith in expert knowledge. She points to evidence that the paradigm of expert knowledge is itself failing, for example, in mental health. If, as John and Legge claim, the quest for democratization of health is a fruit of the French Revolution and the Enlightenment, so too is the scientific paradigm of knowledge. Both Milewa and O'Donovan point to the need to reassess the latter but neither adverts to the consequences of such reassessment for the notion of 'rational control' over human affairs, the possibility of which that paradigm formerly guaranteed.

In Chapter 8, Atie Schipaanboord, Diana Delnoij and Roland Bal also plead the case for patients and their support groups to 'capitalize' their experiential knowledge so that they may use it to exercise their rights. However the context for the exercise of such rights is conceptualized by these authors as liberal society, where that philosophy is now interpreted as calling for the marketization of such goods as health care. In this context patients' rights are defined as rights to choose doctors, insurers, hospitals and the like. The problems with this paradigm of rights are the standard ones that arise with the establishment of markets anywhere, such as the asymmetry of information and lack of competition between providers. Democratization in this paradigm would amount to the strengthening of consumer power within the health market. As indicated by the authors, there are problems inherent in the application of the market model to health: difficulties in mobilizing patient choice and ensuring understanding of and access to information. But these authors argue that the failures of some existing mechanisms for mobilizing and consolidating patient involvement in health policy should lead to the design of better mechanisms rather than abandonment of the project. They recommend the use of ethnographic research techniques as one means to this end.

The Dutch contribution highlights a tension in this volume referred to earlier between conceptions of democratization. For Schipaanboord and her colleagues the marketization of health is a form of democratization. For several other contributors, however, health care is not a marketable commodity but a human right that might be undermined by marketization. Democratization in the latter case would entail abolishing the notion of health care as a commodity and reform of its structures to reflect its conception as a human right the value of which cannot be measured in monetary terms. In this perspective market-oriented reforms are viewed sceptically, and the model of health care provision in the postwar welfare states of Scandinavia, the United Kingdom and elsewhere as providing a basis for further democratization. It is of course possible that this tension reflects fundamental ideological differences in the understanding of democracy; if this is so, it will be incapable of resolution, and readers will simply have to choose which ideology they prefer. However, the tension may reflect rather the important differences in the historical, social and political contexts in which the authors are writing. In welfare systems that have become rigid in their procedures and unresponsive to consumers' needs, marketization of health may give consumers some say where previously they had little or none. Health activists might count such an achievement as the best they can do for the moment given the time and effort required to accomplish fundamental reforms.

In Chapter 9, Jens Geissler addresses the problems of governance and representativeness in the German health system. Democratization in the German context, according to Geissler, means the development of the role of consumer groups within the multiple institutional structures of health care. While these are democratic in many of their structures and procedures, this has not always meant, and still does not necessarily mean, that consumers and consumer groups have significant influence in the system. Reforms to the German system reported by Geissler have, in his estimation, at least secured consumer groups a voice that is heard in decision-making fora, and compulsory financial support from insurers. The latter provides an interesting international precedent; provision of arm's-length public funding for consumer groups along such lines could lessen the risk of such groups being drawn into the orbit of the pharmaceutical industry (see Chapter 16). Legislation has even been passed in Germany requiring that training be provided to lay members of decision-making bodies to help bridge the knowledge gap between them and professional members of such bodies. Geissler does not say whether the lay members' experiential knowledge counts for anything at the decision-making table, but he does report that 8 of 182 patient representatives on the Joint Federal Committee on health felt able to influence and support committee decisions.

Rudolf Forster, Gudrun Braunegger-Kallinger and Karl Krajic (Chapter 10) tell us that for historical reasons civil activism is underdeveloped in Austria, but is now developing. Democratization in this chapter, as in the previous one, is seen as the development of the role of consumer/patient groups within a corporate tradition of governance, both political and administrative. Thus the authors focus on strategic concepts for measuring and developing relative power within corporate systems. Here those concepts are 'conflict capability' and 'organizational capability' (Offe 1974; Geissler 2004). The authors also report their own empirical study of the role of consumer groups in Austria. Health activism, like new social movements generally, has been severely constrained in the past by Austria's 'consociationalist' form of democracy. However in the last 25 years this form of democracy has been significantly eroded by 'competition', allowing 'more pluralist modes of interest aggregation' to arise. Openings for exploitation by non-corporate interest groups, including health consumer groups, are now appearing in Austria's democracy. According to Forster and his colleagues, however, these groups need to develop the capabilities prescribed by Offe if they are to exploit these openings.

It has been taken for granted so far in this book that the political context in which the democratization of health is to take place is a Western-style liberal democratic nation, or union of nations, such as the EU. In Chapter 11, however, we are confronted with a case of the democratization of health preceding the democratization in this Western sense of the relevant nation: Malaysia. Indeed, on the evidence provided by authors Simon Barraclough and Phua Kai Lit, the achievements of Malaysian consumer groups have been considerable, particularly in the restraint they have managed to place on government neo-liberal health care reforms. If we were not already so convinced, the Malaysian example might help persuade us that there is no such thing as a perfect democracy, and that genuine democratic progress can be achieved even under relatively undemocratic conditions, whether they be authoritarian regimes or democratic ones dominated by neo-liberal and managerial approaches to health policy. These authors observe that Malaysian consumer groups lack the resources to research and disseminate consumer positions to government consultative bodies. The secrecy of government policymaking processes makes assessment of consumer group influence almost impossible. Consumer groups themselves, the authors argue, need to develop a more sophisticated knowledge of the workings of the policy process in order to engage with it effectively.

In Chapter 12, Hans Löfgren, Michael Leahy and Evelyne de Leeuw assess the democratization of health in Australia. As in other liberal polities, they observe, there has been a division in this country between those who define democracy in terms of the freedom of individuals to achieve self-sufficiency without government interference (referred to earlier as the liberal-individualist stream of the democratic tradition), and those who see it as the solidarity of citizens constituting a state in the pursuit of a common good (the collectivist stream). For the former, democratization of health has meant state support of the efforts of individuals to provide for their own health care, while for the latter democratization has meant the establishment by the state of a system of universal care. The authors note that while consumer groups had a certain incarnation in the many private health insurance cooperatives that flourished until the advent of Medibank in 1975, they were perceived as institutions supporting the dominance of the medical profession over the entire health system. Democratization of health, they argue, has thus come to be seen as the loosening of this dominance so as to universalize access to services and insurance, and particularly to ensure that formerly excluded groups have their needs met.

Consumer/activist groups played a significant role in loosening the dominance of the medical profession. But democratization, as these groups understood it, was impeded because much of the power wrested from the doctors was assumed by the state and the medical bureaucracy. Accordingly, democratization, in consumers' favoured sense of emancipation from the dominance of medical and managerial interests, and the acquisition of genuine power at the policy table, has been thus constrained. Consumer groups are now under pressure to mitigate this quest in return for a place at the table as marginalized participants. In short, the authors conclude, there is a tendency in Australia for consumer groups to be co-opted to the service of the interests of the dominant medical and managerial groups, interests which are often subordinated to the prevailing imperatives of the state. Australia, however, lacks any comprehensive and detailed study of group relations and dependencies that would enable a more definitive assessment of this tendency.

The influence on the democratization of health of neo-liberal and NPM theory is again assessed in Chapter 13, this time negatively. Democratization, as Canadian authors John Church and Wendy Armstrong conceive it, consists in restoring an 'organic' conception of citizenship in place of the 'customer' conception installed in Canada in the era of neo-liberal reform. An organic form of citizenship, they contend, will not be driven merely by individual self-interest but by a process which discerns the rights and responsibilities of citizens as members of a community. People's expectations of government will not, therefore, be able to be determined simply by surveys of individual preferences as the market paradigm suggests, but will need to be established through more deliberative processes. These authors lament the supplanting of the language of local citizen influence in health matters by that of central control under the influence of market-based theories. However, Church and Armstrong are optimistic about the prospects of a restoration of a more 'organic' relationship between government and citizens which might lead to a rollback of such neo-liberal/NPM health reforms.

The authors of the two chapters focusing on the United States agree that democratic reform there has taken the form of incremental responses to periodic clamouring by aggrieved groups of consumers for more equitable access to services. In Chapter 14 Michael H. Fox and Anna Lambertson provide an analysis of those responses. Democratization for these authors consists in the acquisition by consumer groups of some of the authority over health policy and care that is at present dominated in the United States by medical and managerial professionals. The purpose of acquiring such authority is to challenge the 'social, cultural and economic dominance' of biomedical authority. While the problem and the proposed solution to it do not differ significantly from those identified in other Western democracies, the US context, they point out, is significantly different. There is a stronger tradition of individual self-reliance and of antipathy in some quarters to the forms of 'socialized medicine' that are taken for granted in the United Kingdom and Europe. Thus private health insurance dominates the American scene, and government-funded or -subsidized provision is available only to select groups deemed eligible for such support. Despite these formidable obstacles the authors show considerable faith in the ability of the political activist tradition of US voters to achieve the redress they seek in the balance of authority in health matters.

Christina Nuñez Daw, Denise Truong and Pauline Vaillancourt Rosenau, the authors of the second chapter on the United States (Chapter 15), also contrast the US political tradition of individual self-reliance in health with UK and European traditions of collective responsibility. They accept Fox's cyclical/incremental model of the development of US health policy and predict that, while the Obama reforms offer some hope for the consumer movement, its progress will be fragmented and 'specialized': that the US individualist tradition of political activism will give rise to particular campaigns by groups focused on single issues – for example, diabetes care – rather than an organic activism. This individualist concept of democracy differs from the European and UK concepts in that it endorses the use of society to advance individual interests (demanded as a sacred right) but denies any collective responsibility for the welfare of society's members. These authors conclude that rather than advancing social solidarity, the kind of democratization implied in consumers comparing report cards on competing health services imposes unbearable cognitive burdens.

In the final chapter, Chapter 16, Agnes Vitry and Hans Löfgren report on international trends in relationships between consumer groups and the pharmaceutical industry, and on debates about them. They remark on the power asymmetries between the two parties and the potential for exploitation, particularly conflicts of interest, bound up with interdependencies between stakeholders in contemporary health policy systems. For proponents of democratization, conflicts of interest may appear as a second-order issue. It is surely of great consequence, however, that groups claiming to represent patients and their families, and often the citizen interest more broadly, should not be surreptitiously co-opted either by the short-term manoeuvrings of governments or by the powerful pharmaceutical industry. Vitry and Löfgren conclude that transparency in consumer–industry relationships is a necessary condition of consumer groups authentically advocating on behalf of their constituencies and potentially contributing to the democratization of health systems, but that it will not be a sufficient condition if such transparency simply blunts community sensitivity to conflicts of interest.

Democracy, and thus the democratization of health policy and care, is taken by all contributors to this volume to be a moral good. Different conceptions of that good are evident, however, in their contributions, or at least in the polities they describe. In the United States the aversion to what is often perceived as socialism is cause for pessimism about the prospects of consumers as citizens winning a significant say in health policy and care. Notwithstanding the robust American tradition of political agitation, it seems that the liberal-individualist ideology that is so entrenched there will always be bent to the service of the interests of the dominant actors: the medical profession and the providers. The solidaristic or collectivist understanding of the good of democracy, and thus the democratization of health policy and practice, is more widely embraced outside the United States, particularly in countries with a history of strong social democratic parties. The latter, however, are under siege from neo-liberal and NPM theory. In several nations it seems that the possibilities for democratization in the current context are limited to attaining increased rights as consumers of health services, considered as market commodities. But as several authors affirm, citizens in their nations see themselves as more than consumers in markets: they are human beings for whom health is a right demanded by their dignity. That dignity must therefore guarantee the eventual supplanting of the market conception of health consumer rights. The obstacle to the attainment of those rights, according to most contributions, is the power of the dominant actors in the health care system: the medical profession and the providers. Perhaps the most important source of this power is the very conception of reason which was supposed to be a democratizing force: scientific knowledge. The sequestering of this form of knowledge by professionals has rendered it an anti-democratic force. The greatest vulnerability of those actors who resist the democratizing efforts of health consumer groups is the discrediting of the claims of science to the status of paradigm of knowledge. Philosophers and sociologists have long exposed the inability of science to deliver the certainty promised by that status. Several contributors press the claims for accreditation of the 'experiential knowledge' of consumers and their supporters in the shaping of health policy and care. Perhaps the advancing of those claims should be a major focus of future democratization strategies and research.

ACKNOWLEDGEMENT

The editors wish to thank sincerely Alison Caddick and Crissene Fawcett for their skilful and patient efforts in preparing the manuscripts for publication.

NOTES

1. For a critical appraisal of the French Revolution and its consequences for Western politics, see Elshtain (2008, especially chapters 6 and 7). A more general history of the period and appraisal of the role of revolutions in it appears in Brown and Tackett (2006: i) who write: 'Finally revolution, the political and social upheavals of the late eighteenth and early nineteenth centuries, challenged established ideas of divine-right monarchies and divinely ordained social hierarchies, and promoted more democratic government, notions of human rights, and religious toleration.'
2. The pathogenic paradigm is opposed to the 'salutogenesis' paradigm (Antonovsky 1984) in which the health disciplines have the causes of positive health as their focus and its promotion as their aim.

REFERENCES

Alford, R.R. (1975), *Health Care Politics: Ideological and Interest Group Barriers to Reform*, Chicago, IL: University of Chicago Press.

Antonovsky, A. (1984), 'The sense of coherence as a determinant of health', in J.D. Matarazzo, C.M. Weiss, J.A. Herd, N.E. Miller and S.M. Weiss (eds), *Behavioral Health: A Handbook of Health Enhancement and Disease Prevention*, New York: John Wiley and Sons, pp. 114–29.

Baggott, R., J. Allsop and K. Jones (2005), *Speaking for Patients and Carers: Health Consumer Groups and the Policy Process*, Basingstoke: Palgrave Macmillan.

Beck, U. (1998), 'Politics of risk society', in J. Franklin (ed.), *The Politics of Risk Society*, Cambridge: Polity Press, pp. 9–21.

Brown, S.J. and T. Tackett (eds) (2006), 'Frontmatter', *Enlightenment, Reawakening and Revolution 1660–1815*, Cambridge Histories Online, Cambridge University Press, DOI:10.1017/CHOL9780521816052.001.

Brown, P. and S. Zavestoski (2004), 'Social movements in health: an introduction', *Sociology of Health & Illness*, **26** (6): 679–94.

Dryzek, J. (2002), *Deliberative Democracy and Beyond: Liberals, Critics, Contestations*, Oxford: Oxford University Press.

Elshtain, J.B. (2008), *Sovereignty: God, State and Self*, New York: Basic Books.

Geissler, J. (2004), *Organisierte Vertretung von Patienteninteressen: Patienten-Organisationen als gesundheitspolitische Akteure in Deutschland, Großbritannien und den USA*, Hamburg, Germany: Verlag Dr Kovac.

Giddens, A. (2000), *Runaway World: How Globalization Is Re-shaping Our Lives*, New York: Routledge.

Goodin, R. (1996), *The Theory of Institutional Design*, Cambridge: Cambridge University Press.

Kuhn, T.S. (1970), *The Structure of Scientific Revolutions*, Chicago, IL: University of Chicago Press.

Lakatos, I. (1970), 'Falsificationism and the methodology of scientific research programmes', in I. Lakatos and A. Musgrave (eds), *Criticism and the Growth of Knowledge*, Cambridge: Cambridge University Press, pp. 91–195.

Mulkay, M. (1979), *Science and the Sociology of Knowledge*, London: George Allen & Unwin.

Offe, Claus (1974), 'Politische Herrschaft und Klassenstrukturen – Zur Analyse spätkapitalistischer Gesellschaftssysteme', in H.P. Widmaier (ed.), *Politische Ökonomie des Wohlfahrtsstaates. Eine kritische Darstellung der Neuen Politischen Ökonomie*, Frankfurt am Main, Germany: Fischer, pp. 264–93.

Taylor, C. (1985), *Philosophy and the Human Sciences: Philosophical Papers 2*, Cambridge and New York: Cambridge University Press.

Wade, R. (2008), 'Financial regime change?', *New Left Review*, **53**: 5–21.

2. Health activism in the age of governance

Timothy Milewa

User-oriented mobilizations in and around health care and health policy are diverse in nature and intent. At a more general level they reflect an interpolation of the private, individualized sphere of the self, body and illness experience into the political, regulatory and organizational realms where issues of entitlement, service funding, quality and the nature and parameters of expertise are contested. A focus on the sociological or social-psychological dimensions of these mobilizations thus needs to be balanced by consideration of some of these broader contexts and influences. This chapter reflects on the emergence and activities of health activist groups within the context of multi-actor forms of governance and networked policy interventions involving diverse stakeholders in the public, private and third sectors. These developments constitute more than the context or backdrop to health-related activism. By their nature, health activist groups are consciously or unconsciously engaged in a politics of institutional design through which narratives of inclusion, exclusion, fragmentation and legitimacy are formulated and enacted. They both reflect and co-constitute (often asymmetrically) new, fluid instances of the public sphere – the ground on which dialogue takes place beyond formal institutional arenas and prescribed forms of expression and communication. These instances not only facilitate engagement and dialogue but may also offer opportunities to question fundamental precepts (such as those to do with distributive principles related to goods like health care) and the viability of established and emerging modes of decision-making. The extent to which health activist groups engage with, challenge or even begin to co-produce the principles on which health care might be delivered goes some way towards helping us assess whether these mobilizations constitute more than run-of-the-mill interest group interventions.

EXPLAINING HEALTH ACTIVISM?

One prominent register of patient advocacy and protest organizations in the United Kingdom lists nearly 2000 such groups – a considerable underestimate because the list is composed largely of groups that have formal charitable status, a website or sustained publicity (Patients UK 2010). The rate at which such groups have been established also appears to have increased. A survey in 1997 of 197 condition-specific patient associations in the United Kingdom (such as the British Liver Trust, the Cleft Lip and Palate Association, and the Depression Alliance) found that over 72 per cent of the 197 groups had been established after 1975. Indeed, 55 per cent of groups were founded after 1980 (Wood 2000: 36). Similarly, a questionnaire survey of 123 groups in 1999 found that 66 per cent were established after 1981; the corresponding figure for 'umbrella' groups based on formal alliances between user-oriented organizations was 73 per cent (Baggott et al. 2005: 82). In the area of mental health, results of a survey by the Sainsbury Centre for Mental Health (2003) suggest that of 318 groups identified, 89 per cent were established within 15 years of the survey, with 42 per cent established in the previous 5 years.

At one level these trends might be explained in terms of patients' and citizens' rising expectations and the supposed demystification of orthodox medical expertise. Medical advances, their media representations and the explosive dissemination of information on the internet have perhaps served to focus popular attention on health, illness and mortality. These developments have rendered the body and its workings more transparent. This is, however, a double-edged development. In positive terms, individuals, depending on their circumstances and priorities, can attempt to use techniques of 'self-surveillance, body maintenance and discipline' to 'assess, manage and control risks to their health, thereby "taming uncertainty" ' (Chrysanthou 2002: 473). But at the same time, discoveries in genetic science–genetic engineering both before and after birth, developments such as magnetic resonance imaging, and home screening tests for conditions like bowel cancer, have undoubtedly added to our awareness about what can go wrong both physiologically and psychologically (Kerr and Shakespeare 2002; Shilling 2002). The new complexity has emerged at the same time as increased fragmentation and specialization in orthodox medicine. Medicine is no longer a monolithic entity. Increasingly patients can choose from among high-technology interventions, traditional doctor–patient consultations, internet discussion groups, holistic therapies and a huge range of alternative and complementary therapies. The emphasis has thus shifted from decisions imposed on a docile body by an unquestioned source of medical expertise to a situation where the patient can, if so inclined, sift, evaluate and act on a huge amount of information from different sources (Giddens 1991). And it is this reality that underpins two phenomena that may fuel or limit the politicization of health and illness in relation to health activism – namely, uncertainty and trust.

In terms of uncertainty, beyond the most straightforward instances of treatment and cure, there is always a potential for fear and doubt on the part of patients with regard to health, illness and medicine. As Talcott Parsons recognized over half a century ago, ambivalence is discernible in modern Western medicine's most basic relationship – that between the patient and the clinician. This relationship is sometimes characterized by a known inability to offer a cure (or even treatment) for specific conditions, or an awareness of gaps in diagnostic and therapeutic options:

> On the one hand there are cases, a good many of them, where the upshot of a competent diagnosis is to expose a condition which is known, in the given state of medical knowledge, to be essentially uncontrollable ... [On the other hand the] absolute limits to the physician's control – which of course are relative to the state of medical science at the time and his own assimilation of it – are not the only source of frustration and strain. Within these limits there is a very important area of uncertainty. As in so many practical situations, some of the factors bearing on this one will be well understood, but others are not. The exact relation of the known to the unknown elements cannot be determined. (Parsons 1951: 448–9)

Against this background Parsons goes on, more contestably, to argue that limited medical knowledge and uncertainty might explain, from a scientific perspective, the 'non-rational', 'irrational' and even 'magical' emotional and psychological responses on the part of patients, and, occasionally, on the part of clinicians (Parsons 1951: 450–1). But for our purposes, the most telling argument rests on the assertion that cultural norms and practices often help to shape the means by which incomplete or ambiguous knowledge (the basis of uncertainty) is expressed and dealt with in the relationship between clinician and patient. These practices are not social theoretical abstractions. They can be found today, for example, in clinical judgements where information is withheld from patients, in patients' and carers' tacit avoidance techniques and, more recently, the 'evidence-based', almost actuarial, presentation by doctors of probabilistic prognoses and data pertaining to the clinical effectiveness and side-effects of different medical interventions (Timmermans and Berg 2003: 88–9).

Such practices and modes of expression may serve to mediate, articulate, downplay or obscure uncertainty in the clinical encounter, but this uncertainty can also have a profound impact on how patients see themselves and their relationships with others. Such re-evaluations may be a potential basis for 'illness identities', affiliation with others in the same position and, potentially, politically oriented collective protest and self-advocacy (Prior 2003; Allsop et al. 2004; Brown et al. 2004). However, we can move beyond Parsons's focus on the patient–clinician encounter. Our bodies – whether healthy, ill, young, old, biddable or impaired – are more than shells we try to preserve and treat. They are 'interactive and relational' in everyday life and therefore inhere in our dealings with family, friends, strangers and the wider society (Lyon and Barbalet 1994: 55). In other words the apparent locus of individual identity, the body, transcends a supposed division between the public sphere and a 'private' sphere usually depicted as 'the domain of the household ... of sexuality and reproduction, and of care for the young, the sick and the elderly' (Benhabib 1992: 91).

Specifically, this interweaving of the private into the public sphere has implications for the constitution of a 'public-ized' politics of health. As Parsons suggested, patterns of authority and passivity in the individual patient–clinician encounter, together with representations of and reactions to uncertainty, can change in different contexts and over time. But given the fact that the body is omnipresent in both the private and public spheres, such change is not confined to individual patient–clinician interactions. Uncertainties around individualized health care are increasingly encroaching on broader debates and conflicts within health policy, for example when assumptions about entitlement or the state's health care responsibilities come up against patients' and citizens' perceptions and calculations. Equity in the distribution of resources, the manner in which health services are configured, the 'right' to certain treatments and demands to participate in strategic or operational decision-making (Salter 2004) are examples of this kind of encounter. And, as debate moves further away from individual episodes of diagnosis and treatment to more general issues about authority and the validity of different forms of knowledge, the power invested in clinicians' recognized expertise and the status of policymakers becomes more open to challenge from non-experts and lay experts. In short, the body – as a site of identity, surveillance, maintenance and uncertainty in relation to illness and health care – has a latent political dimension that can focus individual and collective mobilization.

Clearly the degree to which this latent embodied politics develops and is expressed depends on the specific polity, principles of welfare provision (if any) and systems of health care in place, together with the opportunities and resources that facilitate or obstruct collective mobilization. Aspects of the work of T.H. Marshall, although very clearly developed in the shadow of British history, provide a broad indication of the domains and interstices in which activism may either develop or be stymied. Writing in 1950, Marshall (1963) identified three forms of citizenship rights. There are civil rights (such as those concerned with freedom of expression and equality before the law) and the political rights most often associated with being able to vote in and contest elections. Social rights are a third, far more complex and contextually contingent set of rights. In the United Kingdom and other so-called welfare states, these rights most obviously include health care entitlements, social services and the maintenance of income at specified minimum levels. These entitlements, which may be drawn upon regularly by all citizens, form a residual safety net for the poorest or least fortunate in society and a fallback option for others.

Alternatively (or concurrently) social rights can be contested, constituted or developed around less prescriptive measures and practices than welfare entitlements. These include non-statutory standards and practices in and around health and social care, such as the right to informed choice in relation to medical treatments, courtesy and the protection of patients' dignity. Practices and conventions around the governance, planning, delivery, evaluation and funding of health and social care are also of direct relevance to many health activist groups. These mediate conflict and collaboration in relation to the uncertainty that attends gaps in knowledge and treatment related to particular medical conditions. This is perhaps best illustrated by briefly examining two of the better-known fields of health activism, namely HIV/AIDS and physical impairment.

Writing in the Canadian context about HIV/AIDS, Brown (1997) suggests that protest and self-help organizations represent more than just interest groups within an extant political system. By using the body (and indeed the sexualized body) as a focus of activism, groups expand and modify the political arena to include what have previously been seen as private spaces (spaces previously treated as if they are beyond or even in opposition to the public sphere of governance). With regard to HIV/AIDS, the notionally private sphere of sexual and familial relations meshes with public issues of disclosure, exposure and debate, as well as 'political' legislation in the anti-discrimination field. As controversies around employment, insurance, discrimination and stigma suggest, the supposedly private nature of chronic illness transcends the distinction between the public and private spheres. Indeed, HIV/AIDS activism – albeit in the relatively comfortable environs of North America and Western Europe – might even be the basis of a *new* form of radical democratic politics (Brown 1997: 11). As early as 1981 in the United States, the Gay Men's Health Crisis organization was established. By the early 1990s it had an annual budget of nearly US$20 million and coordinated the work of about 2000 volunteers (Small 1997: 19). And in 1987 the first branch of a particularly visible network, the AIDS Coalition to Unleash Power (ACT UP) was established. Its initial approach echoed that of the 1960s American civil rights movement. ACT UP, which now has groups all over the United States, held protests and demonstrations highlighting HIV/AIDS as a major public health issue, challenging discrimination against people with HIV/AIDS and attempting to persuade government and pharmaceutical companies to pursue particular lines of clinical research. Concurrently an ACT UP offshoot, the Treatment Action Group, and other activist groups began to engage directly with government and commercial decision-makers by sitting on committees, responding to official consultations and helping to shape research priorities and funding allocations (Milewa and Barry 2005: 507).

A similar form of embodied politics can be seen in the field of disability rights, in particular physical disabilities, where activists are concerned about

more than just the efficacy and availability of medical interventions. Their
activities are political in the sense that they often reflect a particular discourse
of physically impaired people's position in society. A ubiquitous, though not
wholly uncontested, demarcation is routinely drawn in relation to physical
impairment (such as paralysis below the waist) – that between the medicalization of conditions and the social model of disability. According to the latter
many of the difficulties faced by people with physical impairments are seen to
reflect wider social attitudes and prejudices, avoidable physical impediments
and limited legal and material support. Examples include buildings that are
unnecessarily difficult to access for people with mobility problems, poorly
designed public transport, prejudice on the part of employers and poorly
funded educational provision for people with severe physical impairments. As
with HIV/AIDS activism, the struggle for disability rights has been compared
to African-Americans' struggle for civil rights. Protests and sit-ins in relation
to public transport and welfare payments reflect a marked increase in the
number of activist groups.

By 2000 the British Council of Disabled People encompassed over 130
organizations, claiming to represent more than 400 000 people with physical
impairments (Barnes 2002: 314). This growth in consumer representation
seems to have had an impact. In 1982 the UK Labour Party attempted to introduce the first significant anti-discrimination legislation but was defeated by
the Conservative government. Between 1982 and 1995 there were 12 more
unsuccessful attempts to introduce anti-discrimination legislation. Finally, in
1995 the Disability Discrimination Act was introduced. Its official aim was to
give disabled people specific rights and protection in the fields of employment; access to goods, facilities and services; and the buying or renting of
property (in 2002 the legislation was extended to include education).

It is clear from the examples of activism around HIV/AIDS and physical
impairment that the uncertainty that can vitiate mobilization does not preclude
dialogue and collaboration with existing centres of political or medical power.
Indeed activism without such dialogue can only ever constitute empty postur-
ing or quixotic appeals for revolutionary change. Accordingly, health activist
groups can be seen as mobilizations that attempt, with varying degrees of
success and durability, to change and co-produce the environments in which
they exist. This will vary in terms of magnitude and fragility. One example in
this last respect is the campaign for access by women to legal abortions in the
United States. Before the US Supreme Court ruling in 1973 that a total ban on
abortion was an unconstitutional invasion of personal choice and privacy in
family matters, a plethora of organizations had campaigned for change. One,
the Abortion Counselling Service ('Jane'), part of the Chicago Women's
Liberation Union, not only campaigned for abortion rights but also provided
terminations. Between 1969 and 1973 Jane conducted approximately 11 000

illegal abortions, many of them being performed by activists themselves – a twin assault, both on legal restrictions and on the demesne of the medical profession (Joffe et al. 2004: 787). But the contested and fragile nature of this changed reality has been evident ever since the Supreme Court ruling. There has been a succession of legal (and sometimes violent) attempts to curb access to legal terminations, to the extent that a constitutional 'about-face' remains conceivable (Francome 2004).

But not all such changes are as open to challenge and reversal. Klawiter (2004) masterfully demonstrates this in charting the experience of an American woman, 'Clara', who was diagnosed with breast cancer in the late 1970s and who had to resume treatment in the late 1990s:

> In the [late 1970s] regime her experience of breast cancer was relentlessly individ-
> ualised … Surgeons were the undisputed sovereigns within the medical setting, and
> structurally speaking, the only role available to women with breast cancer was that
> of the duly compliant patient … By 1997, however, a new regime of breast cancer
> had emerged in the San Francisco Bay Area. Not only had the clinical contours of
> disease changed, but the public face of breast cancer had undergone a remarkable
> transformation. Clara was treated in a feminist and lesbian-friendly cancer centre.
> She decided between medical alternatives, attended patient education workshops,
> participated in her treatment as a member of a 'healthcare team' … Women with
> breast cancer had become a visible presence in the public domain … Breast cancer
> had been politicised along multiple dimensions and reframed, among other things,
> as a feminist issue. (Klawiter 2004: 865–6)

The experience of feminist campaigns around access to abortion and the trajectory taken by activism around physical impairment and HIV/AIDS tells us that health-related mobilizations can sometimes bring about significant change in the social, political and legal aspects of health care. However, there is no explanation thus far for why health activism has become such a notable phenomenon in the last three or four decades. Why have the issues of uncertainty and trust, as phenomena that can vitiate and delimit health activism, moved from the background to the foreground? It is to this question that I now turn.

GOVERNANCE, AFFORDANCES AND HEALTH ACTIVISM

The idea of 'governance' provides a routine if often hazy refuge for those seeking explanations for the social change of recent decades. But if the body and attendant uncertainties straddle the private and public spheres in such a way as to imbue health, illness and health care with a political dimension, then changes in the relationship between the public sphere and the wider polity could help us understand the evolution of contemporary health activism. Debates around the congested state, multi-level governance, deliberative politics and Third Way ideology reflect an accentuation in the modern state's complexity, a move away from hierarchical models of public administration and the increasing role of non-government actors in the articulation of public policy (Skelcher 2000; Stoker 2006). The economic and political developments and enhanced linkages associated with a global economy, the unprecedented flow and speed of information and a diminution in class-based politics have, from this perspective, contributed to a situation where nearly all governments have had to deal with 'a complex cluster of arrangements of power and accountability that can no longer be – if they ever were – captured by the formal institutions of government' (Davies 2007: 48). At one extreme, a (repressive) state might struggle to suppress the internet's potential for furthering transparency and the flow of politically inconvenient information (Terranova 2004; Chen and Zhu 2009). Alternatively, public institutions, their various actors, and mobilizations within civil society can try to adapt existing decision-making processes or establish new and distinct collaborative spaces for dialogue to reflect the changing nature of governance (McKie 2003; Marks and Hooghe 2004; Callaghan and Wistow 2006).

The implications for health activism and other forms of collective mobilization thus depend on the orientation and substance of such a shift away from government towards governance. As Fox and Ward (2008) argue, the impressively elastic idea of governance can be framed in at least three ways. 'Interest-based' accounts of governance simply reframe conventional models of political pluralism and fluidity, seeing health activist groups as just another set of stakeholders defending and promoting their material and political interests. It is the complexity of contemporary governance, rather than the changed nature of interest group behaviour, that casts their activities in a new light. Interest groups now operate in a more diverse and fluid environment that in itself offers no guarantee that traditionally marginalized sections of society will find a seat at the table. Other explanations of the rise of governance centre on evolving institutional structures and the opportunities they have presented for health activist groups. The institutional arrangements used to assess the case for public funding of new health technologies, for example, vary markedly between countries in terms of opportunities for participation by lay actors. Greß et al. (2005) compared organizations across countries, including the Federal Committee of Physicians and Sickness Funds (Germany), the National Institute for Health and Clinical Excellence (England and Wales) and the Federal Commission for General Health Insurance Benefits (Switzerland). The breadth and number of interests represented and consulted in decision-making was seen as relatively high in Switzerland and England and Wales when compared with the pyramidal, corporatist approach evident in Germany.

The situation in Germany was said to reflect a historical background in which the German medical profession, with the aid of the state, had grown progressively stronger, and in which control of sickness (insurance) funds had become increasingly remote from the workers for whose benefit they were originally established (Busse and Riesberg 2004).

Neither of these interpretations of governance can be discounted, and there is indeed no reason why they cannot, for our purposes, coexist with a third conception concerning *governmentality*. The complex multilevel and multinodal institutions and networks of governance have, from this perspective, afforded a space for the development of new ways in which we (individuals, families and collective mobilizations) are governed. Although punitive and coercive aspects of 'traditional' hierarchical government undoubtedly continue to exist there is now also an emphasis on self-governance. This idea of governance, in addition to denoting hierarchical direction and control, encompasses a variety of institutions and techniques that encourage individuals and self-interest groups to make choices and pursue aims within broad normative parameters. This differs from government as there is a recognition that sources of expertise and answers to complex questions (such as those to do with health and welfare) may reside not only in the state, but also in the market sector and civil society, or all three simultaneously (Sibeon 2000). The notion of unitary and hierarchical policy governance in fields such as health, based on a clear distinction between the governors and the governed, is thus brought into question. The analytical focus in relation to the place and impact of health activism may become explicable, in part, by focusing on

> the ways in which, by drawing citizens into more direct and involved relationships with governance practice, collaboration and participation [dispersed expertise] may serve to enable the production of new forms of governable subject; but also, how the spaces which are opened up may form points around which social identity and agency is mobilised. (Newman 2005: 120)

The impact of health activist groups in relation to particular issues like women's access to abortion, anti-discrimination legislation for physically impaired people, or the promotion of rights for people with HIV/AIDS may therefore depend on more than the availability of resources, their ideological appeal or the degree of success in framing messages to reach a wider audience (Snow and Benford 2005). The instruments and mechanisms that facilitate or impede transformation of the 'visions, metaphors, models, knowledge, facts, judgements, presuppositions, hypotheses, convictions, ends and goals' of health activist movements into effective change are central (Kooiman and Jentoft 2009: 820). The most fundamental of these instruments is based on conceptions of how change can or should be brought about in a democratic manner. Should decisions of direct interest to health activist groups, such as the funding, reach and quality of specialist health services, be the product of 'back room, brokered compromises among private interests', street demonstrations and protest, or of 'reasoned public debate about the common good' (Fraser 1992: 113) balanced by consideration of the needs of particular groups with specific requirements?

If, normatively and practically, this last approach to decision-making is seen to offer the most to health activist groups then another question arises. How is such democratic dialogue to be realized? From one perspective, the ideal has already been attained within modern representative democracies. Universal adult suffrage and stable systems of representative government can be seen as a bulwark against the opaque backroom deals and the street demonstrations spoken of by Fraser. This system provides a necessary distance between elected representatives and functionaries within state institutions and individual citizens and interest groups (Posner 2003). Indeed Posner suggests that it is unrealistic for voters to do any more than assess media reports, speak to significant others and, should the opportunity arise, interrogate politicians when deciding how to cast their ballots. Some voters (such as people with chronic illnesses and their carers) are indeed experts on particular issues. But are they in a position to balance their objectives (possibly in a domain such as health care) against the myriad other claims on the state – for example, foreign aid, defence expenditure and investment in infrastructure? Posner certainly does not attribute omniscience to representative government in this respect. Instead he argues that reasoned, persuasive argument is less likely to emerge if the decision-making powers of representative government are devolved to self-interested individuals and groups in civil society. Their principal power rests on universal suffrage and regular elections – a means to check politicized elements within the state (who might otherwise govern primarily in their own interests) and to ensure the continuity of a stable, orderly, process for changing political regimes.

HEALTH ACTIVISM, REPRESENTATION AND NEW DEMOCRATIC PRACTICES

But if this electorally based 'business as usual' was sufficient in terms of representation for groups such as the physically impaired there would be no rationale at all for health activist groups. Their existence reflects, consciously or otherwise, five broad criticisms of reliance on aggregative democracy (vote counting) and representative government. First, the state is a multiplicity of complex, related, emergent and sometimes unforeseen policy domains. This, in tandem with the reality of electorates that frequently run into many millions of people, means that elections are a very imprecise means for reflecting societal preferences about particular aspects of policy. Individual votes are more likely to reflect an expression of more or less coherent worldviews, disaffection with one or more electoral contestants, or cultural or family traditions (Caplan 2007). Second, the multiplicity and complexity of policy domains means that it is difficult for electors either to authorize individual political representatives to pursue a particular course around specific policies or to hold representatives to account for discrete decisions (Pitkin 1967). Third, the emphasis on voting by individuals means that there is no procedure for citizens to communicate directly with each other to assess respective points of view, state and reflect critically on the reasons for their personal preferences or, through reasoned argument, be persuaded to revise their preferences (Dryzek 2000). Fourth, and relatedly, if democratic legitimacy is founded primarily on the opportunity to vote and the quantitative aggregative principle, there is no inherent link between the democratic process and the quality of reasoning that might underpin particular policy decisions – individuals simply identify their personal preferences and try to realize them (Fraser 1992). This is linked to a fifth criticism of aggregative democracy. Aggregative models are often seen to be premised on the idea of rational choice on the part of voters, interest groups, personnel within state institutions and politicians. Individuals are assumed to have a clear idea of their self-interest and a proclivity to realize it by whatever means available. But this seems as much an article of faith as an empirically based fact.

Accordingly, so-called difference democrats reiterate these criticisms but add that aggregative democratic approaches alone may reinforce or ignore more fundamental social divisions and inequalities that are likely to marginalize certain groups (such as mentally ill people). Fraser (1992) and Young (2000), for example, argue that truly democratic practice has to acknowledge the diverse nature of multiple public spheres and modes of political expression and public discourse. Some marginalized groups are 'differentiated from others by cultural form, practices, special needs or capacities, structures of power and privilege' and this is reflected in specific modes of expression (Young 2000: 90). Such forms are not inimical to reasoned argument but may contribute to an a priori diminution in the perceived status of some participants in the public discourse that precedes and accompanies the processes of aggregative democracy. Most forums and contexts are governed by norms and expectations of discourse allied to penalties of one form or another for their infraction. Yet some forms of discourse reflect 'affective, embodied and stylistic aspects of communication' – as is evident, for example, in cultural celebrations like 'Mad Pride' or protests by disability rights activists designed to disrupt inaccessible forms of public transport (Crossley 1998). As such protests illustrate, political communication can occur beyond formal political arenas and begin to challenge the inequalities that disadvantage or exclude some groups within the structures and procedures often associated with 'official' political debate.

Patients' and citizens' growing influence through the role and impact of health activist groups and more individualized forms of consumerist leverage is, then, premised, at least in part, on a substantive re-articulation of what is meant by democracy and democratic practice. But the practicability of such change is, as intimated, shaped by historically specific factors like the behaviour of key organized interests, the organizational structure of decision-making institutions and entrenched perspectives in the understanding and enactment of democratic practices. It is to this politics of institutional design that, in conclusion, I now turn.

CONCLUSION: HEALTH ACTIVISM AND THE INSTITUTIONAL DESIGN OF NEW DEMOCRATIC FORMS

The suggestion that uncertainty and interdependence are increasingly undermining hierarchical approaches to government in favour of policymakers, 'civil servants, citizens and private sector actors who act as "entrepreneurs" or "problem solvers" in policy networks of their own making' certainly appears to offer fertile ground for health activist groups (Hajer 2003: 8). But such narratives do not necessarily provide a means of addressing the individual and collective uncertainties around health care and health policy discussed above. If the 'new' democratic practices are to be anything more than an aspirational narrative it will require (as Parsons might have suggested) a significant level of trust between policymakers, service providers, citizens, service users and health activist groups. Such trust will have to be premised on 'authentic dialogue', where parties engage in good faith, honestly represent the constituencies for whom they claim to speak and recognize the dialogical principles and procedures that typify the arenas of the new governance (Cohen 1997: 74; Innes and Booher 2003: 38).

In other words, health activist groups are in the business of attempting to produce (or co-produce), dialogical procedures and spaces of a particular 'actionable form' that point to, but do not determine roles, norms and appropriate behaviours in connection with desired outcomes (Goodin 1996: 31). The parameters of such institutional design are, by definition, elastic. But as Skelcher et al. (2005) suggest, admittedly in a context outside health activism, political manoeuvres in this regard are likely to take three ideal-typical 'actionable forms'. The managerial form, which is often influenced by new public management precepts of managerial discretion and efficiency in pursuit of given goals, tends to regard users of health and welfare as individual consumers or clients rather than stakeholders acting through collective mobilizations. Individual consumers in turn focus on improving the quality of services rather than on developing new ideas of democratic practice and dialogue. A second actionable form centres on asymmetrical co-option. The emphasis here is quasi-corporatist in nature, with elite representatives of different interests coming together to reach agreement or to develop plans for broader constituencies. Clearly the degree to which such representatives can truly claim to speak for wider interests (for example, mental health service users) would vary considerably and, again, the role of self-advocacy and collective mobilization on the part of stakeholder groups would be marginalized. But there is a third actionable form, an 'emancipatory' form oriented towards more fluid, expansive and reconstituted democratic forms which, as I have shown in this chapter, are associated with autonomous health activist groups who see themselves as more than pressure groups.

In this respect their ambition to change the nature and terms of democratic practice may appear fanciful. But health activist groups exist only because their aims have not been met in the context of the political, bureaucratic and medical status quo.

REFERENCES

Allsop, J., K. Jones and R. Baggott (2004), 'Health consumer groups in the UK: a new social movement?', *Sociology of Health & Illness*, **26** (6): 737–56.

Baggott, R., J. Allsop and K. Jones (2005), *Speaking for Patients and Carers: Health Consumer Groups and the Policy Process*, Basingstoke: Palgrave Macmillan.

Barnes, C. (2002), 'Introduction: disability, power and politics', *Policy and Politics*, **30** (3): 311–18.

Benhabib, S. (1992), 'Models of public space: Hannah Arendt, the liberal tradition and Jürgen Habermas', in C. Calhoun (ed.), *Habermas and the Public Sphere*, Cambridge, MA: MIT Press, pp. 73–98.

Brown, M. (1997), *RePlacing Citizenship: AIDS Activism and Radical Democracy*, London: Guildford Press.

Brown, P., S. Zavestoski, S. McCormick, B. Mayer, R. Morello-Frosch and R. Altman (2004), 'Embodied health movements: new approaches to social movements in health', *Sociology of Health & Illness*, **26** (1): 50–80.

Busse, R. and A. Riesberg (2004), *Health Care Systems in Transition: Germany*, Copenhagen: European Observatory on Health Systems and Policies.

Callaghan, G. and G. Wistow (2006), 'Governance and public involvement in the British National Health Service: understanding difficulties and developments', *Social Science & Medicine*, **63** (9): 2289–300.

Caplan, B. (2007), 'Beyond conventional economics: the limits of rational behaviour in political decision making', *Public Choice*, **127** (3): 505–7.

Chen Gang and Zhu Jinjing (2009), 'Behind the "Green Dam": internet censorship in China', East Asian Institute background brief no. 474, National University of Singapore.

Chrysanthou, M. (2002), 'Transparency and self-hood: utopia and the informed body', *Social Science & Medicine*, **54** (3): 469–79.

Cohen, J. (1997) 'Deliberation and democratic legitimacy', in J. Bohman and W. Rehg (eds), *Deliberative Democracy: Essays on Reasoning and Politics*, Cambridge, MA: MIT Press, pp. 67–91.

Crossley, N. (1998), 'Transforming the mental health field: the early history of the National Association for Mental Health', *Sociology of Health & Illness*, **20** (4): 458–88.

Davies, C. (2007), 'Grounding governance in dialogue? Discourse, practice and the potential for a new public sector organizational form in Britain', *Public Administration*, **85** (1): 47–66.

Dryzek, J. (2000), *Deliberative Democracy and Beyond: Liberals, Critics, Contestations*, Oxford: Oxford University Press.

Fox, N. and K. Ward (2008), 'What governs governance, and how does it evolve? The sociology of governance in action', *British Journal of Sociology*, **59** (3): 519–38.

Francome, C. (2004), *Abortion in the USA and the UK*, Aldershot: Ashgate.

Fraser, N. (1992), 'Rethinking the public sphere: a contribution to the critique of actually existing democracy', in C. Calhoun (ed.), *Habermas and the Public Sphere*, Cambridge, MA: MIT Press, pp. 109–42.

Giddens, A. (1991), *Modernity and Self-Identity*, Cambridge: Polity Press.

Goodin, R. (1996), 'Institutions and their design', in R. Goodin (ed.), *The Theory of Institutional Design*, Cambridge: Cambridge University Press, pp. 1–53.

Greß, S., D. Niebuhr, H. Rothgang and J. Wasem (2005), 'Criteria and procedures for determining benefit packages in health care: a comparative perspective', *Health Policy*, **73** (1): 78–91.

Hajer, M. (2003), 'A frame in the fields: policymaking and the reinvention of politics', in M. Hajer and H. Wagenaar (eds), *Deliberative Policy Analysis: Understanding Governance in the Network Society*, Cambridge: Cambridge University Press, pp. 88–110.

Innes, J. and D. Booher (2003), 'Collaborative policymaking: governance through dialogue', in M. Hajer and H. Wagenaar (eds), *Deliberative Policy Analysis: Understanding Governance in the Network Society*, Cambridge: Cambridge University Press, pp. 33–59.

Joffe, C., T. Weitz and C. Stacey (2004), 'Uneasy allies: pro-choice physicians, feminist health activists and the struggle for abortion rights', *Sociology of Health & Illness*, **26** (6): 775–96.

Kerr, A. and T. Shakespeare (2002), *Genetic Politics: From Eugenics to Genome*, Bristol: New Clarion Press.

Klawiter, M. (2004), 'Breast cancer in two regimes: the impact of social movements on illness experience', *Sociology of Health & Illness*, **26** (6): 845–74.

Kooiman, J. and S. Jentoft (2009), 'Meta-governance: values, norms and principles, and the making of hard choices', *Public Administration*, **87** (4): 818–36.

Lyon, M. and J. Barbalet (1994), 'Society's body: emotion and the "somatization" of social theory', in T. Csordas (ed.), *Embodiment and Experience: The Existential Ground of Culture and Self*, Cambridge: Cambridge University Press, pp. 48–67.

Marks, G. and L. Hooghe (2004), 'Contrasting visions of multi-level governance', in I. Bache and M. Flinders (eds), *Multi-level Governance*, Oxford: Oxford University Press, pp. 15–30.

Marshall, T. (1963), 'Citizenship and social class', originally published 1950, in T. Marshall (ed.), *Sociology at the Crossroads and Other Essays*, London: Heinemann, pp. 67–127.

McKie, L. (2003), 'Rhetorical spaces: participation and pragmatism in the evaluation of community health work', *Evaluation*, **9** (3): 307–24.

Milewa, T. and C. Barry (2005), 'Health policy and the politics of evidence', *Social Policy & Administration*, **39** (5): 498–512.

Newman, J. (2005), 'Participative governance and the remaking of the public sphere', in J. Newman (ed.), *Remaking Governance: Peoples, Politics and the Public Sphere*, Bristol: Policy Press, pp. 119–38.

Parsons, T. (1951), *The Social System*, London: Routledge and Kegan Paul.

Patients UK (2010), 'Support Groups', accessed 2 January 2010 at www.patient.co.uk/selfhelp.asp.

Pitkin, H. (1967), *The Concept of Representation*, Berkeley, CA: University of California Press.

Posner, R. (2003), *Law, Pragmatism and Democracy*, Cambridge, MA: Harvard University Press.

Prior, L. (2003), 'Belief, knowledge and expertise: the emergence of the lay expert in medical sociology', *Sociology of Health & Illness*, **25** (3): 41–57.

Sainsbury Centre for Mental Health (2003), 'The mental health service user movement in England', Sainsbury Centre for Mental Health, policy paper 2, London.

Salter, B. (2004), *The New Politics of Medicine*, Basingstoke: Palgrave Macmillan.

Shilling, C. (2002), 'Culture, the "sick role" and the consumption of health', *British Journal of Sociology*, **53** (4): 621–38.

Sibeon, R. (2000), 'Governance and the policy process in contemporary Europe', *Public Management*, **2** (3): 289–309.

Skelcher, C. (2000), 'Changing images of the state: overloaded, hollowed-out, congested', *Public Policy and Administration*, **15** (3): 3–19.

Skelcher, C., N. Mathur and M. Smith (2005), 'The public governance of collaborative spaces: discourse, design and democracy', *Public Administration*, **83** (3): 573–56.

Small, N. (1997), 'Suffering in silence? Public visibility, private secrets and the social construction of AIDS', in P. Aggleton, P. Davies and G. Hart (eds), *AIDS: Activism and Alliances*, Bristol: Taylor & Francis, pp. 15–24.

Snow, D. and R. Benford (2005), 'Clarifying the relationship between framing and ideology', in H. Johnston and J. Noakes (eds), *Frames of Protest: Social Movements and the Framing Perspective*, Lanham, MD: Rowman & Littlefield, pp. 205–12.

Stoker, G. (2006), 'Public value management: a new narrative for networked governance?', *American Review of Public Administration*, **36** (1): 41–57.

Terranova, T. (2004), *Network Culture: Politics for the Information Age*, London: Pluto Press.

Timmermans, S. and M. Berg (2003), *The Gold Standard: The Challenge of Evidence-Based Medicine and Standardization in Health Care*, Philadelphia, PA: Temple University Press.

Wood, B. (2000), *Patient Power? The Politics of Patients' Associations in Britain and America*, Buckingham: Open University Press.

Young, I. (2000), *Inclusion and Democracy*, Oxford: Oxford University Press.

3. Health consumer groups in the United Kingdom: progress or stagnation?

Kathryn Jones and Rob Baggott

Improving patient and public involvement (PPI) in health care has been a declared aim of recent British governments (Department of Health 1996, 1999, 2004a). The objective has been to develop services that are more responsive to the needs of patients and the public by strengthening their role in decision-making at individual, service and policy levels. Timothy Milewa in this volume argues that new governance arrangements bringing multiple actors – including patients, the public, professions and commercial interests – into negotiation, design and implementation of health policy have opened new avenues for interaction and activism. Even so, there is ongoing concern about a 'democratic deficit' in the National Health Service (NHS), particularly the lack of representation of public and patient interests at the policy level (Cooper et al. 1995; House of Commons Health Committee 2007).

As voluntary sector organizations seeking to promote or represent the interests of users and carers in the health arena, UK health consumer groups play an important role in redressing this deficit. These groups have long been involved in providing support and services to patients and the public (Lock 1986). However, academic interest in health consumer groups developed from the late 1980s, reflecting a growing awareness of their activities (Hogg 1999; Wood 2000). In 1999 the United Kingdom's Economic and Social Research Council (ESRC) funded a study of health consumer groups which showed that groups engaged with different policy actors and undertook various policy activities. The study concluded that they were becoming more involved in the policy process and that for some groups at least the traditional view that they were invariably weak and lacked influence was inaccurate (Baggott et al. 2005).

Since this study the PPI agenda has shifted, with policy now emphasizing individual choice, local accountability and representation, as well as a greater role for the voluntary sector in service provision. Another important development has been new devolved government arrangements giving Wales, Scotland and Northern Ireland greater authority over the design and operation of their health care systems. In addition the European Union (EU) has taken a closer interest in health matters, even though the financing and provision of health care remains the responsibility of member states. These developments are likely to have an impact on health consumer groups organizing at the national level.

In this chapter we explore how UK health consumer groups have fared under changed conditions. The first part of the chapter provides a brief overview of the ESRC project. This is followed by an examination of recent developments in the health care policy arena and their likely impact on groups. Finally, the chapter considers whether health consumer groups are likely to gain influence relative to other interests in health care.

THEORIES AND METHODS

The ESRC project was undertaken between 1999 and 2001 (see Baggott et al. 2005 for full details of the research design). It involved a postal questionnaire survey of health consumer groups, semi-structured interviews with group leaders and officers, and semi-structured interviews with politicians, civil servants and representatives of research charities, professional groups and the pharmaceutical industry.

The study took a 'multiple lens' approach (Sabatier 1999; Allsop et al. 2004) and drew on theories of social movements, group formation and the lay challenge to dominant biomedical scientific discourse (Brown et al. 2003; Epstein 1996; Jennings 1999). In addition, theories of social capital gave us insight into how health consumer groups develop social and political resources, public trust and membership (Anheir and Kendall 2002; Putnam 2000). To understand the extent to which these groups were challenging other interests we drew on Alford's (1975) model of structural interests, which posits that representatives of community interests lack power and influence compared with other policy actors, such as professions, managers and corporate interests, mainly because they face institutional bias and can exert influence only by mobilizing extraordinary political resources. We also considered theories of pressure groups and policy networks to understand groups' campaigning strategies (Marsh and Rhodes 1992). The typologies developed by Whiteley and Winyard (1987) and Grant (1995) prompted us to investigate differences in the tactics and status of groups. In particular, the concepts of 'insider' and 'outsider' groups were useful in understanding why some groups developed close relationships with government while others focused on lobbying parliament and the media (Maloney et al. 1994).

KEY CHARACTERISTICS OF UK HEALTH CONSUMER GROUPS

We identified key similarities and differences between groups, which led us to develop the following typology:

- Formal alliance organizations – groups whose membership consisted of other autonomous national organizations.
- Population-based groups – groups representing all patients, or a specific population subgroup (for example, the elderly, ethnic minorities).
- Condition-based groups – groups representing people with particular conditions (for example, arthritis, cancer, heart disease).

Table 3.1 summarizes the key characteristics of the groups that responded to the questionnaire. The majority were membership organizations, but included individuals and other health consumer groups. Those without a membership maintained strong links to their client group or were run by activists with experience of the health condition their organization represented. Most groups were registered charities. Although most groups focused on a single condition, a quarter of them were interested in issues across condition areas. Around two-thirds had formed since 1981, suggesting that the patients' movement was still in its infancy compared with other social movements (Byrne 1997). More than half survived on an income of £100 000 a year or less. Resources were a critical issue for groups, affecting staffing levels and capacity.

In addition 82 per cent of groups stated that influencing national policy was 'very important' or 'important'. And 63 per cent rated influencing local policy as 'very important' or 'important'. Groups believed opportunities for involvement in policymaking were improving. A more recent study of patient organi-

Table 3.1   UK health consumer groups' key characteristics

	%
Membership organization	92
Registered charity	91
Focused on a single condition	75
Formed since 1981	66
Income £100 000 or less	54
Headquarters in London	38

Source: ESRC Questionnaire 1999.

zations representing chronic conditions suggests a push towards policy advocacy has continued, with 66 per cent reporting policy activity (Posner 2009). In our study, groups valued interaction with patients and the public. They used this to understand patient experience and to identify policy issues and research priorities, thus providing a source of legitimacy in their inter-action with policymakers. They saw this experiential knowledge as a key factor in their policy role.

INTERACTION WITH OTHER HEALTH CONSUMER GROUPS

The questionnaire established that 86 per cent of groups had links or alliances with other user/carer organizations, and three-quarters identified these as a 'very important' or 'important' facilitator in the policy process, while 46 per cent were in 'at least monthly contact' with other groups. There was evidence of networks between organizations, often involving the same people meeting in different fora, which developed trust and mutual understanding. However, joint work was stronger for some health conditions than others. Three levels of cooperation were found: ad-hoc projects and collaborative networks; informal alliances; and formal alliances. Alliances played a key role in supporting and developing policy activity. Incentives to collaborate included the ability to present a united voice to policymakers and strength in numbers. Alliances were also promoted by external factors (Jones 2007) and the government often encouraged groups to work together on common issues, in some cases by providing financial support.

INTERACTION WITH GOVERNMENT AND PARLIAMENT

Table 3.2 summarizes the frequency of contact between groups and the government and parliament. Many had regular contact with key government actors, in particular Department of Health civil servants. Interviewees suggested that the policy arena had opened up in recent years, in part due to the government's PPI reforms and its NHS modernization agenda. Groups also argued that they had pushed their own agendas, helping to shape and redefine policy problems. They identified a number of avenues of influence, including participation on National Service Framework external reference committees, representation on Modernization Action Teams and direct lobbying of government bodies such as the National Institute of Health and Clinical Excellence, which assesses the cost effectiveness of treatments and recommends their use in the NHS.

Table 3.2   UK health consumer groups' contact with the Department of Health and Parliament

	'At least monthly'	'At least quarterly'	'At least annually'	'Not in the past three years'
	%	%	%	%
Department of Health Ministers	13	30	67	33
Department of Health Civil Servants	25	48	72	28
MPs	23	45	72	28

Source: ESRC Questionnaire 1999.

The ability of groups to represent patients, users and carers and to reflect patient experience affected their standing with government. Both ministers and civil servants were keen for groups to demonstrate active engagement with their constituency and bring experiential knowledge to policy discussions. They believed that involving health consumer groups in policy would build consensus and provide new perspectives on existing policy problems.

Groups adopted various strategies. A number, particularly the larger, better-resourced organizations, had good links with ministers and civil servants. These were more likely to employ specialist policy staff and to be able to respond to requests for participation. Alliances both among health consumer groups and with other policy actors were considered important channels of policy activity. Groups also made use of the media to place additional pressure on policymakers. They lobbied parliament, persuading MPs to table parliamentary questions or contribute to debates, and provided written or oral evidence to parliamentary committees.

INTERACTION WITH OTHER STAKEHOLDERS

The study explored groups' relationships with other health care stakeholders, including professional and commercial interests, regarded as powerful interests in health care (Moran 1999; Baggott 2007). Relationships with these stakeholders varied in their scope and content between little or no involvement; involvement in 'one-off' projects; and longer-term, more fruitful relationships.

At least quarterly contact with doctor organizations was reported by 48 per cent of health consumer groups, 68 per cent had individual professionals among their membership and 34 per cent included professional associations as affiliates. In addition, 49 per cent believed that a lack of support from professionals was a key barrier in the policy process. Some argued that since professionals dominated policy discourse they needed to understand patient experiences.

Most groups valued professionals' expertise and suggested that they had more extensive and positive relationships with them. Professionals valued health consumer groups' expertise, acknowledging that user experience was increasingly important as a supplement to professional knowledge. They also commented that they were under pressure from government to involve the 'lay perspective'.

Health consumer groups also developed links with commercial interests, particularly medical technology manufacturers and the pharmaceutical industry. Thus 45 per cent were in at least quarterly contact with industry. However, 38 per cent had had no contact with industry in the past 3 years. Recent research reveals continuing relationships between the two sectors; in 2007, 29 pharmaceutical companies working in the United Kingdom listed financial or in-kind support to 246 health consumer groups on their website (Jones 2008). Despite concerns about organizational capture and possible conflicts of interest, groups in the study argued that they shared mutual interests with industry and that it was legitimate to accept funding as long as they remained independent. However, they were reluctant to accept funding for policy-related activity, instead using it for member support services. Health consumer groups were wary of any accusation of dancing to the industry's tune. They did acknowledge dilemmas, for example when promoting access to the best available treatment might involve advocating the use of particular drugs. Some groups established guidelines for good practice and rules of cooperation. On the other hand, the pharmaceutical industry recognized the particular expertise of health consumer groups and claimed it worked with them so as to share information and develop mutual understanding (Jones 2008).

Impact on Policy

The ESRC study identified instances where health consumer groups had influenced policy, noting that some groups were evolving from policy outsiders to policy insiders. However, this was the case only for those with good-quality access to decision-makers (involving good political contacts, sufficient resources and an understanding of policy processes). While health consumer groups were a growing presence, they lacked the heavyweight political contacts of other policy actors. Subsequent research on the UK policy process by Baggott (2007) confirms this view. His interviewees suggested that groups were becoming more professionalized and displayed a greater understanding of the 'rules of the game', but in their view they lacked power relative to other actors and were influential only on specific issues rather than strategic decisions.

THE EVOLVING POLICY AGENDA

The ESRC study demonstrated that health consumer groups are being accepted as the voice of patients, users and carers by government and other stakeholders. However in the past few years health consumer groups have been forced to adapt to an evolving health policy agenda, combined with new challenges emerging from changes in health policy processes. These factors have been matched by other pressures from within the voluntary health sector.

Changes in the Structure of PPI and Other Policy Developments

Since the ESRC project was completed the structure of PPI in England has changed significantly. In 2003 Patient and Public Involvement Forums were created in every NHS Trust to represent patients and the public at the local level (Baggott 2005). At the national level the Commission for Patient and Public Involvement in Health was established to ensure consistency and coherence in local arrangements. However, the Commission struggled to develop productive relationships with government and other stakeholders and lacked credibility among key PPI activists (Hogg 2009).

The following year, as part of a programme of reducing the number of public bodies, the government proposed abolishing it (Department of Health 2004b). Ministers appointed an expert panel to review evidence on PPI and make recommendations for its future direction. For national health consumer groups, further reform raised two key issues: government emphasis on individual patient choice in health care meant that the collective representation of consumers' needs might be undervalued in the new system (Hogg 2009); and there was no systematic approach to the incorporation of health consumer groups into the development of national policy. The expert panel argued that 'choice' made 'voice' more, not less, important and that PPI structures needed to ensure the collective patient voice was heard. It recommended that government should not lose sight of PPI at the national level and backed efforts by groups to establish a formal alliance to support engagement with patients, users and carers (Department of Health 2006a). In 2007 a House of Commons Health Committee inquiry into PPI recommended the development of a national strategy, concluding that 'at a national level, patient and public involvement is fragmented and lacking a coherent strategy; we recommend that government addresses this as a priority' (House of Commons Health Committee, 2007: 92).

By April 2008 both the Commission and Patient and Public Involvement Forums had been abolished and a new system of Local Involvement Networks (LINks) established. LINks exist in all local authorities that have social services responsibilities. They are charged with promoting and supporting public involvement in the commissioning, provision and scrutiny of health and social care, and with obtaining people's views on local health and social services and presenting them to those responsible for health and social care (Department of Health 2006b). However, the new model has attracted criticism on such grounds as governance frameworks and accountability structures not being made explicit in the legislation (Hogg 2009). Health consumer groups raised concerns about the lack of clear guidance for LINks. Nonetheless they have begun addressing how they may influence local structures, believing they can support LINks by providing access to their user/member networks, using local branches to build a national body of evidence, and helping to coordinate local activity (Cook 2009).

Another innovation relates to the establishment of new foundation trusts. From 2003, NHS service providers were encouraged to achieve foundation trust status, lured by the promise of more autonomy over finances and management. This status entailed new structures of governance, enabling local people and patients to become trust members and participate in elections for their governing bodies. Although ostensibly democratic, these arrangements did not fit well with other PPI structures and have not produced the level of engagement promised (House of Commons Health Committee 2003; Santry 2009).

The Department of Health claimed that changes in PPI reflected the growing connection between health and social care and an increasing focus on local commissioning of services (Hogg 2009). Indeed government has indicated that PPI is an essential element of the commissioning of services by local Primary Care Trusts (PCTs). A core competency of the World Class Commissioning framework, which guides how PCTs commission local services, is public and patient engagement (Department of Health 2007). A 2009 review of patient and public engagement at the local level suggested that commissioning was encouraging NHS managers to see PPI as a 'must do' element of their work (Picker Institute Europe 2009). However, the extent to which local health consumer groups have been involved in commissioning remains in doubt (PatientView 2009).

The past decade has also seen a strengthening of the legal and regulatory framework for PPI. NHS trusts are now assessed against core standards for PPI in inspections by the Care Quality Commission, the regulatory body for health and social care services in England specifically. Section 11 of the

Health and Social Care Act 2001 required NHS bodies to involve and consult the public in the planning and provision of services, and on proposals for change. Following criticism in the 2007 Health Committee's PPI inquiry about how this statutory duty had been operationalized, and as a result of court cases that exposed a lack of clarity in the wording of the current law and associated guidance, the government sought to clarify service providers' responsibility. The Local Government and Public Involvement in Health Act 2007 stated that service providers need consult only on 'significant' changes to the manner of delivery or range of services to be provided, making it difficult for the public to challenge changes which simply involved the contracting of existing services from non-NHS suppliers (Hogg 2009). Each Strategic Health Authority and PCT is now bound to report on any consultation relating to commissioning decisions and on how the views of patients and the public are represented in these deliberations.

The Department of Health also encouraged the development of an evidence base to support PPI. Between 2006 and 2009 the NHS Centre for Involvement – a consortium of academics, consumer groups and local government – helped identify, share and promote best practice in PPI to NHS staff and organizations. Other national institutions have also been established to support PPI, such as the Picker Institute Europe which coordinates the NHS national patient survey in England for the Care Quality Commission. In addition a PPI specialist collection has been established on the National Electronic Library for Health, which provides access to to the best available evidence on PPI.

Reforms in the NHS have provided further avenues for interaction with government. A number of health consumer groups are represented on the Department of Health's National Stakeholder Forum. Its role is to provide 'feedback and early advice on emerging policy' (Department of Health 2010). Yet there has been a shift in emphasis away from national service frameworks and clinical guidelines to locally driven change. In 2007 Health Minister Lord Darzi set out plans for reform of the English NHS in the *NHS Next Stage Review*. The focus was on locally led reorganization around eight clinical pathways (maternity and newborn; children's health; planned care; mental health; staying healthy; long-term conditions; acute care; end of life). Lord Darzi identified the need for PCTs to involve patients and the public in developing local plans. The review also announced a formal constitution for the NHS setting out principles and values, as well as the rights and responsibilities of patients, the public and staff. Several health consumer groups submitted proposals to the review and were involved in national stakeholder events, in particular seeking reassurance that the review would not lead to variations in care across England.

The development of the National Institute of Health and Clinical Excellence has also affected the health consumer group sector. Its role in approving access to particular drugs and treatments has provided a key focus for activity. While groups are formally engaged in its decision-making processes, they have also been involved in external campaigns to overturn decisions and in research to assess the implementation of guidance.

Organizational Change

The health consumer group sector has undergone a restructuring of its formal alliances. In 2006 a working group was formed to produce a proposal for a national level formal alliance for health and social care organizations (Taggart 2007). In 2007–8, National Voices was launched. The organization, which covers England, is a coalition of more than 200 groups and has four key areas of work: advocacy for patients, carers and service users through events, research, surveys and campaigns; work with government, the NHS, politicians, professionals and regulators to improve services and strengthen the voice of service users; hosting and supporting a service user panel, bringing together a wide range of current service users; and providing information, help and support to its members together with opportunities for them to influence the health and social care agenda (National Voices 2009).

There had been little consensus within the sector about the need for such a body (Baggott et al. 2005), but health consumer groups now clearly see a purpose for National Voices. Indeed two key formal alliances, the Long-term Medical Conditions Alliance and the Patients Forum, have merged with it. The new organization announced that its initial focus would be on influencing policy:

'National Voices' will be a success if, within a couple of years of its inception, service user involvement is a pre-requisite to policymaking and a systematic approach to engagement means that no policy or strategic direction can emerge without voluntary sector engagement. (Taggart 2007:11)

One core consumer group activity is developing strategies for organizational maintenance and survival. Given the state of flux within the voluntary sector it is difficult to determine how many organizations there are at any one time (Kendall 2003). The ESRC interview sample provides an indication of the extent to which organizational circumstances change. Of the 39 groups previously interviewed only 22 were still operating under the same name in Autumn 2010, four had rebranded/relaunched, six had merged with other health care organizations and six had closed. The remaining group, though still registered with the UK Charity Commission, was nearly nine months overdue in sending accounts and its website had closed down.

For some groups rebranding/relaunching was necessary to reflect changes to the original remit of the charity. Indeed, it has been argued that rebranding is a sign of an increasingly professionalized sector (Fearn 2007). For example, in 2002 the National Schizophrenia Fellowship rebranded itself Rethink, because many of its service users and members did not have a diagnosis of schizophrenia and there was concern that the stigma associated with schizophrenia might dissuade people from contacting the organization (Batty 2002).

Other groups merged, creating stronger organizations. In the cancer field, the UK Breast Cancer Coalition merged in 2003 with Breakthrough Breast Cancer, a high-profile charity focusing on fundraising for research and education. Breakthrough was able to access the Coalition's grassroots advocacy experience while the Coalition gained from Breakthrough's fundraising and research expertise (Shifrin 2003). In 2002 Cancerlink, a support network of local self-help groups, merged with specialist nursing provider Macmillan Cancer Support (Macmillan 2009). In 2008 Cancerbackup, which campaigned and provided information for people affected by cancer, also merged with Macmillan.

In the field of heart-related illness, the Family Heart Association merged in 2002 with the British Hyperlipidaemeia Association, a professional body for scientists and health professionals working on inherited high-cholesterol conditions. Weiner (2008) argues this was a strategic move to reinforce their legitimacy with policymakers and funders. Aiming to strengthen their position in the policy arena, the United Kingdom's two largest support groups for older people, Help the Aged and Age Concern, merged in 2010 and relaunched under the new name Age UK.

The closures of the College of Health (2003) and the Maternity Alliance (2005) were due to financial constraints (Gould 2003; Volresource 2005). Established in 1994 to campaign on mental health, the Zito Trust closed down in 2009, stating that it had achieved its original objectives. While its trustees saw a need for continuing advice and support services, attracting funding in a competitive environment was difficult (Zito Trust 2009). However, new groups also appeared; for example in 2008 Maternity Action formed to continue some of the work of the Maternity Alliance (Maternity Action 2009).

This sector remains in flux, making it difficult for health consumer groups to maintain momentum in the policy process and often affecting the balance of power between organizations representing particular health conditions. For example, in the cancer area three new formal alliances have been established over the past decade. Cancer52, an alliance of groups 'working to address the inequalities that exist in policy, services and research into the less common cancers', evolved out of work for the National Clinical Director for Cancer on the Department of Health's Cancer Reform Strategy (Cancer52 2010). In 2002 the Cancer Campaigning Group and the Rarer Cancers Forum also formed. Both groups have a policy agenda around access to services. This suggests the sector is developing a more structured approach to campaigning. It reflects a significant change since the ESRC study, in which fragmentation within the cancer sector had raised concerns about the cancer groups' ability to cooperate in lobbying and campaigning (Jones 2007).

Cross-condition alliances have also formed, often as a result of new policy directives galvanizing action. In 2009 Rare Disease UK formed as an alliance of academics, patient organizations, industry and individuals working to promote national strategies for rare diseases as a result of the European Council's recommendation for action in this area. The Specialised Healthcare Alliance formed in 2003 to campaign for people with rare diseases and other complex conditions requiring specialized medical care. In addition, new bodies like the National Institute of Health and Clinical Excellence may act as a catalyst for groups. In 2002 the Medical Technology Group, a coalition of patient groups, research charities and developers and manufacturers of medical technologies, formed to secure 'patient access to the best diagnostic, imaging, surgical and supported living technology' (Medical Technology Group 2009). These formal alliances encompass other health care stakeholders, including the medical technology industry, perhaps suggesting that health consumer groups still rely to some extent on other more powerful actors.

A key factor in organizational survival and maintenance is funding. In recent years government has sought to build formal relationships with the voluntary sector, bringing it into service delivery and developing guidelines and frameworks to reflect this new relationship (Department of Health 2004c). This is something of a double-edged sword for health consumer groups. On the one hand groups providing services may gain greater access to decision-makers. But at the same time their contractual obligations may constrain their ability to represent patients and the wider public. Their independence may be further limited by threats to future funding should they speak out on the impact of policies.

Changes in Policy Processes

Since devolution, the United Kingdom's four constituent countries are increasingly adopting different policy priorities, policymaking processes and PPI structures (Greer 2009a). For groups established to serve the needs of patients, users and carers across the United Kingdom, devolution adds to resource pressures. Influencing policy in, say, Scotland may require different strategies than in England. Larger charities in particular have restructured their operations to reflect devolution, but for smaller organizations whose resources are already stretched devolution risks diluting their already meagre resources for influencing policy. There has been no research into the impact of devolution on the representation of patient and public interests, and on health consumer groups in particular, something which needs urgent remedy.

Another important development in recent years is that health consumer groups are looking more towards Europe than previously. For example, the UK Stroke Association is a member of the Stroke Alliance for Europe (SAFE), formed in 2004 to represent the interests of patients and carers and to advocate for stroke prevention and care across Europe. Despite the fact that the delivery of health services remains a national competency, European involvement in health policy is likely to increase, particularly in relation to the pharmaceutical industry, the setting of research priorities, cross-border health care, and disease prevention (Baggott 2007; Greer 2009b). While the links UK groups have developed with Europe have not yet been studied systematically, there are strong indications that groups are working at this level, either lobbying EU institutions directly or by forming or joining pan-European alliances. The ESRC study found that even by 1999 a fifth of groups had had contact with the EU in the previous 3 years. Recent scoping work by the authors on pan-European health consumer groups – formal alliances whose membership comprises national level groups – suggests that this sector has evolved significantly over the past decade, with over half of groups listed in a directory of EU-level organizations having formed since 2000 (PatientView 2008).

For some groups, lobbying at this level is a vital part of their role; for example one of the Genetic Interest Group's policy aims is to engage 'with European initiatives that can benefit the patients of inherited conditions in the UK' (Genetic Interest Group 2010). It has lobbied for regulations to promote the development and registration of 'orphan' medicinal products (for diseases affecting less than five of every 10 000 EU residents) at EU level and is a founding member of the European Alliance of Genetic Support Groups and a member of the European Organisation for Rare Disorders (EURORDIS). For other organizations, the implications of EU policy for the UK health system can raise concerns: for example the Patients Association has commented on the effect of the EU Working Time Directive, which limits the hours junior doctors can work. Working at a supranational level is likely to affect the aims and activities of groups. For example, Baker (2005: 762), citing the example of the Parkinson's disease sector, argues the need for horizontal and vertical integration of policy aims to ensure there is a 'consistent message that reflects the needs of patients'.

In the UK the health consumer group sector appears more highly developed in its depth, resources and involvement in the policy process than in most other EU countries (Baggott and Forster 2008). However there is limited comparative research at the international level for assessing how the UK experience compares with other advanced health systems (see Wood 2000 and this volume for notable exceptions). This variation may be due to the way health systems and the voluntary sector have evolved in different countries and warrants further research.

CONCLUSIONS

The ESRC study concluded that by the early years of the twenty-first century the health consumer group movement in the United Kingdom was beginning to challenge the perspectives of other actors in the national policy process. Have health consumer groups been able to build on these achievements and more readily challenge other interests?

Although there remains a strong rationale for the involvement of health consumer groups in policymaking, there is little evidence they have strengthened their position in the national policy process. Those within the sector recognize that despite two decades of PPI policy, the majority of groups still struggle to exert influence, compared with other interests. In 2003 the chief executive of Breakthrough Breast Cancer commented: '[It's] only really since the NHS Plan that there has been the beginnings of strategic relations between voluntary organizations and the Department of Health and the NHS. We've a long way to go before we are sitting at the table as equals' (Shifrin 2003).

In 2008 the former National Director for Patients and the Public also suggested that patients' interests were subordinate to those of more powerful actors:

> When user interests come to the fore, as they have done on occasions under both Conservative and Labour Governments, the interests of health professionals, NHS institutions, the research and pharmaceutical industries and the Department of Health have all combined to nullify change. The NHS has sixty years experience of successfully avoiding the impact of government policies and the preferences of patients. (cited in LGA Health Commission 2008: 47)

We would not argue that health consumer groups have regressed. Rather, PPI strategy has shifted its focus towards the local level and this may have limited groups' opportunities to build on their early success at the national level. The extent to which local groups (and the branches of national consumer organizations) will have more opportunities to exercise influence is unknown, as the full implications of changes in local systems of PPI remain unclear. While there are some signs from the sector that national health consumer groups are working to promote local involvement, early indications are that they have concerns about the new PPI mechanisms (Cook 2009; PatientView 2009). More research is needed on the role and influence of health consumer groups at the local level – an area of activity excluded from the ESRC study – and the impact of devolution on these organizations, particularly because many changes outlined above affect only England.

In England, National Voices has the potential to strengthen the sector and may provide the means by which the views of patients, users and carers continue to be heard at national level. As Hogg (2009: 174) argues, 'a strong national voice for patients and citizens is essential in formulating health policies'. National Voices' stated priority is policy influence. It has already responded to government consultations and hosted workshops on behalf of the Department of Health. It has also begun pushing its own policy agenda – together with the Royal College of Nursing it recently funded a review of local involvement in commissioning (PatientView 2009). While the sector recognizes the value of coming together, the closeness of National Voices to government may lead some to question its independence. It remains to be seen if it can build on the work of previous alliances in challenging government policy.

Given the number of organizations coming together at the international (especially the European) level, it would also be timely to explore the role, activities and impact of these groups, particularly how they incorporate the different traditions, philosophies and agendas of national-level health consumer groups. Further research is warranted on how internal and external pressures prompt or hinder the formation of groups and their involvement in the policy process within and across different health systems. Comparative research is also warranted on the extent to which groups at all levels reflect citizen or consumerist perspectives in their policy activities. In order to assess whether or not health consumer groups constitute an independent and influential interest group there is a pressing need to research the extent to which these groups are influencing policy at the supranational level, particularly against professional and commercial interests.

REFERENCES

Alford, R. (1975), *Health Care Politics: Ideological and Interest Group Barriers to Reform*, Chicago, IL: University of Chicago Press.

Allsop, J., K. Jones and R. Baggott (2004), 'Health consumer groups in the UK: a new social movement?', *Sociology of Health & Illness*, **26** (6): 737–56.

Anheier, H.K. and J. Kendall (2002), 'Interpersonal trust and voluntary association: examining three approaches', *British Journal of Sociology*, **53** (3): 343–62.

Baker, M. (2005), 'Challenges for patient organisations: focus on Europe', *Journal of Neurology, Neurosurgery and Psychiatry*, **76** (6): 762–3.

Baggott, R. (2005), 'A funny thing happened on the way to the Forum', *Public Administration*, **83** (3): 533–51.

Baggott, R. (2007), *Understanding Healthcare Policy*, Bristol: Policy Press.

Baggott, R., J. Allsop and K. Jones (2005), *Speaking for Patients and Carers: Health Consumer Groups and the Policy Process*, Basingstoke: Palgrave.

Baggott, R. and R. Forster (2008), 'Health consumer and patients' organizations in Europe; towards a comparative analysis', *Health Expectations*, **11** (1): 85–94.

Batty, D. (2002), 'Brand new approach', *The Guardian,* 3 July, accessed 10 December 2009 at www.guardian.co.uk.

Brown, P., B. Mayer, S. Zavestovski, T. Luebke, J. Mandelbaum and S. McCormick

(2003), 'The health politics of asthma: environmental justice and collective illness experience in the United States', *Social Science & Medicine*, **57** (3): 453–64.

Byrne, P. (1997), *Social Movements in Britain*, London: Routledge.

Cancer52 (2010), 'About us', accessed 15 January 2010 at www.cancer52.org.uk.

Cook, B. (2009), *LINks – A Real Opportunity for National Voluntary Organizations*, London: National Voices.

Cooper, L., A. Coote, A. Davies and C. Jackson (1995), *Voices Off: Tackling the Democratic Deficit in Health*, London: Institute of Public Policy Research.

Department of Health (1996), *Patient Partnership: Building a Collaborative Strategy*, Leeds: Department of Health.

Department of Health (1999), *Patient and Public Involvement in the New NHS*, London: Department of Health.

Department of Health (2004a), *Patient and Public Involvement in Health: Evidence for Policy Implementation*, London: Department of Health.

Department of Health (2004b), *Reconfiguring the Department of Health's Arm's Length Bodies*, London: Department of Health.

Department of Health (2004c), *Making Partnership Work for Patients, Carers and Service Users*, London: Department of Health.

Department of Health (2006a), *Concluding the Review of Patient and Public Involvement. Recommendations to Ministers from Expert Panel*, London: Department of Health.

Department of Health (2006b), *A Stronger Local Voice: A Framework for Creating a Strong Local Voice in the Development of Health and Social Care*, London: Department of Health.

Department of Health (2007), *World Class Commissioning: Competencies*, London: Department of Health.

Department of Health (2010), 'The national stakeholder forum', accessed 15 January 2010 at www.dh.gov.uk.

Epstein, S. (1996), *Impure Science: Aids, Activism, and the Politics of Knowledge*, Berkeley, CA: University of California Press.

Fearn, H. (2007), 'What's in a name?', *Charity Times* (January/February), accessed 26 November 2009 at www.charitytimes.com.

Genetic Interest Group (2010), 'Policy', accessed 15 January 2010 at www.gig.org.uk/policy.ht .

Gould, M. (2003), 'Unfinished business', *The Guardian*, 29 October, Society Pages, p. 4.

Grant, W. (1995), *Pressure Groups, Politics and Democracy in Britain*, London: Harvester Wheatsheaf.

Greer, S. (2009a), *Territorial Politics and Health Policy*, Manchester: Manchester University Press.

Greer, S. (2009b), *The Politics of European Health Policies*, Maidenhead: Oxford University Press.

House of Commons Health Committee (2003), *Patient and Public Involvement Seventh Report 2002–3*, London: The Stationery Office.

House of Commons Health Committee (2007), *Patient and Public Involvement in the NHS. Third Report 2006–7*, London: The Stationery Office.

Hogg, C. (1999), *Patients and Power*, London: Sage.

Hogg, C. (2009), *Citizens, Consumers and the NHS*, Basingstoke: Palgrave.

Jennings, M.K. (1999), 'Political responses to pain and loss', *American Political Science Review*, **93** (1): 1–15.

Jones, K. (2007), 'Building alliances: incentives and impediments in the UK health consumer group sector', *Social Policy and Society*, **6** (4): 515–28.

Jones, K. (2008), 'In whose interest? Relationships between health consumer groups and the pharmaceutical industry in the UK', *Sociology of Health & Illness*, **30** (6): 929–44.

Kendall, J. (2003), *The Voluntary Sector: Comparative Perspectives in the UK*, London: Routledge.

LGA Health Commission (2008), *Who's Accountable for Health?*, London: Local Government Association.

Lock, S. (1986), 'Self-help groups: the fourth estate in medicine?', *British Medical Journal*, **293** (6562): 1596–600.

Macmillan (2009), 'Our history', accessed 17 November 2009 at www.macmillan.org.uk.

Maloney, W.A., A.G. Jordan and A.M. McLaughlin (1994), 'Interest groups and the policy process: the insider/outsider model revisited', *Journal of Public Policy*, **14** (1): 17–38.

Marsh, D. and R. Rhodes (1992), *Policy Networks in British Government*, Oxford: Clarendon.

Maternity Action (2009), 'Maternity Alliance', accessed 12 November 2009 at www.maternityaction.org.uk/maternityalliance.html.

Moran, M. (1999), *Governing the Health Care State*, Manchester: Manchester University Press.

Medical Technology Group (2009), *Medical Technology and Innovation*, **21**: 1.

National Voices (2009), 'About us', accessed 19 November 2009 at www.national voices.org.uk.

PatientView (2008), *European Patients Groups Directory*, Brussels: Burson-Marsteller.

PatientView (2009), *Local Healthcare Commissioning: Grassroots Involvement?*, London: National Voices/Royal College of Nursing.

Picker Institute Europe (2009), *Patient and Public Engagement: The Early Impact of World Class Commissioning*, Oxford: Picker Institute Europe.

Posner, N. (2009), 'Patient organizations for long term conditions', *RCN Research Institute Newsletter*, **1** (4): 1.

Putnam, R. (2000), *Bowling Alone*, New York: Simon & Schuster.

Sabatier, P. (1999), 'The need for better theories', in P. Sabatier (ed.), *Theories of the Policy Process*, Boulder, CO: Westview, pp. 3–19.

Santry, C. (2009), 'Voters halve as governors win elections uncontested', *Health Service Journal*, 5 November, p. 11.

Shifrin, T. (2003), 'Target conscious', *The Guardian*, 29 October, accessed 17 November 2009 at www.guardian.co.uk.

Taggart, E. (2007), *National Voices*, London: National Voices Working Group.

Volresource (2005), 'Mergers and closures', accessed 5 June 2006 at www.vol resource.org.uk/kcnews/news3432.htm.

Weiner, K. (2008), 'Lay involvement and legitimacy', *Journal of Contemporary Ethnography*, **38** (2): 254–73.

Whiteley, P.F. and S.J. Winyard (1987), *Pressure for the Poor: The Poverty Lobby and Policy Making*, London: Methuen.

Wood, B. (2000), *Patient Power? The Politics of Patients' Associations in Britain and America*, Buckingham: Open University Press.

Zito Trust (2009), 'The closure of the Zito Trust: statement by the trustees', accessed 17 November 2009 at www.zitotrust.co.uk/closure%20statement.doc.

4. Citizens, consumers and stakeholders in European health policy

Meri Koivusalo and Jonathan Tritter

In this chapter we track emerging issues in public participation and involvement in European policymaking. We focus on the politics, legitimacy and accountability of different actors as well as exploring how European participation processes relate to globalization in general and global and regional governance in particular. Health policies tend to be understood as national or even local, yet they are often shaped and defined by regulatory decisions and policies that are determined globally and regionally.

EUROPEAN UNION AND HEALTH

Governance in the European Union (EU) is based on legal treaties and founded on the protection and promotion of the 'Four Freedoms' – the free movement of goods, capital, services and persons – which are understood as fundamental to the maintenance of a common market. These treaties define the basis on which the European Commission can undertake initiatives and propose regulatory action in the form of directives. While the European Commission can initiate actions, these need to be approved by the Council of the European Union and the European Parliament. In principle, citizens in the EU are represented both through their own governments, which are members of the Council of the European Union, and their elected representatives in the European Parliament. However in terms of democratic governance a deficit can be identified at the European level, particularly in relation to executive powers. This has been part of a European discourse on civil society since the Maastricht Treaty of 1992.

Health policies have traditionally been part of national policy. While some aspects of health were raised in the Treaty of Rome, which established the European Economic Community, health was not understood as a matter for European-level policy. This situation has slowly changed but remains contentious. Article 129 of the Maastricht Treaty included provisions on health, but these were more explicit in the Amsterdam Treaty of 1997.

Since consumer issues have become prominent in domestic markets they have also inevitably emerged in and demanded responses from the EU. Thus particular European civil society actors have been present from an early stage in the history of the EU. The European Consumers' Organisation, established in 1962, was one of the first European-level civil society groups. In health a range of non-governmental actors seeks to influence the European agenda, including those with a specific focus, such as the European CanCer Organisation (ECCO), and more general groups like the European Public Health Alliance (EPHA). The first EU health programme was focused on cancer. Initiated in 1984, it sought European engagement in areas and issues closer to citizens; this programme led later to campaigns on tobacco and cancer (Greer 2009; Boessen and Maarse 2009).

Health was originally part of the brief of the Directorate-General responsible for Employment, Social Affairs and Equal Opportunities (DG Employment). The establishment of the Directorate-General Health and Consumer issues (now DG Sanco) gave health issues a higher profile within the European Commission. Some health-related activities, such as services of general interest, the open method of coordination of care of the elderly, and occupational health care issues, have remained under the auspices of the DG Employment, which has close links to NGOs active in the social and employment field – including trade unions and disability organizations – as well as discrimination and equality focused organizations. Another aspect of European health policy concerns trade- and development-related health issues, such as HIV/AIDS care and access to medicines, which were also raised in the recent consultation on global health under the auspices of the Directorate-General Development (European Commission 2009b).

In the late 1990s the legal and constitutional aspects of the EU were more prominently articulated as part of European health policymaking. While the European Court of Justice (ECJ) had made decisions on health-related matters prior to the Kohll (ECJ 1998a) and Decker (ECJ 1998b) cases, the political context and process of policy development on such matters changed in response to them. While the ECJ deals with individual cases, its judgements have wider significance, since case law is the basis for further action by the European Commission and politics determines which legal decisions become policy initiatives. For example political influence exerted by the tobacco industry resulted in rejection of an approved European directive (Boessen and Maarse 2008). Interest groups use three strategies to shape policy: test case litigation, sequential litigation and simultaneous litigation to further a case (McCown 2009).

EUROPEAN GOVERNANCE AND CITIZEN PARTICIPATION

Owing to the nature of its governance the EU's role and relationship to citizens in general remain contested, with the EU often being accused of creating a 'democratic deficit'. In health this is reflected in opinion surveys showing that while citizens value health provision highly they are against EU engagement in health policy. The European Commission aimed to address this problem in its *White Paper on European Governance* (European Commission 2001), which included recommendations on the setting of minimum requirements for consultation. Treaties have also introduced new mechanisms for citizen participation, such as the European Citizens' Initiative (European Commission 2009a). Another aspect of governance is the evolving relationship between citizens' rights and European policies, and the revision of the European Social Charter (Council of Europe 1996), although the impact of such measures has been compromised by some countries, such as the United Kingdom, specifying exclusions from some of the Charter's commitments.

The European Commission has the right to initiate policies. This has led to efforts to understand the role of participation in the initial phase of policy-making – shaping and influencing what is proposed (Carboni 2009; Greer 2009). While there is broad scope for participation in the European policy process, how an issue emerges and is framed is important. The Commission's crucial role in setting the agenda adds weight to its relevance in the policy-making process, but treaties have enhanced the role of the European Parliament. Introduced by the Lisbon Treaty (2007), the EU's ordinary legislative procedure is now 'co-decision': that is, based on the principle of parity, meaning that neither the European Parliament nor the Council of the European Union may adopt legislation without the assent of the other body (Lisbon Treaty Article 294). This new procedure creates scope to make changes to Commission proposals in the European Parliament.

European multi-level governance also offers scope for scrutiny by various actors. The European Council and the European Parliament are the most important actors in the decision-making process. It is mandatory to consult the Economic and Social Committee on issues defined in the Treaty of Rome, but consultation can be made based on the initiative of institutions, including the Economic and Social Committee (Economic and Social Committee 2010).

Citizen engagement with the work of the Council of the European Union is limited to conferences or issue-based meetings. The influence of citizens on member governments remains primarily through national mechanisms for participation and accountability, and thus varies across the EU. While in some countries for some issues this may take the form of referenda or a popular vote, issues tend to be debated as part of broader decision-making measures on European policies. More informal dialogue and debates about European-level policies have been sought in the context of annual meetings and gatherings, such as the annual European Health Forum, Gastein, which has been referred to as 'a kind of Davos' for European health policymaking.

CONSUMERS, PUBLIC HEALTH ORGANIZATIONS AND STAKEHOLDERS

Consumer and public health organizations have a presence in the European Parliament in intergroup work and secretariats. For example the EPHA and the European Consumers' Organisation share responsibility for the secretariat to the European Parliament's Health Intergroup. The Health and Consumer Intergroup aims to provide 'regular opportunities for MEPs [Members of the European Parliament] to exchange views with public health and consumer experts, Commission officials, NGOs and other relevant stakeholders' (Health and Consumer Intergroup 2004). The Consumer Intergroup has been active since 1989, the Health Intergroup since 1994. In January 2010 the EPHA reported that, after an unsuccessful attempt by the Secretariat to secure a health intergroup, the EPHA would pursue the creation of a health forum within the European Parliament (European Public Health Alliance 2010). Current discussions within the Parliament focus on a small number of meetings a year on key topics and dossiers. Other health-related arrangements with civil society secretariats include, for example, the Working Group on Reproductive Health, HIV/AIDS and Development, for which Marie Stopes International acts as the secretariat.

The EU Health Forum can be described as a means of formalizing and creating structural dialogue between the European Commission and NGOs. In the 1990s the relationship between the European Commission and public health organizations had a mutually supportive agenda. One aspect of this was the joint battle over tobacco, where DG Sanco, supported by the NGOs, was confronted by other more prominent Directorate-Generals, as well as the lobbying machinery of the tobacco industry. That DG Sanco now seems less willing to challenge more powerful Directorate-Generals on the causes of health problems may be the consequence of this experience. Today it focuses on ensuring that health policy complies with internal market obligations. This would go some way to explaining also why DG Sanco has shifted towards stakeholder-type participation in the establishment of platforms as well as creating further scope for patient group participation in policymaking. As a result, effective participation in these platforms has become more difficult for NGOs and networks active in public health as it requires resource commitments that NGOs funded on a short-term basis find difficult – certainly much more so than 'stakeholder' corporations (see European Public Health Alliance 2005).

Health issues are dealt with under several Directorates other than DG Sanco. Perhaps the most important is the Directorate-General Enterprise (DG Enterprise). A study of European pharmaceutical policies and advocacy coalitions by Carboni (2009: 31) concluded by emphasizing 'the role played by the commission as both policy broker and entrepreneur in a process'. As DG Enterprise controlled pharmaceutical policy instead of DG Sanco, this resulted in an industry-oriented agenda and easy access for the pro-industry coalition to policymaking. This is in accordance with other research and studies, which have shown a bias towards industrial policy, rather than public health or health care policy priorities in EU health policies (Permanand 2006; Adamini et al. 2009). This has been accompanied by longer-term calls and efforts to strengthen the public health aspects of pharmaceutical policy. These aims emerged when it was realized, with the announcement by the European Commission Chair in November 2009, that DG Sanco's responsibility would include pharmaceutical products and medical devices. However it remains to be seen how this shift will affect European policy content or engagement with citizens and civil society.

GLOBALIZATION AND EUROPEAN UNION HEALTH POLICY PROCESSES

Globalization influences many policy processes and often feeds into regional and national debates on regulation, standard-setting and policy priorities. In the EU the implications of globalization for health are most evident in relation to trade and development policies, but also in relation to more general European policy aims such as innovation, competitiveness and 'better' regulation. The Lisbon Strategy, and more recently the EU 2020 Agenda, represent broad political approaches shaping and legitimizing EU action and thus have crucial relevance in shaping all policy areas, including health policy.

Particular networks and organizations illustrate and promote particular forms of globalization. For instance the Transatlantic Consumer Dialogue (TACD) provides 'a forum of US and EU consumer organisations which develops and agrees on joint consumer policy recommendations to the US government and the EU to promote the consumer interest in EU and US policymaking' (TACD 2010). Access to medicines has become a part of this dialogue, in particular as a result of the efforts of the Consumer Project on Technology (now known as Knowledge Ecology International), which has followed intellectual property rights debates from a broad perspective. TACD has become part of the EU's formal external dialogue, but still remains the poor relation of the TransAtlantic Business Dialogue (TABD), which defines itself as 'the leading voice promoting a barrier-free transatlantic market for growth, innovation and sustainability in the global economy' (TABD 2010).

The Lisbon Treaty introduced new powers and an important shift in the work of the European Commission in strengthening competence in trade policies and opening up the scope for common external policies. The European Commission has been quick to envisage an EU role in global health, including a variety of areas and issues. EU engagement with global health issues should be considered not merely a matter of solidarity with developing countries, but also in relation to power-sharing between the European Commission and member states. It has particular relevance for health, where the burden of costs and accountabilities remains strongly at member state level.

Influencing EU trade policies remains a challenging task and while the European Commission has established consultations, including a Directorate-General Trade Issue Group on Trade and Health, its role in influencing decisions has been limited at best (Dur and De Bievre 2007). Health issues related to trade policy have predominantly been dealt with in the context of development and the interests of developing countries. Yet most civil society organizations involved in trade policy work under a development mandate rather than a broader policy mandate. This has resulted in health issues and health NGOs being focused primarily on health and development rather than on health issues within the EU.

THE POLITICS OF CIVIL SOCIETY PARTICIPATION

Increasingly, the EU language of 'civil society participation' is being replaced by that of 'stakeholder participation', which has a different connotation and focus and tends to lend greater prominence to interest groups and representatives of parties affected by proposed changes rather than to citizens or citizen groups. From a health promotion perspective, tobacco or alcohol industry associations would not be seen as the most appropriate civil society participants in health-related standard-setting or regulatory action, or in identifying health policy priorities. As 'stakeholders', industry associations have a more legitimate presence in health policymaking. The emphasis on stakeholder participation emerges from the context of industrial policies and changes in EU legislation that have enabled and strengthened such stakeholders' inclusion in policymaking.

A case in point can be found in the *White Paper on European Governance*, which deals with engagement with civil society, regional organizations and citizens. Early consultation and sharing with civil society groups was the primary emphasis (European Commission 2001). Requirements for early and effective participation of interested parties in policymaking became established as part of 'better regulation' measures in the Mandelkern report (Mandelkern 2001). Thus:

> To be effective, consultation must start as early as possible. Interested parties should therefore be involved in the development of a policy at a stage where they can still have an impact on the formulation of the main aims, methods of delivery, performance indicators and, where appropriate, the initial outlines of that policy. Consultation at more than one stage may be required. (EU Commission 2002)

While this emphasis on consultation and governance includes NGOs, public interest actors and participants, the ways in which actual measures have been implemented seem to have especially enabled corporate engagement and lobbying. The importance of early-phase lobbying has also been emphasized by pharmaceutical industry lobbyists, one of whom was reported as saying 'the earlier you are in the process, the more chances you have to be successful' (Carboni 2009: 11).

The traditional role of lobbyists and interest groups has been prominent in EU policymaking, and in health this has been particularly clear in relation to pharmaceutical policies. In the late 1990s pharmaceutical and biotechnology industries were perhaps the most prominent and effective interest group representatives at the European level, having the capacity to change substantially the direction of European Commission regulatory aims and measures (Greenwood 1997; 2007). There is also evidence of tobacco industry success in shaping regulatory efforts at the European level (Hastings and Angus 2004). A large share of this influence has been based on informal mechanisms and not mediated through formal European Commission or European Parliament forums. Networking, seminars and other activities continue to provide opportunities to influence policymaking within the EU. The tobacco industry has also been shown to have broader influence on the ways in which impact assessment and regulatory policies have become shaped in the EU (Smith et al. 2010).

European Commission policymaking increasingly uses web-based consultations. While these 'open consultations' are a method that can create transparency and provide opportunities for broadly based participation, they also give the Commission scope to define the extent and nature of support for proposals and, where active advocacy groups exist, benefit from their contributions. This is also reflected in the way consultations are framed, as they often tend not to focus on the actual content of a document or proposed measure but instead pose a series of questions chosen by the Commission. The 'answers' to consultation questions are then analysed and drawn together by the Commission. There is potential to create transparency in the development of policy by making available the answers that are lodged and details of those who participate, which could also provide the basis for an evaluation of the process and outcomes of such consultations. The Commission's guidance on the matter states that: 'contributions to open public consultations will be made public on the single access point' (European Commission 2002). However it is unclear whether all the answers submitted are made public. For instance the Commission did not commit to post all the submitted responses to the recent consultation on global health on its website (European Commission 2009b), making it difficult to evaluate or judge the legitimacy of the Commission's findings.

A case in point is apparent in the Commission's recent consultation on the EU 2020 Agenda. In response to the Commission's overview of the views expressed, social NGOs – as part of the Social Platform – stated (Reuter 2010):

> We represent 42 pan-European social NGO networks, and find that the overview of the responses to the EU2020 consultation totally mischaracterises the position of our sector. It claims that we 'broadly support the Commission's proposed priorities', yet our response to the consultation explicitly said the opposite: that the proposed text represented a step back for social cohesion and social inclusion in Europe.

The Social Platform's response also expressed concern over the Commission's portrayal of citizens and fundamental rights, specifically the way the EU 2020 Agenda considers citizens to be consumers: 'Citizens must be empowered to play a full part in the single market. This requires strengthening their ability and confidence to buy goods and services cross-border, in particular on-line' (European Commission 2009c: 10). The result, the Social Platform suggests, is that fundamental rights are considered merely in the context of civil rights and the right to security (Social Platform 2009).

The legitimacy and focus on participation and involvement of consumers beyond EU common markets has proved difficult. Despite expectations that a social rights approach would mean greater access to health care and social security across borders, this has not necessarily been realized. The Patient Rights draft directive has, in spite of its name, less to do with patient rights than with the expansion of choice and markets in the EU (Tritter et al. 2009). Even in the more clear-cut area of consumer rights, recent efforts to harmonize such rights have caused concern. While harmonization was earlier based on minimum levels of requirements, the new proposal is based on maximum levels, set at the current minimum level of protection. The European Consumers' Organisation has argued that this would lead in many member states to the removal or reduction of important consumer protection rights (European Consumers' Organisation 2008). A recent Parliament report indicates a shift and backing-off from full harmonization towards a targeted harmonization approach, which would imply more scope to keep a higher level of consumer protection at least in some areas of consumer rights (Schwab 2010). While this implies that campaigning and consumer voice can make some difference, it remains to be seen whether the balance in the process will in future tilt towards the benefit of consumer rights or represent more adjusting of consumer rights to better fit the needs of stakeholders and internal markets.

POLICIES AND POLITICS OF HEALTH AND CONSUMER GROUPS – ISSUES OF CONCERN

In health care there are concerns about the way NGOs have become important as means for creating demand for particular medicines, thus shaping pharmaceutical policies. Public health groups, with their distinct role, may come to be marginalized with the emergence of groups that support more liberalized and commercialized service provision – groups and actors that are more industry advocates than health advocates.

The rising cost of pharmaceuticals has drawn attention to the assessment of the cost effectiveness of new treatments, as well as the comparison of new treatments to existing ones on the market. The UK National Institute for Health and Clinical Excellence has led in this area in terms of implementation, drawing on mechanisms to integrate the views of NGOs and members of the public in their judgements. At the centre of the debate is the recognition that globally the majority of new pharmaceuticals are based primarily on the incremental innovation of products already on the market, often with very limited additional clinical benefits (OECD 2008). Many new pharmaceutical products are geared to small patient groups, but often with very high prices. This has made patient groups and NGOs important in terms of creating demand and influencing policy and purchasing decisions.

The 'use' of patient groups and NGOs to further the goals of industry is not new. At one end of the spectrum are the 'front groups' supported by corporations that take part in 'astroturf lobbying', a 'grassroots program that involves the instant manufacturing of public support for a point of view in which either uninformed activists are recruited or means of deception are used to recruit them' (Stauber and Rampton 1995a: 23). This term was originally coined by US Senator Lloyd Bentsen, a Texan, first appearing in the *Washington Post* where he said of the huge number of cards and letters he had received from opponents to insurance provision: 'A fellow from Texas can tell the difference between grass roots and Astro Turf' (quoted in Stauber and Rampton 1995b).[1] Such practices, particularly apparent around environmental issues, are also widespread in health and have been documented extensively in the United States, Australia and the United Kingdom:

> Front groups enable corporations, such as pharmaceutical companies, to take part in
> public debates and government hearings behind a cover of community concern.
> Corporations could do this openly and in their own names but it is far more effec-
> tive to have a group of citizens or a group of experts – preferably a coalition of such
> groups – which can publicly promote the outcomes desired by the corporation
> whilst claiming to represent the public interest. (Gosden and Beder 2001: 148)

For instance in the United States grassroots groups demanding access to
hepatitis C vaccine were found to have been initiated and funded by industry
(O'Harrow 2000). While all patient groups or campaigns demanding access to
new medicines or other technologies should not be dismissed as 'astroturf' or
'front' groups, it is important to recognize how patient groups and NGOs can
have a mutually beneficial relationship with industry in calling for access to
medicines, increasingly put in terms of 'rights to health'. While it may be
easier to focus attention on the role of industry in establishing, supporting and
financing patient groups, corporate interests are broader than this, extending to
the articulation of 'rights to health' and choice of health care and patient
mobility within the EU.

According to official accounts the establishment of the European Patients'
Forum by DG Sanco was a response to the lack of a joint platform for the various patient groups involved with the Pharmaceutical Forum during the G10
process (European Patients' Forum 2010). Clearly it makes sense to avoid situations where a multitude of single-disease organizations swamps the
Commission in an effort to influence policy. But the European Patients' Forum
– established as a platform for patient organizations and interests – has been
criticized for the proportion of its funding derived from corporate sources and
for a lack of focus on the conflict of interests this entails (Health Action
International 2005). Analysis of responses to a public consultation regarding
the pharmaceutical industry as an information-provider about prescription
medicines (direct-to-consumer advertising) showed a substantial division
between consumer organizations, which were all against the proposal,
compared with patient organizations and patient information organizations,
which were more favourable towards it (Carboni 2009).

In addition to NGOs and formal and informal networks, Brussels also hosts
a substantial number of think tanks and lobbyists (Coen 2007), many of which
receive funding from the pharmaceutical industry. Recognizing the pervasive-
ness of funded organizations and lobbying, the European Parliament has
proposed a framework for the activities of lobbyists (European Parliament
2008).

Consumer Powerhouse is one example of such entrepreneurial activity
around health policymaking. With a background in the Swedish industry association TIMBRO, it has better links to corporations, think tanks and networks
than to consumer associations, yet Consumer Powerhouse has sought to

present itself as the voice of the consumer and a key source of information. The word 'consumer' in the corporation's title is problematic because little of its work represents, informs or derives from actual consumer views or perspectives. The presence and role of groups associated with pro-corporate views and policies like Consumer Powerhouse, other well-funded networks and think tanks is important, but as in the case of Consumer Powerhouse it is also problematic because there is confusion about whose voice it is and thus about its legitimacy as a source of information about consumers, citizens and service users at the European level. Furthermore, as organizations working on health and consumer issues rarely have equal resources for this type of action, a bias exists in favour of the lobbying power of corporate actors.

Conflicts of interest and sources of funding are important considerations in judging the position, publications and views of organizations that seek to participate in shaping European policy. In light of commercialization and interest group politics, it is necessary to emphasize that one of the major sources of funding for European NGOs, think tanks and networks is the European Commission itself. This has been particularly important for environmental policy, but is also reflected in some public health campaigning. One of the first anti-tobacco measures supported by the Commission was to provide funding for the European Bureau for Action on Smoking Prevention (Boessen and Maarse 2009).

CONCLUSIONS

The development of EU health policies has taken place against the backdrop of the evolution of general modes of European governance and particular modes of group participation in European policymaking. A wide variety of interests are now taking part in participatory processes at the European level, making procedures for explicit, transparent information about participants, their funding sources and the perspectives they claim to represent more necessary than ever.

We have sought to identify a range of ways in which participation in policy processes provides avenues for interest groups, and in particular commercial interests, for influencing the politics, policies and regulatory approach of the EU. The problem is not that participation and consultations take place, but that the promotion of particular forms of participation and the context in which they occur can serve to legitimize certain practices, as well as demands for specific products, regulatory interventions or policy measures.

The use and abuse of participatory approaches and democratic avenues in regulation or standard-setting, or in health or pharmaceutical policies, is not new. However it is important that such processes entail sufficient transparency, breadth and political and technical accountability so that new mechanisms to enhance participation do not primarily benefit special interest groups and industrial concerns. This is particularly salient for health policies within the EU as the costs and consequences of policies at the European level are borne primarily at a national level.

EU policies involve some consultation and are the result of the codecision process which permits checks and balances, and can go beyond the forms of involvement and level of transparency in policymaking of many member states. However the purpose of these consultative measures is not always clear. Nor is what takes place always evident. The lack of clarity in these matters becomes particularly problematic in areas where there are conflicts of interest between health or social issues and the broader economic goals of the EU.

Citizens are in danger of becoming defined as consumers within a market, limiting not only the scope and nature of participation in policy processes but also the ways in which EU policies concerning rights might evolve. EU measures adopted under the rubric of consumer and patient rights have not delivered such rights. Rather, the 'better regulation' the EU was supposed to deliver has come to be cynically regarded, if not as a facade for industry and market-driven measures, at least as undermining rather than strengthening citizens' rights. As the EU is increasingly likely to exert regulatory power in health and pharmaceutical policy, European policies must be subject to critical analysis if we are to avoid being sold astroturf rather than participatory processes that connect with the grassroots.

NOTES

1. Any reader not seeing the relevance here of 'a fellow from Texas' may like to know that the first well-publicized laying of the material was at the Houston Astrodome.

REFERENCES

Adamini S., H. Maarse, E. Versluis and D. Light (2009), 'Policymaking in data exclusivity in European Union: from industrial interests to legal realities', *Journal of Health Politics, Policy and Law*, **34** (6): 979–1010.

Boessen, S. and H. Maarse (2008), 'The impact of the treaty basis on health policy legislation in the European Union: a case study on the tobacco advertising directive', BMC Health Services Research, 8: 77, doi:10.1186/1472-6963-8-77, accessed 12 June 2010 at www.biomedcentral.com/1472-6963/8/77.

Boessen, S. and H. Maarse (2009), 'A ban on tobacco advertising: the role of interest groups', in D. Coen and J. Richardson (eds), *Lobbying the European Union: Institutions, Actors and Issues*, Oxford: Oxford University Press, pp. 212–32.

Carboni, N. (2009), 'Advocacy groups in the multilevel system of the European Union:

a case study in health policy-making', European Social Observatory paper 1, November, Brussels.

Coen, D. (2007), *Lobbying in the European Union*, November, PE 393.266. Directorate-General Internal Policies, Citizen Rights and Constitutional Affairs, Brussels: European Parliament, accessed 12 June 2010 at www.eurosfaire.prd.fr/7pc/doc/1211469722_lobbying_eu.pdf.

Council of Europe (1996), *European Social Charter* (revised), Strasbourg, France: Council of Europe.

Dur, A. and D. de Bievre (2007), 'Inclusion without influence? NGOs in European trade policy', *Journal of Public Policy*, **27** (1): 79–101.

Economic and Social Committee (2010), 'How the European Economic and Social Committee works', accessed 12 June 2010 at www.eesc.europa.eu/organisation/how/index_en.asp.

European Commission (2001), *European Governance. A White Paper*, Brussels: European Commission.

European Commission (2002), *Towards a Reinforced Culture of Consultation and Dialogue – General Principles and Minimum Standards for Consultation of Interested Parties by the Commission*, COM(2002) 704 final, Brussels: European Commission.

European Commission (2009a), *Green Paper on a European Citizens' Initiative*, Brussels 11.11. 2009. COM (2009) 622 final, Brussels: European Commission.

European Commission (2009b), 'The EU role in global health. Issue paper', accessed 15 June 2010 at www.ec.europa.eu/development/icenter/files/europa_only/EU_role_global_health_issue_paper_en.pdf.

European Commission (2009c), *Commission Working Document Consultation on the Future of 'EU 2020' Strategy*, Brussels: European Commission.

European Consumers' Organisation (2008), The Future of European Consumer's Rights – BEUC's Reaction to the Fundamental Issues Raised by the Proposal for a Directive of Consumers Rights, COM (2008) 614. Brussels: BEUC, accessed at www.docshare.beuc.org/docs/3/KOBPJEPDBHLMOMKDKLGOEHPMPDBG9DBY7Y9DW3571KM/BEUC/docs/DLS/2009-00291-01-E.pdf.

European Court of Justice (ECJ) (1998b), C-158/96 European Court of Justice judgment, Kohll vs Union des Caisses maladie, 28 April.

European Court of Justice (1998b), C-160/196 European Court of Justice judgment. Decker vs Caisse de maladie des employés privées, 28 April.

European Parliament (2008), *Report on the Framework for the Activities of Interest Representatives (Lobbyists) in the European Union*, Brussels: European Parliament.

European Patients' Forum (2010), 'Why was EPF created?', accessed 2 April 2010 at www.eu-patient.eu/About-EPF/What-is-EPF/Why-was-EPF-created/.

European Public Health Alliance (2005), 'The EU platform on action on diet, physical activity and health – an insider's perspective', accessed 2 March 2010 at www.epha.org/a/2344.

European Public Health Alliance (2010), 'Secretariat news', Winter, accessed 15 June 2010 at www.epha.org/a/3822m.

Gosden, R. and S. Beder (2001), 'Pharmaceutical industry agenda settings in mental health policies', *Ethical Human Sciences and Services*, **3** (3): 147–59.

Greenwood, J. (1997), *Representing Interests in the European Union*, London: Macmillan.

Greenwood, J. (2007), 'Review article: organised civil society and democratic legitimacy in the European Union', *British Journal of Political Science*, **37** (2): 333–57.

Greer, S. (2009), 'The changing world of European health lobbies', in D. Coen and J. Richardson (eds), *Lobbying the European Union: Institutions, Actors and Issues*, Oxford: Oxford University Press, pp. 189–211.

Hastings, G. and K. Angus (2004), 'The influence of the tobacco industry on European tobacco-control policy', in The ASPECT Consortium (ed.), *Tobacco or Health in the European Union Past, Present and Future*, Luxembourg: Office for Official Publications of the European Communities, pp. 195–226.

Health Action International (2005), *Does the European Patients' Forum Represent Patient or Industry Interests? A Case Study in the Need for Mandatory Financial Disclosure*, Amsterdam, Netherlands: Health Action International.

Health and Consumer Intergroup (2004), *Health and Consumer Intergroup Terms of Reference*, accessed 15 June 2010 at www.epha.org/IMG/pdf/HCI_ToR.pdf.

Mandelkern (2001), *Mandelkern Group on Better Regulation. Final Report*, Brussels: European Commission, accessed 12 June 2010 at www.ec.europa.eu/governance/better_regulation/documents/mandelkern_report.pdf.

McCown, M. (2009), 'Interest groups and the European Court of Justice', in D. Coen and J. Richardson (eds), *Lobbying the European Union: Institutions, Actors and Issues*, Oxford: Oxford University Press, pp. 89–104.

O'Harrow, R. (2000), 'Grass roots seeded by drugmaker', *Washington Post*, 12 September, A1.

Organisation for Economic Co-operation and Development (OECD) (2008), *Pharmaceutical Pricing Policies in a Global Market*, OECD Health Policy Studies, 24 September, Paris: OECD.

Permanand, G. (2006), *EU Pharmaceutical Regulation. The Politics of Policy Making*, Manchester: Manchester University Press.

Reuter, C. (2010), media release of the 'Social Platform, EU2020' consultation, accessed 12 June 2010 at www.socialplatform.org/News.asp?news=23862.

Schwab, A. (2010), 'Working document on the proposal for a directive on consumer rights', Brussels: European Parliament, accessed 12 June 2010 at www.europarl.europa.eu/meetdocs/2009_2014/documents/imco/dt/807/807372/807372en.pdf.

Smith, K.E., G. Fooks, J. Collin, H. Weishaar, S. Mandal and A.B. Gilmore (2010), '"Working the system" – British American Tobacco's influence on the European Union Treaty and its implications for policy: an analysis of internal tobacco industry documents', *PlosMedicine*, **7** (1), e1000202, doi:10.1371/journal.pmed.1000202, accessed at www.plosmedicine.org/article/info%3Adoi%2F10.1371%2Fjournal.pmed.1000202.

Social Platform (2009), 'Social platform does not buy into this Europe 2020 agenda and make four proposals for improvement', accessed 12 June 2010, www.cms.horus.be/files/99907/MediaArchive/Policies/Lisbon_Strategy/091217_Social%20Platform%20Letter%20EU%202020.pdf.

Stauber, J. and S. Rampton (1995a), 'Deforming consent: the public relations industry's secret war on activists', *CovertAction Quarterly*, **55**: 18–25.

Stauber, J. and S. Rampton (1995b), *Toxic Sludge is Good for You: Lies, Damn Lies, and the Public Relations Industry*, Monroe, ME: Common Courage Press.

TransAtlantic Business Dialogue (TABD) (2010), accessed 25 February 2010 at www.tabd.com.

Transatlantic Consumer Dialogue (TACD) (2010), accessed 25 February 2010 at www.tacd.org.

Tritter, J., M. Koivusalo, E. Ollila and P. Dorfman (2009), *Globalisation, Markets and Healthcare Policy: Redrawing the Patient as Consumer*, London: Routledge.

5. The People's Health Movement: health for all, now!

Prem Chandran John and David G. Legge

INTRODUCTION

Avoidable Disease Burden

The avoidable disease burden of developing countries is huge. Half a million young women die in childbirth each year, almost all in resource-poor settings and with almost all the deaths completely preventable (WHO 2007). This is a global challenge for all: experts, governments, corporations and civil society; but it demands action to address inequality and injustice, including the greed, insecurity and power relations which perpetuate an unbalanced allocation of resources. It is not just about mobilizing a few extra dollars of charity; it is about developing a system which provides fairer access to resources as a matter of right.

The Social Movement/Health Activist Perspective

Our focus is on the role of civil society in the struggle for health. The People's Health Movement (PHM) brings together individuals and organizations (mainly in the developing world) that share a concern about the avoidable disease burden, who criticize inequities in health care, and who demand structural reform to underpin the right to health.

The people's health movement (as a broad social movement) reflects the concern and action of ordinary people and groups (health activists). It both provides the vehicle for and is constituted by the claims and actions of those who gather, speak and act. PHM (the global organization and network of organizations) provides channels and opportunities for communication across the wider social movement and a platform for coordinated action.

Integral to the PHM perspective is the Alma-Ata vision of primary health care (WHO 1978) linking the local and the global; linking the diagnosis of community needs with an understanding of the wider economic and political determinants of health; and working with communities to address immediate and local needs in ways which also contribute to structural change.

Purpose

In offering this PHM perspective on the democratization of global health governance, we aim to:

- challenge the conventional construction of global health governance as solely the prerogative of world leaders, funding officials and global experts;
- challenge the passivity and fatalism which arise when we construct the determinants of global health only in terms of the big structures; 'it is all too big; I could have no influence';
- demonstrate the practicality and potential of health activism and the social movement strategy;
- illustrate the forms of action which are close at hand for ordinary people and communities, in both the rich world and the poor world.

Outline of this Chapter

We start with a brief discussion of civil society, its place in the structures of global governance and the activist tradition (the ethic of citizen engagement). This detour is necessary because it highlights some key features of the ideological context of social movement activism.

Having sketched the political and ideological context, we describe the origins of PHM; how it engages with the prevailing regime of global economic and health governance; and how it is positioned in relation to the nihilism of the various fundamentalisms.

We then turn to health and sketch some elements of the PHM analysis of the determinants of population health in the era of neo-liberal globalization. In the neo-liberal paradigm the continued poverty of the excluded billion is a necessary condition for the continued affluence and waste of the global middle class.

From the determinants of health we move to the drivers of change and forms of action that lie within the reach of the activist and the social movement. These drivers of change include delegitimation, inspiration and 'glocalization'. Forms of action include analysis, critique and advocacy, community engagement, service development, behaviour change and movement-building (including spiritual practice).

It will be evident that while this chapter is prepared for a wider audience it also serves our purpose as activists within the people's health movement in terms of standing back and reflecting on our work, our context, our strategies and forms of action. In this respect readers will be part of an internal discussion of the people's health social movement.

CIVIL SOCIETY ACTIVISM

Global Governance

The concept of global governance (see, for example, Rhodes 1996) provides a useful framework for contextualizing the role of civil society, the social movement and the health activist. This involves conceiving of a system of global governance and mapping the various players and dynamics onto that system. It is out of such a system that we may expect the immediate resource transfers, the medium-term initiatives which will map pathways and change attitudes, and the longer-term structural changes which will create a more equitable (and sustainable) world. The global governance system includes but goes beyond national governments and intergovernmental organizations. Other key players include transnational corporations, peak bodies, conferences, the media and academics. This listing of generic players (governments, corporates, academics and so on) should not obscure the role of specific countries such as the United States, Japan and China; federations such as the European Union; and groupings such as the OECD, the G8, the G20 and the G77.

Civil Society

'Civil society' refers to an important set of players in this system of global governance (Hettne and Odén 2002). It does not have a seat at the top table but influences the political context within which decisions are taken. Civil society is very heterogeneous and not very tightly organized. It is bottom-heavy in the sense that most action takes place at the local level, reflects local concerns and seeks to impact on local-level structures. However, civil society does have a presence in the deliberations of global governance, a presence mediated by international civil society organizations and social movements.

A social movement is a collectivity that shares in some degree a common set of concerns, understandings and claims and a sense of shared identity. It is bigger than but includes formal organizations. Examples include the environmental movement, the women's movement and the people's health movement. Fundamentalist religions are also social movements in this sense.

The people's health movement is a social movement in that it encompasses many different people in different settings who share a commitment to community health and who understand that they are working beside others who share this commitment. It includes a variety of organizations that reflect this commitment in some degree, but encompasses a much broader collectivity than simply the members of such organizations.

Citizen Engagement

The idea that citizens can and should participate in their own governance reflects the individualist ethic which emerged with early capitalism and the European Enlightenment. It reflects the confidence of the Enlightenment in the power of rational analysis, civil deliberation and collective action. It is not a universal norm. In more authoritarian cultures there is less space for and less confidence in the power of citizen engagement.

Citizen engagement, democratic governance and freedom of expression are linked, but it is necessary to distinguish between them to understand the anti-democratic impulse of modern liberalism. In the European tradition democratic forms of government are commonly traced back to ancient Greece. This was a democracy of the elite and did not include women or slaves. This kind of elitist construction of democracy was shaken by the French Revolution and subsequent revolutionary movements which rejected the kings and popes in favour of democratic structures and procedures which involved everyone. The democracy of revolutionary Europe was strongly influenced by the confidence of the Enlightenment in the power of rational analysis and collective deliberation in human affairs.

Modern liberalism, understood in terms of freedom of expression, freedom of association and, most importantly, the freedoms of the marketplace, has a different genealogy. Weber (1930) described how the dynamism of early capitalism broke through the privileges of the aristocracy and how a new individualism and a new claim for individual freedoms were a necessary part of this. Weber points out how the development of Protestantism provided a religious language and rationale for this movement.

In revolutionary America the construction of freedom was shaped by hostility to the English king, which led to a strong connotation of freedom *from* government. This is reflected in the US construction of democracy as providing scope for popular participation in collective decision-making while at the same time entrenching structures designed to limit the capacity of government to interfere with the freedom of the individual. This remains a powerful discourse in US politics and is expressed clearly in the new liberalism, which is an explicit reference to the earlier fight against government for market freedoms. However, the vision of revolutionary democracy from eighteenth- and nineteenth-century Europe continues to inspire, including in the United States.

Europe is a small domain of human civilization and it would be wrong to construct a history which fails to respect the revolutionary and democratic traditions of Asia, Africa and Latin America. However, the dominance of European, Japanese and US imperialisms in the period before the Second World War meant that these were largely traditions of local resistance rather than of engagement in any kind of global discourse.

This changed with decolonization and the independence movements that followed the Second World War and led to a flowering of confidence in the possibilities for freedom, democracy and independence. At the global level this confidence was expressed in the Bandung Conference of 1955 (Encyclopaedia Britannica 2010) and the birth of the Non-Aligned Movement (NAM) in 1961 (Non-Aligned Movement 2010). The kind of freedom celebrated by NAM was not restricted to the marketplace and the democracy of the independence movements was not constrained to protect business from the will of the people.

The new confidence of the NAM set the tone for the Declaration of Alma-Ata (WHO 1978), which recognized the structured unfairness of the global economy in its reference to the NAM's call in 1973 for a 'new international economic order' (Wikipedia 2010a). It recognized the social and environmental determinants of health and affirmed the importance of intersectoral collaboration in any health sector initiative to address such determinants. The Declaration affirmed the role of primary health care practitioners in working with communities to address the locally specific as well as the more widely pervasive determinants of health. The Declaration of Alma-Ata occupies a unique place in the people's health movement because of its clear recognition of the structural determinants of health and the critical role of the primary health care sector. It has inspired generations of practitioners with a vision of primary health care which addresses the social determinants of health as part of providing decent health care, and which addresses the immediate health issues in people's lives in ways that also contribute to changing the larger structures.

The tragedy of the 1970s was that even while NAM was calling for a new international economic order and Alma-Ata was calling for primary health care, new imbalances in the global economy were emerging that would make these goals much more difficult to achieve. The first of these imbalances was the oil price rise of 1973, which led to massive revenue increases for the oil-producing countries. These revenues were deposited in the commercial banks, which initiated a massive lending spree to countries and corporations alike (SAPRIN 2002). Here lie the origins of the debt trap. The second of these imbalances was the gradual emergence of global stagflation – a slowing of economic growth (stagnation) associated with intractable inflation. After some dithering the governors of the global economy elected to 'fight inflation first' by raising interest rates until inflation was brought under control. The prolonged period of high interest rates made the economic contraction more severe and more long-lasting. The period of high interest rates had a devastating impact on the many developing countries that had borrowed (or guaranteed private borrowings) when interest rates were very low (in the early to mid-1970s) but then found themselves facing massive interest rate increases as their loans rolled over in the early 1980s. Thus the debt trap was sprung and the era of IMF-mandated 'structural adjustment' was launched (Korner et al. 1986).

The 1980s was a 'lost decade' in terms of economic development in low- and middle-income countries. Developing countries faced escalating debt and pressure from the IMF to radically restructure their economies, away from protectionism and import substitution to small government and export development. Associated with these structural adjustment policies were increased living costs and the de-funding of public services, including food subsidies and health care (SAPRIN 2002).

The optimisms of the revolutionary democratic tradition in the North and the decolonizing tradition in the South were rapidly deflated. The ascendancy of neo-liberalism and the so-called Washington Consensus (Wikipedia 2010b) promoted the 'invisible hand' of the market to cult status, with amplified warnings about the adverse outcomes of humans seeking to take charge of their own destiny (Mihevc 1995). The nihilism of the market fundamentalists was matched by the emergence of religious fundamentalisms, with a radical return to God and a rejection of rational secularism – perhaps in part because of the negative message of the market fundamentalists.

These discursive waves and currents constitute the ideological context of civil society activism and progressive social movements like the people's health movement. A 'modernist' confidence in (perhaps faith in) the possibility of rational collective control over human destiny is integral to civil society/social movement activism. Market and religious fundamentalisms represent a salient challenge to this confidence.

The Disempowerment of Scale

A second challenge to civil society activism is the 'disempowerment of scale': 'It is all too big; I could have no influence over the global structures that shape my life.' This perception is a continuing challenge for progressive social movements, especially for the people's health movement, and particularly for PHM, which emerged as a response to neo-liberal globalization and its impact on health.

In part this is a problem of mechanistic thinking which constructs the 'big structures' (the global economy, trade regulation, nuclear weapons) as independent realities separate from the lived experiences and agency of ordinary people. As many thinkers, in particular Foucault (Layder 1994) and Giddens (1984), have pointed out, the big structures are in fact constituted through participation in and acceptance of them by ordinary people. In this respect the ideas of legitimation and legitimation crisis (Habermas 1975) are critical links in thinking about the influence of ordinary citizens on the stability and transformation of the big structures. The 2008 global financial crisis has seen a serious weakening in the standing of neo-liberal orthodoxy as the dominant paradigm for global economic policymaking. The *legitimacy* of neo-liberalism's claims to have all of the necessary answers for global policymaking has been shaken. In this respect, neo-liberalism faces a legitimation crisis.

The idea of delegitimation recognizes that the authority and reach of structures like the IMF depend on the acceptance of their legitimacy by millions of ordinary people who are willing to participate in their projects and thus act to sanction them. The story in Box 5.1 illustrates the dance of legitimation: the delegitimation of the TRIPS (Trade Related Intellectual Property Rights) regime by the Treatment Action Campaign and its re-legitimation with funding provided through the Global Fund.

The need for global solidarity in confronting structures and dynamics which are global in their reach is self-evident, but building a shared position is complicated by the different manifestations through which the global structures are expressed in the different regions, countries and sectors and at different levels. Developing a shared analysis across a broad social movement is an organic process, and common perceptions cannot be imposed without regard to context. Rather, participants from different settings need to share experiences and gradually build an analysis and strategy which focuses on what is common in ways that do not do violence to what is locally unique. The story in Box 5.1 illustrates the power of local and international solidarity.

BOX 5.1   ACCESS TO DRUGS AND THE DANCE OF LEGITIMATION

The World Trade Organization (WTO) was established in 1994 (WTO 2010b). Among the agreements it was to administer was the TRIPS agreement, which included provision for extended patents and patenting products as well as processes (WTO 2010a).

In 1997, 39 international pharmaceutical companies brought a case against the South African government saying that its 'parallel importing' legislation (designed to improve access to cheaper versions of brand-name drugs) was against its TRIPS commitments. At this stage the cost of a treatment with brand-name antiretrovirals for one year was around $10 000 while the Indian generics manufacturer Cipla was selling generic versions of the same drugs to Médecins Sans Frontières (MSF) for US$350 per treatment year (Oxfam 2002).

Over the next 4 years a powerful civil society action emerged against the drug companies. This involved street action in South Africa (the Treatment Action Campaign), high-level policy analysis (Knowledge Ecology International and MSF) and solidarity action in the United States (in particular through Health GAP and ACT UP).

In May 2001 the companies withdrew their action and paid the costs of the South African government (for a summary of this story see Raghavan 2001). In December 2001 in Doha the Ministerial Council of the WTO adopted its Statement on Public Health (WTO Ministerial Council 2001) and agreed to amendments to the TRIPS Agreement that, in theory, would make compulsory licensing more flexible.

From 2001 to 2003 the United States stonewalled the adoption of workable protocols for implementing more flexible compulsory licensing ('t Hoen 2009). Meanwhile (1999–2000) a new body, the Global Fund to fight AIDS, Tuberculosis and Malaria, was established (mainly through G8 funding but also with Gates Foundation support) with a brief to support wider access to expensive medications (although without compulsory licensing).

THE PEOPLE'S HEALTH MOVEMENT

Where It Came From

The People's Health Movement (PHM), as an organized network, was formed in December 2000 following the first People's Health Assembly (PHA) in Bangladesh. PHA 2000 was convened by eight global civil society networks concerned that the slogan 'Health for all by the year 2000' – which the World Health Organization (WHO) had promoted during the 1980s and 1990s – had not been achieved. The People's Health Assembly, was named with reference to the annual World Health Assembly, where ministers of health gather in Geneva as the governing body of the WHO. However, this was to be a *people's* health assembly. PHA 2000 was attended by 1453 participants from 75 countries (largely developing countries) and lasted 5 days. It included formal speeches, workshops, cultural programmes, exhibitions, films and testimonies. The programme canvassed the experience of primary health care since Alma-Ata; reviewed the impact of structural adjustment and World Bank policies on health; explored a wide range of social determinants of health; and shared the experiences of the wider social movement for health around the world (see PHM 2010a).

PHA 2000 was preceded by a series of events held across the world. The most dramatic of these was the mobilization in India. For nearly 9 months prior to the assembly, local and regional initiatives took place, including people's health enquiries and audits; health songs and popular theatre; subdistrict- and district-level seminars; policy dialogues and translations into regional languages of national consensus documents on health; and campaigns challenging medical professionals and the health system to become more 'health-for-all'-oriented. Finally, over 2000 delegates travelled to Kolkata, most of them riding on five converging people's health trains, where they brought forth ideas from 17 state and 250 district conventions. After 2 days of simultaneous workshops, exhibitions, two public rallies for health and a myriad of cultural programmes, the assembly endorsed *The Indian People's Health Charter*. About 300 delegates then travelled to Bangladesh, mostly by bus, to attend PHA 2000. Similar preparatory initiatives, though less intense, took place in Bangladesh, Nepal, Sri Lanka, Cambodia, Philippines, Japan and other parts of the world, including Latin America, Europe, Africa and Australia.

PHA 2000 adopted *The People's Charter for Health*, which outlined the global health situation, identified the main barriers to health for all and adopted a set of principles, priorities and strategies to guide the people's health social movement globally. The Charter (since translated into many languages) has proved to be a powerful leadership document in the years since December 2000. It states that:

> Equity, ecologically-sustainable development and peace are at the heart of our vision of a better world – a world in which a healthy life for all is a reality; a world that respects, appreciates and celebrates all life and diversity; a world that enables the flowering of people's talents and abilities to enrich each other; a world in which people's voices guide the decisions that shape our lives. (PHM 2010b)

People's Health Assembly 2

The second People's Health Assembly (PHA 2) followed in July 2005, in Cuenca, Ecuador, with 1492 participants from 80 countries. PHA 2 was organized around nine streams, including issues of equity and people's health care; intercultural encounters on health; trade and health; health and the environment; gender, women and health sector reform; training and communicating for health; the right to health for all in an inclusive society; health in people's hands; and PHM affairs (PHM 2010d). Planning is underway for the third People's Health Assembly in South Africa in 2012.

The Components of the People's Health Movement

The foundation of the PHM are the networks of civil society organizations

operating locally, nationally (see Box 5.2 for the Indian network) and internationally working towards health for all along the lines articulated in *The
People's Charter for Health*. These include health centres, community-based
organizations, special-interest networks, health care practitioners and students,
research centres and think tanks. These are the groups and organizations that
make up the broad social movement for people's health. Insofar as they see
themselves as linked together through the organized PHM, they are its
constituent base.

BOX 5.2   PHM IN INDIA – JAN SWASTHYA
ABHIYAN

PHM in India is known as Jan Swasthya Abhiyan (JSA). JSA is a
coalition of 22 national networks, resource groups and federations of NGOs working towards equity in health and development
with a value base of social justice and health as a human right. It
was established as a formal body after participants at the first
National Health Assembly, held in Kolkata in 2000, decided to
create a broad national platform to continue collective work on
health and health care.

Member organizations of JSA have had several decades of
involvement in people's movements, community-based work and
progressive thinking. Besides 12 networks and federations working in health-related areas, there is strong participation from the
women's movement, science movement and the national alliance
of people's movements. The growing dalit and environmental
movements and trade unions participate sporadically. JSA is
present in 22 states, with varying levels of activity at district and
subdistrict levels.

The strength of the coalition is its diversity, its experience and
the willingness of its members to work together. The plurality of
perspectives is both a strength and a weakness. It is significant
that a large number of non-health or non-medical networks with a
clear political stance associate themselves with the JSA and
actively participate in or support various campaigns. However, as
would be expected, it is the health groups who maintain the continuity and momentum of JSA's work.

JSA has undertaken several campaigns since 2000 to influence health-related policies in India. Using a number of strategies, it has addressed different constituencies, including state and

national governments, corporations, WHO and the public in relation to socially embedded issues like gender, caste and commu-
nalism. These engagements include:

- policy analysis and policy advocacy (partly responsible for
  the development of the National Rural Health Mission);
- campaigns on gender issues (sex-selective abortion,
  violence);
- access to medicines and reform of intellectual property
  rights;
- HIV/AIDS and the rights of people living with AIDS;
- the right to food campaign.

As well as these national campaigns, JSA has developed a very
wide range of projects and campaigns through its state and
district chapters.

While PHM is especially strong in India the general pattern
described above is replicated in many other countries.

PHM is organized on the basis of 'country circles' which come together in
regional networks, represented on the PHM Steering Council. The other main
group on the Council are the representatives of the international networks,
including but going beyond the eight founding networks from PHA 2000.
Between meetings of the Steering Council, the PHM is coordinated by its
global Coordinating Commission, which works under the guidance of the
Steering Council.

PHM has a small staff, its Global Secretariat, which is based in Capetown,
Cairo and Delhi, and is heavily dependent on modern communications tech-
nology. The secretariat is guided on a day-to-day basis by the Coordinating
Commission.

PHM's funding partners are a critical component of the overall movement.
They are generally based in the North and raise money through donations and
other fundraising. These funding partners are a very real expression of
North–South solidarity.

What the People's Health Movement Does

The core work of PHM is that of its constituent parts, in particular, the country circles and the international networks. As an organization, it provides
communication channels and opportunities that link the very diverse elements
of the larger movement. It supports a number of activities at global and

regional levels that integrate the efforts of the country circles and global networks. One of these is the International People's Health University, which offers a programme of short courses for health activists, mainly in developing countries (PHM 2010c).

PHM Global also supports ad-hoc policy work and campaigning on various issues and topics on the global policy agenda. There has been a continuous flow of publications, submissions and statements arising from this kind of policy coordination. The Right to Health campaign (see Box 5.3) has been the flagship campaign of recent years.

BOX 5.3   THE RIGHT TO HEALTH CAMPAIGN

The Right to Health Campaign was initiated in 2004 by the Jan Swasthya Abhiyan (JSA), the PHM's coordinating body in India, in collaboration with the Indian Human Rights Commission.

The campaign includes participatory surveys of public health care facilities, from village to district levels. On the basis of these surveys, status reports are prepared for different regions in the country, including reports on the different tiers of the public health system – from primary to tertiary. Each level of care is surveyed according to a specially designed questionnaire for that level.

The campaign collects and documents cases of denial of health care. The cases are systematically recorded in line with a detailed protocol that identifies different forms of denial, including non-availability of essential health care equipment, mass-scale tubectomy operations, non-availability of transport facilities to enable patients to be referred to better health services, and non-availability of essential drugs and equipment for essential testing.

Public hearings are a critical part of the campaign, at sub-district, district, state, regional and national levels. The status reports and cases of denial are presented at the public hearings as testimonies before a joint panel, which includes representatives from the Human Rights Commission and civil society as well as eminent persons. The hearings are also attended by public health officials, who get a chance to reply to the reports and cases presented. A panel then pronounces recommendations.

The campaign aims to mobilize communities around the right to health care; to document and highlight specific instances of denial of health care; and to present testimonies that detail these instances of denial while also emphasizing structural and system deficiencies.

The testimonies are not just individual cases of denial but are chosen as examples of common kinds of health care denial in public health care. The objective is not to target individuals or facilities but to focus on structural problems. However, testimonies can be very personal: for example one about a 2½-year-old boy losing his vision owing to delayed diagnosis and inadequate treatment.

The recommendations of the hearings are followed up with joint monitoring (involving the Human Rights Commission and the JSA), stressing the systemic gaps in the public health system that led to the reported cases of denial.

In the first phase of the campaign in 2004 several districts and most states organized public hearings following the same format. These culminated in five regional hearings and finally a national hearing in New Delhi in December 2004. The national hearing was attended by India's minister for health and senior Ministry of Health officials. At this hearing the National Action Plan to Operationalize the Right to Heath Care was jointly presented by the Human Rights Commission and the JSA.

The Right to Health campaign has continued ever since, with widespread mobilization around the action plan, including the JSA National Health Assembly in March 2007, attended by over 2500 activists.

Following the success of the Right to Health campaign in India, the PHM launched a global campaign. In many countries the campaign focus has included the right to health (meaning a focus on the social determinants of health) as well as the right to health care.

Engagement with the World Health Organization

PHM representatives have attended every World Health Assembly since 2001, with a view to building links with WHO staff, members of ministerial delegations and other international NGOs. PHM has advocated for:

- Health system strengthening, in particular, overcoming fragmentation caused by the proliferation of disease-specific funding programmes, and a return to comprehensive primary health care with a focus on the social determinants of health.
- A stronger role for the WHO in global health governance vis-à-vis the World Bank, private foundations and transnational corporations,

including stronger advocacy of population health outcomes in relation to trade agreements and intellectual property regulation.

The PHM worked closely with the WHO Commission on the Social Determinants of Health (2004–8), in particular supporting the Commission's civil society consultation. The PHM also works closely with other global civil society networks that advocate the health-for-all agenda at the WHO.

The WHO is subject to a range of pressures beyond those coming from civil society, in particular from member states, including the rich countries who channel much of their funding to the WHO through specific ('extra-budgetary') projects. The WHO also needs to maintain working relationships with the World Bank 'family', private donors (such as the Gates Foundation) and the proliferating global health initiatives (public–private partnerships). In this context its engagement with civil society, including the PHM, is a further source of pressure, but it also potentially provides a constituency of support. There are clear limits to the WHO's financial and regulatory power but the WHO could play an important leadership role if it was willing (and able) to project such leadership towards health for all, and if there was a stronger constituency of support at the country level and in civil society.

BOX 5.4   THE UNIVERSITIES ALLIANCE FOR ESSENTIAL MEDICINES

The Universities Alliance for Essential Medicines (UAEM) started at Yale in 2000 at the height of the South Africa stand-off over the drug stavudine – an anti-retroviral used in the treatment of HIV – which the MSF wanted to use for its projects in South Africa. The drug had been developed by a scientist at Yale University, which had licensed it to the drug company Bristol-Myers Squibb. The MSF had approached both Yale and the company but had been unable to convince them to make the drug available. It then contacted some students at Yale and asked them to take on the issue. The students launched a powerful campaign at the university (including a 'TB die-in') and managed to persuade Yale and Bristol-Myers Squibb to export the drug at much lower prices – almost 95 per cent lower. That success inspired students elsewhere in the United States, and the UAEM was set up 2 years later. Now over 50 universities are involved.

Three universities in the United States and Canada have since

embedded the UAEM's core principles into their university consti-
tutions, and numerous other universities are now considering how
to better integrate these principles into their work. Those universities that have signed up still grant exclusive licences to pharmaceutical companies for their discoveries, but written into these
licences is the requirement that any drug or medical technology
relevant to developing countries be made accessible to them. For
example, the University of British Columbia is currently ensuring
a drug they have developed for leishmaniasis is available to
developing countries (UAEM 2010).

GLOBAL HEALTH INEQUITY: A PHM ANALYSIS

Health inequalities continue to flourish more than 30 years after Alma-Ata.
The life expectancy of a black male in Baltimore is less than that of a
Bangladeshi male. A Japanese woman will live 42 years longer than a woman
in Lesotho. The odds of a woman in Afghanistan dying in childbirth are 1 in
8, as compared with 1 in 17 400 in Sweden. An Indigenous Australian male
can expect to live 17 years less than other men in the same country, while
maternal mortality is 3 to 4 times higher among poor women in Indonesia
compared with rich women (WHO 2009).

These statistics largely reflect the social determinants of health, including
poverty, environmental degradation, conflict and violence, poor housing, sanitation and various forms of discrimination and exclusion (Commission on
Social Determinants of Health 2008). Of course which social determinants are
in play is highly specific to particular places and groups of people, as are the
institutional forms through which remedies might be sought.

Health care is also in crisis, including financial barriers to access; underfunding of public sector health care; hospital-centric care and neglect of
primary health care; 'vertical' disease programmes which offer higher salaries
and draw human resources away from the public and generalist health system;
dependence on transnational pharmaceutical companies which set prices to
maximize profits rather than access; brain drain; and 'aid' programmes with
huge transaction costs.

We must recognize also the rising threat of global warming, and its impact
on the poor in particular. Extreme weather events will have a greater impact
on informal settlements than well-constructed cities. Changes in rainfall
patterns will damage agricultural productivity in many regions. People in the
poor world will be very disadvantaged in adapting to such changes (Core
Writing Team 2007).

The Causes of the Causes

PHM is committed to working towards more equitable access to the social conditions for good health, for universal access to decent health care and for effective action on global warming and other forms of environmental degradation. This project calls for an analysis of the structures which stabilize and reproduce health inequities and for a set of strategies and forms of action through which the broad people's health movement might effect change.

Understanding the *structures* that reproduce health inequities and the possible *drivers of change* provides a basis for selecting *forms of action* through which *we* can contribute to driving change. These forms of action include:

- information strategies that embolden the forces for change and delegitimize the dominant ideologies;
- cultural action which throws new light on the familiar and helps to articulate alternatives;
- networking and dialogue leading to stronger alliances and more coherent action;
- community engagement, such as right-to-health initiatives, through which people and communities gain new confidence in their power to change;
- policy critique and advocacy;
- service development reforms, creating health systems that address the structural determinants of health, as well as biomedical factors;
- institutional reform, creating institutions that are accountable and responsive and which clear the path for progressive change;
- personal behaviour change (for example, away from patriarchy, away from materialism), changes that are both individual and collective; are both personal and political;
- movement-building (ranging from leadership development to spiritual practice).

These forms of action comprise the repertoire of the broad social movement for people's health.

Sometimes the causes of the causes are local and specific (for example, the specific circumstances of Palestine or Cuba or the island states of the Pacific); others are more general and pervasive (for example, neo-liberal globalization and global warming). The interplay of the local/specific and the global/general means that health issues present themselves in myriad ways in different localities, countries, regions and for different income strata, classes, genders and ethnicities.

Where the structures that reproduce health inequalities are local and specific, the key drivers of change will be local and specific; the relevant strategies and forms of action will be most appropriately determined by local activists. These are the local people's health movements, operating at local, national and regional levels. Insofar as these are local and specific struggles the role of the PHM Secretariat is to support and learn from these struggles.

However, the precipitating factors which led to establishing the formal PHM were about more general factors, in particular the structures and dynamics associated with neo-liberal globalization and the judgement that these could not properly be addressed through isolated local or specific struggles. The consensus at PHA 2000 was that the local and specific movements and the more narrowly focused global networks needed to work more closely together to build a stronger capacity globally to address those causes of the causes which are global and general.

Globalization

Widening inequalities in income and wealth are direct reflections of deep imbalances in the global economy. Most important among these is the growing capacity to produce goods (including food) with less and less labour, which means fewer people receiving decent wages to buy such goods. Farmers in developing countries are forced to leave the land because industrialized agriculture supported by subsidies can undercut them. Auto workers are unemployed in rust-belt cities around the world because fewer and fewer factories are needed to supply the global market (which itself is stagnating because unemployed workers don't buy new cars). This is the crisis of overproduction (Bello 2006).

Free trade and global economic integration – presented by neo-liberalism as the solution to global health (see Feachem 2001) – enable the rich countries to maintain living standards by intensifying the exploitation of the poor. Debt-financed consumption in the North is supported by a net flow of resources from the South to the North (Globalisation and Health Knowledge Network 2007). Meanwhile, 1 billion marginalized people are both unable to sell their labour and unable to buy the necessities of life: a 'reserve army' of unemployed non-consumers. The continued destabilization of the global environment and the refusal to mitigate global warming also reflect the precarious imbalances of the global economy.

The global economy does not have to be structured in this way. The current structures and dynamics of the global economy are set by a specific governance regime which maintains the flow of value from South to North and reproduces the health inequalities discussed above. This governance regime is constituted by states and empires (and their armies and foreign policies); by intergovernmental organizations (such as the IMF and the WTO); by transnational corporations (such as the large transnational pharmaceutical corporations); and by particular structures of information and communications (for example, News Limited). A critical element of the regime of global economic governance is ideological, specifically the ideology of neo-liberalism with its hostility to the modernist vision of rational democratic control over human destiny.

Globalization from Below

The emergence of PHM is an illustration of 'globalization from below' (Brecher et al. 2002). This move, which corresponds to the image of globalization as a global village, draws upon globalization's possibilities for solidarity and collaboration. PHM provides a shared platform for reflection, analysis, advocacy and campaigning. Through communication and sharing, it supports the emergence of a stronger solidarity across both national borders and the boundaries of class, race, gender and religion.

CONCLUSIONS

Global governance (including the governance of both global health and global economics) is not the sole prerogative of world leaders, funding officials, global experts and CEOs. Civil society activism includes strategies and practices which ordinary people and community groups can deploy to exert influence on the direction of humanity. However, the success of social movements like the people's health movement is not guaranteed; it depends on individuals and groups choosing to become part of it.

ACKNOWLEDGEMENTS

The authors gratefully acknowledge the assistance of several PHM colleagues who contributed to the development of this chapter. We are also grateful to the various organizations that provided information about their activities for inclusion in this chapter, as well as those whose contributions, for reasons of space, were not able to be included.

REFERENCES

Bello, W. (2006), 'The capitalist conjuncture: over-accumulation, financial crises, and the retreat from globalisation', *Third World Quarterly*, **27** (8), 1345–67.
Brecher, J., T. Costello and B. Smith (2002), *Globalisation from Below: The Power of Solidarity*, Cambridge, MA: South End Press.
Commission on Social Determinants of Health (2008), *Closing the Gap in a*

Generation: Health Equity Through Action on the Social Determinants of Health, Geneva: World Health Organization.

Core Writing Team, R.K. Pachauri and A. Reisinger (eds) (2007), *Climate Change 2007: Synthesis Report*, Geneva, Switzerland: Intergovernmental Panel on Climate Change.

Encyclopaedia Britannica (2010), 'Bandung Conference', *Encyclopaedia Britannica online*, accessed 29 March at www.britannica.com/EBchecked/topic/51624/ Bandung-Conference.

Feachem, R.G.A. (2001), 'Globalisation: from rhetoric to evidence', *Bulletin of the World Health Organization*, **79** (9): 804.

Giddens, A. (1984), *The Constitution of Society: Outline of the Theory of Structuration*, Cambridge: Polity Press.

Globalisation and Health Knowledge Network (2007), *Towards Health-Equitable Globalisation: Rights, Regulation and Redistribution: Final Report to the Commission on Social Determinants of Health*, Ottawa: University of Ottawa, accessed 29 March 2010 at www.who.int/entity/social_determinants/resources/ gkn_final_report_042008.pdf.

Habermas, J. (1975), *Legitimation Crisis*, Boston, MA: Beacon Press.

Hettne, B. and B. Odén (eds) (2002), *Global Governance in the 21st Century: Alternative Perspectives on World Order*, Studia Latina Stockholmiensia no. 48, Stockholm: Almqvist & Wiksell International.

Korner, P., G. Maass, T. Siebold and R. Tetzlaff (1986), *The IMF and the Debt Crisis: A Guide to the Third World's Dilemmas*, London: Zed Books.

Layder, D. (1994), *Understanding Social Theory*, London: Sage.

Mihevc, J. (1995), *The Market Tells Them So: The World Bank and Economic Fundamentalism in Africa*, Penang, Malaysia and Accra, Ghana: Third World Network.

Non-Aligned Movement (2010), 'Background', accessed 29 March at www.nam. gov.za/background/index.html.

Oxfam (2002), 'US bullying on drug patents: one year after Doha', London: Oxfam, accessed 29 March 2010 at www.oxfam.org.uk/resources/policy/health/downloads/ bp33_bullying.pdf.

PHM (2010a), accessed 29 March at www.phmovement.org/pha2000/index.html.

PHM (2010b), accessed 29 March at www.phmovement.org/cms/en/resources/ charters/peopleshealth.

PHM (2010c), accessed 29 March at www.phmovement.org/iphu.

PHM (2010d), 'People's Health Assemby 2', accessed 29 March at www.phmovement. org/pha2.

Raghavan, C. (2001), 'Pharmaceutical TNCs beat a tactical retreat', *Third World Economics*, **256**: 11–13.

Rhodes, R.A.W. (1996), 'The new governance: governing without government', *Political Studies*, **44** (4): 652–67.

SAPRIN (2002), 'The policy roots of economic crisis and poverty: a multi-country participatory assessment of structural adjustment', Washington DC: SAPRIN, accessed at www.saprin.org/global_rpt.htm.

't Hoen, E.F.M. (2009), *The Global Politics of Pharmaceutical Monopoly Power, Drug Patents, Access, Innovation and the Application of the WTO Doha Declaration on TRIPS and Public Health*, Dieman, Netherlands: AMB Publishers.

Universities Alliance for Essential Medicines (2010), 'Universities allied for essential medicines', accessed 29 March at www.essentialmedicine.org/.

Weber, M. (1930), *The Protestant Ethic and the Spirit of Capitalism*, London: Allen & Unwin.

World Health Organization (WHO) (1978), 'Primary Health Care', Alma-Ata conference, Geneva: WHO, accessed 29 March at www.who.int/hpr/NPH/docs/declaration _almaata.pdf.

WHO (2007), 'Maternal mortality in 2005: estimates developed by WHO, UNICEF, UNFPA and the World Bank', Geneva: WHO, accessed 28 March at www.who.int/reproductivehealth/publications/monitoring/9789241596213/en/index.html.

WHO (2009), 'The World Health Report 2008 – Primary Health Care (Now More Than Ever)', Geneva: WHO, accessed 29 March 2010 at www.who.int/whr/2008/en/index.html.

Wikipedia (2010a), 'New international economic order', accessed 29 March at www.en.wikipedia.org/wiki/New_International_Economic_Order.

Wikipedia (2010b), 'Washington Consensus', accessed 29 March at www.en.wikipedia.org/wiki/Washington_Consensus.

World Trade Organization (WTO) (2010a), 'TRIPS material on the WTO website', accessed 29 March at www.wto.org/english/tratop_e/trips_e/trips_e.htm.

WTO (2010b), 'What is the WTO?', accessed 29 March at www.wto.org/english/thewto_e/whatis_e/whatis_e.htm.

WTO Ministerial Council (2001), 'Doha ministerial declaration', accessed 29 March 2010 at www.wto.org/english/thewto_e/minist_e/min01_e/mindecl_e.htm.

6. Aboriginal community control and decolonizing health policy: a yarn from Australia

Bronwyn Fredericks, Karen Adams and Rebecca Edwards

Before colonization Australian Aboriginal people lived in a complex society, with high levels of self-determination in all aspects of their lives, including ceremony, spiritual practices, medicine, social and kinship relations, management of land and systems of law. Aboriginal peoples were, as sovereign peoples, able to determine, monitor and evaluate individual, family and community well-being: something their descendants strive to maintain and restore today.

Aboriginal people have the worst health of any population group in Australia. Puggy Hunter states that this is 'the result of the past 200 years of dispossession and dislocation of Aboriginal families and communities' and argues that 'the right of native title holders to negotiate over developments on their land is intrinsically linked to improved Aboriginal health in Australia' (Hunter 1998: 2). It is testament to Aboriginal people's strength and endurance that cultural, social and spiritual practices have survived and continue to be maintained and revived. This chapter provides an overview of Aboriginal history since 1788 and gives an account of the current health of Aboriginal people in Victoria. It then analyses Aboriginal health policy more generally, and lastly highlights the role of the Victorian Aboriginal Community Controlled Health Organisation (VACCHO) in supporting and advocating for improving the development and implementation of health policy through increasing levels of participation by the Victorian Aboriginal community.

ABORIGINAL HEALTH STATUS IN VICTORIA

Aboriginal people experienced a relatively healthy lifestyle and quality of life before colonization in 1788 (Saggers and Gray 1991: 59). At the time that Australia was invaded by white settlers in 1788, Aboriginal Australians were 'physically, socially and emotionally healthier than most Europeans of that time' (Thomson 1984: 939; Moodie 1973). This is reiterated in the National Aboriginal and Torres Strait Islander Health Strategy Consultation Draft (NATSIC 2001: 5) and also in Engels (1892 [1973]: 130–3). Views on pre-colonization and the health of the Australian Aboriginal population are based on historical records based on impressions and observations by British and European explorers. These reflect a consistent picture regarding the health of Aboriginal people at that time. On several occasions James Cook (said to have 'discovered Australia') observed that the Aboriginal people were 'of middle stature straight bodied slender-limb'd the Colour of Wood soot or of dark chocolate ... Their features are far from disagreeable' (Clark 1966: 51). Australia's first governor, Governor Arthur Phillip, made similar assertions to those of the European explorer Edward Eyre, as outlined in Stone (1974: 20). Eyre, in writing about the Murray River area, described the local Aboriginal people as 'almost free from diseases and well-shaped in body and limb' (quoted in Cleland 1928). There are also other accounts in the historical records (Elphinstone 1971: 295; Dampier in Abbie 1976: 5).

At the time these British and European observations were made there were hundreds of Aboriginal nations, each living within a distinct geographic area of the landmass now known as Australia. Descendants of these nations are today accustomed to referring to their own geographical area as 'country'. A map available from the Australian Institute of Aboriginal and Torres Strait Islander Studies (Horton 1999) shows the 500 indigenous nations and their country. To many Aboriginal Australians, country means place of origin – in the literal, spiritual and cultural sense. It refers to specific clans, tribal groups or nations and encompasses all the knowledge, cultural norms, values, practices, stories and resources within that particular area – that particular Indigenous place – and underpins the particular ontologies, epistemologies and axiologies of the Aboriginal people in that place.

In New South Wales (initially the only mainland colony) colonization saw the introduction of infectious diseases, such as smallpox, which spread to Aboriginal people causing death and disability (Koori Heritage Trust 2009). By 1830 Europeans had begun to arrive in Victoria, causing the destruction of the Aboriginal way of life and culture through killings, massacres, starvation, introduction of disease, removal of children and the claiming of lands (Blainey 1994; Lippmann 1994; Rintoul 1993; Rosser 1985). Past government policies and practices, intervention and abuses focused on denying Aboriginal people basic human rights, that is, the right to live and practise culture and to exist as Aboriginal peoples on and within their countries. Such policies were premised on assumptions that Aboriginal people were uncivilized heathens, primitive and immoral (Henderson 2000). There are many accounts of resistance and protests by Victorian Aboriginal people in the face of colonization. Such resistance included retaliation against massacres, walking off missions, petitions, letters of protest, establishment of Aboriginal-led organizations and, in 2004, the 'Long Walk' to Canberra (Koori Heritage Trust 2009; Nelson et al. 2002; Vickery et al. 2005).

Even today Aboriginal people in Victoria experience significant health inequalities compared with non-Aboriginal people. The 2006 census (ABS and AIHW 2008) recorded 33 517 people as indigenous Australians (Aboriginal and Torres Strait Islanders) in Victoria, with a non-indigenous population of 5 093 023. The life expectancy of Aboriginal people in Victoria is 17 to 19 years less than that of non-Aboriginal Victorians (ABS 2007; ABS and AIHW 2008). The mean weekly income for Aboriginal and Torres Strait Islander families in 2006 was AUS$395 compared with AUS$665 for other Australian families (AHMAC 2006), while 17.1 per cent of Aboriginal house-holds had five or more people compared with 10.1 per cent of all Victorian households (ABS 2007). Aboriginal and Torres Strait Islander people experi-ence racism at double the rate of other Australians (Paradies et al. 2008). Aboriginal children in Victoria are 11 times more likely to come into contact with the child protection system than other Victorian children (ABS and AIHW 2008). The destruction that began in 1788 continues to impact on Victorian Aboriginal people's lives, culture, health and well-being to varying degrees. There may be some reported improvements in certain areas but it is widely recognized that

> the health and well-being of Indigenous Australians has failed to keep up with the overall improvements in the health and well-being of non-Indigenous Australians, so that the level of disadvantage faced by Indigenous Australians has continued to grow over time. (Australian House of Representatives Standing Committee on Family and Community Affairs 2000: 3)

ABORIGINAL HEALTH POLICY

Historically, the development of Aboriginal health policy has seen the involve-ment of many groups and individuals – governments, churches, special inter-est groups, health professionals and corporations. Most policy decisions have been made by governments and the state bureaucracy, although this can be broadened to include churches and charitable welfare organizations, which have also been involved in the delivery of health programmes to Aboriginal communities. Past policies in Aboriginal health focused primarily on repro-duction, prostitution, venereal disease and reducing the transmission of such to the non-indigenous population. Policies on reserves and missions were developed and implemented by missionaries and managers, controlling living arrangements, marriage, travel, food allocation (primarily through rations) and the type of education provided (Evans et al. 1988; Kidd 1997; Manne 2001). Institutions were founded specifically for children (Beresford and Omaji 1998) which implemented a range of policies with significant impacts on individual and community health and well-being.

These institutions generally prohibited the practice of cultural ceremonies and the use of Aboriginal language. Others agents, including health professionals, police officers and government administrators, instituted questionable practices and 'operated in concert to suppress local Aboriginal sovereignty, steal their lands, and destroy their languages, cultures and social cohesion'. Further, 'colonisation produced situational traumatisation, such as seeing relatives shot or taken away, but it also produced cumulative trauma as a result of shame and self-hate, and intergenerational trauma as a result of unresolved and unaddressed grief and loss' (Phillips 2003: 23). Evidence shows that past events, practices and policies have an ongoing impact on Aboriginal people and communities (Fredericks 2008, 2007), particularly as some policies are still in practice today in various forms (Fredericks 2009a, 2009b). These policies have contributed to the attitudes that Aboriginal people currently have towards health service professionals, law-and-order workers, religious people, teachers, and bureaucrats who implement new policies (Fredericks 2008).

Involvement by the Aboriginal community in decision-making in health policy was, until recently, virtually non-existent. In Victoria a working party was established in 1980 as a result of lobbying by the Aboriginal Community Controlled Health Organisations and their advocates to improve the situation of Aboriginal people in decision-making about Aboriginal health. The working party consisted of government and Aboriginal community representatives and undertook the first state-wide health consultation with the Aboriginal community. The working party made several recommendations, some of which were implemented (Vickery et al. 2005). The National Aboriginal Health Strategy (NAHS) was instituted in 1989 and was the first national policy providing a process that enabled Aboriginal people's collective input. Aboriginal communities felt for the first time that they were being listened to and that notice would be taken of their views and wishes (Anderson 1997). Some Aboriginal people expressed optimism that this was finally a change in the way that government worked with Aboriginal communities. Through participation and empowerment, governments have recognized that Aboriginal communities can be active contributors to policy decisions. For the non-Aboriginal population it may be difficult to understand the significance of these policy consultations for the Aboriginal community, as most non-Aboriginals take the ability to articulate views for granted. This was a substantive step towards decolonizing health policy when, 'for the first time, all stakeholders seemed to share some consensus about strategic directions in Aboriginal health' (Anderson 1997: 120).

The NAHS (NAHS Working Party 1989) acknowledged Aboriginal history, its traumas and resultant health problems. It recommended the alleviation of acute existing health problems, along with fundamental changes in preventive health care to achieve long-term improvements in Aboriginal health. It stressed the vital role of Aboriginal community-controlled health services operating alongside mainstream health services, as well as intersectoral collaboration. It insisted that health service provision was not the sole solution in addressing Aboriginal health inequalities. The NAHS was comprehensive in its approach and argued for strategic recommendations, on the basis for example that this would also be a more cost-efficient approach. While some of the positive changes in Aboriginal health can be traced back to the NAHS either directly or indirectly, one of the greatest disappointments was that it was never resourced adequately, leading to it not being fully implemented. There was some improvement in hospital access and reporting through the Aboriginal Hospital Liaison Officer programme, and regular meetings took place between the Aboriginal community and the Victorian government. However Aboriginal health status remains lower than that of other non-Aboriginal Victorians.

The decade following the NAHS has been described at a national level as defying a historical trend in decolonizing policy, with Aboriginal voices in policy development being minimized (Sanders 2006). Protests such as the 'Long Walk' (Schwartz 2004), and Aboriginal people turning their backs on Prime Minister Howard in response to his government's refusal to apologize for past treatment of Aboriginal people (Rintoul 2002), epitomize this decade.[1]

In February 2008 the new Labor prime minister, Kevin Rudd, acknowledged the pain and suffering caused by past Aboriginal child removals and family separations when he offered a national 'Apology to the Stolen Generations'; he also apologized for the inequalities that existed between indigenous and non-indigenous Australians (Rudd 2008). This was followed in August 2008 by the signing of the 'Statement of Intent to Close the Gap on Indigenous Health Inequality' by the prime minister, the premier of Victoria and the chairperson of the Victorian Aboriginal Community Controlled Health Organisation (VACCHO). This statement commits respective governments and organizations to achieve equality of health status and close the gap in life expectancy between Aboriginal and non-Aboriginal people by 2030. This signing followed 2 years of campaigning by the National Aboriginal Community Controlled Health Organisation (NACCHO) and Oxfam Australia through the development of a document detailing both the health problems of Australia's indigenous people and their solution. This development was based on an extensive review of the evidence within Australia and overseas for improving the health outcomes of indigenous populations (NACCHO and Oxfam 2007).

The Close the Gap partners have supported the need to address the social and cultural factors that influence this gap, for example housing, community safety and security, justice, education, culture, language and community development. Key targets include improving housing, reducing levels of smoking, and improving availability and access to fresh food, which all significantly reduce the rates of indigenous death and illness from disease and chronic conditions. The Australian Human Rights Commission (2009) and Tom Calma (2009) highlighted that indigenous Australians must be involved in decision-making about their health to address the health inequalities they experience. Furthermore, Aboriginal people need to be involved in decision- making about all factors that affect their lives, including policy development. This work has been furthered through the support of the Council of Australian Governments (COAG). At a COAG meeting in late November 2008, the federal government committed AUS$4.6 million to closing the gap on indigenous disadvantage. This has progressed the Close the Gap initiative. However there are still gaps in the COAG decision process, particularly its non-engagement with the indigenous community on funding and resource allocation.

THE VICTORIAN ABORIGINAL COMMUNITY CONTROLLED HEALTH ORGANISATION

The Victorian Aboriginal Community Controlled Health Organisation (VACCHO) was established in 1996 and today represents 24 Aboriginal Community Controlled Health Organisations (ACCHOs) in Victoria. Each member is an Aboriginal community-controlled organization. Most provide multiple or a holistic range of services, with health care provision as the core. Some are comprehensive primary health care services. Some have visiting specialist services. A number of ACCHOs were established in the early 1970s in a number of country centres, as well as one in an inner-urban municipality and one in an outer-suburban municipality.

Aboriginal community control refers to Aboriginal people being in control and participating in decision-making structures, administrative procedures and service delivery. Moreover, 'Community control in health is about people owning it, having a say about their own health and having the opportunity to provide feedback' (VACCHO and CRCAH 2007: 1). It is also about 'self-determination, reconciliation and providing culturally appropriate services. But it is also more than that; it is also cultural history, cultural identity and having a "place" to identify with' (VACCHO and CRCAH 2007: 2). Community-controlled health organizations are therefore about Aboriginal people controlling their own destinies and exercising responsibility for decision-making in health with their communities. It enables Aboriginal people to provide health services in the form, structure, setting and language appropriate to their community. In essence ACCHOs embody the notions and practices of community empowerment.

Paulo Freire (1970), Wallerstein and Bernstein (1988: 380) explore empowerment in the context of community and community development. The latter define empowerment as

> a social action process that promotes participation of people, organisations, and communities in gaining control over their lives in their community and larger society. With this perspective, empowerment is not characterised as achieving power to dominate others, but rather to act with others to effect change.

Wallerstein (1992: 198) adds that this social action process is about working 'towards the goals of individual and community control, political efficacy, improved quality of community life, and social justice'. Wallerstein argues that empowerment is an important promoter of health and that powerlessness, or lack of control over destiny, is a broad-based risk factor for disease, and therefore ill health (1992: 197-205). Community empowerment in the Australian Indigenous context is the process by which Aboriginal communities have the opportunity to increase control over their own health services.

There is also a call for the term 're-empowerment' to be used in recognition that indigenous people were once empowered sovereign peoples who through the processes of colonization became disempowered (Fredericks 2010, 2008, 2007; Redbird 1995). Labonte (1989) argues that it is through individual self-empowerment that people can bring about change. He describes in several of his writings how processes of empowerment can be built and how organizations, specifically health and well-being organizations, can work in ways that are more empowering (Labonte 1986, 1989, 1991a, 1991b).

ACCHOs are structured and operated in such a way as to involve individual community members and collectives, an arrangement that empowers their communities. For example, all ACCHOs have their own boards of directors or management committees, either elected or appointed from their community. VACCHO was established by Victorian Aboriginal people to support, represent and advocate for the ACCHO sector. VACCHO is committed to engaging and working with its members to maximize their health and well-being by ensuring participation and community ownership (VACCHO 2006, 2009).

VACCHO represents the ACCHO sector at local, state and national levels and presents a unified voice when working with governments. Its role is to support and advocate for and on behalf of its membership and the Victorian Aboriginal community. The VACCHO vision is that 'Aboriginal people will have a high quality of health and well-being, thus enabling individuals and communities to reach their full potential'. The definition of health in this case is not simply ... physical wellbeing but refers to the social, emotional and cultural wellbeing of the whole community. Aboriginal people have a whole-of-life view of incorporating the cyclical concept of life, death and the relationship with the land. (VACCHO 2009: 10)

VACCHO is a 'peak body' – in Australia, an association of groups – rather than a service provider and allows for differences of opinion among its member organizations. It works through a model of power *for* and on *behalf of* rather than power *over* its members. This empowers all its members as a process that affirms and strengthens the Aboriginal ways of being and working (Wallerstein 1992). VACCHO thus works in solidarity with the sector while recognizing that all member services are individual organizations in their own right. Each member organization elects two representatives to attend quarterly meetings arranged by VACCHO's secretariat. Each year an Annual General Meeting is convened and a new Board elected. The Board provides the overall strategic direction for the organization, including policy direction, programme development and representation. Aboriginal community members through their local ACCHO and then through VACCHO are engaged in defining and managing their own organizations. VACCHO, throughout all its work, is informed by the philosophy of community control and the motto 'By Community for Community'. It also initiates and strengthens networks and partnerships, increases workforce development opportunities and demonstrates leadership on specific health issues. It represents the Victorian ACCHOs at national meetings of the ACCHO sector and to Australian government departments. Advocacy by VACCHO is 'carried out with a range of private, community and government agencies, at state and national levels, on all issues related to Aboriginal health' (VACCHO and CRCAH 2007).

Another way of explaining how VACCHO functions is via the painting *The Story of VACCHO* (Figure 6.1), which illustrates the philosophy of the organization. This illustration uses symbolism to highlight the dynamic way in which VACCHO works with Aboriginal people and its member organizations. For example the figures sitting around in groups across the state of Victoria symbolize the discussion that takes place in communities to achieve better health for Aboriginal people. The tracks that criss-cross the state are inspired by the old tracks Aboriginal people once used and symbolize the connections between VACCHO, its members and Aboriginal people in other states. The figures represent VACCHO members working on behalf of all Victorian Aboriginal people in no one central location in Victoria (VACCHO 2009: 2).

VACCHO is well placed to represent its members and to work in ways that engage Aboriginal people meaningfully in the development of Aboriginal policies and programmes that reflect community knowledge and experience. VACCHO is able to capitalize on knowledge drawn from within Aboriginal

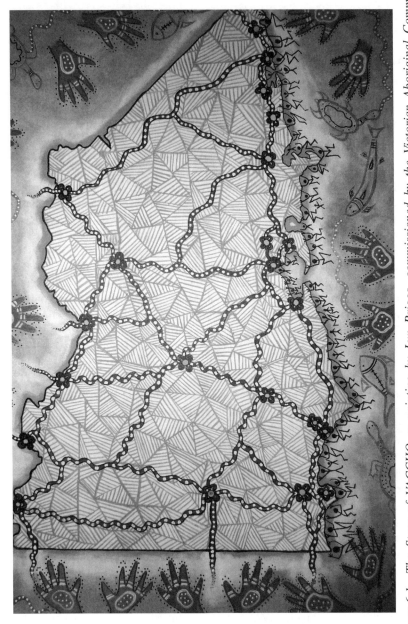

Figure 6.1   The Story of VACCHO, a painting by Lyn Briggs, commissioned by the Victorian Aboriginal Community Controlled Health Organisation (VACCHO)

communities and develop both well-informed criticism of existing policies and achievable directions for the development and implementation of new policies. It is to this work that we now turn.

DECOLONIZING POLICY IN ACTION

Soon after its inception VACCHO began to make significant impacts on Aboriginal health policy and decision-making in Victoria. Without solid part-nerships between VACCHO and its member organizations this would have been an almost impossible task. Much is also owed to VACCHO's form of governance which, while supporting and advocating for and on behalf of the Victorian Aboriginal community, also develops the capacity of others to assist in the promotion of change. In its early establishment VACCHO, in consulta-tion with its membership, developed several policy documents, developed programmes and provided new funding to support VACCHO members. Provision of Aboriginal health worker training began when VACCHO regis-tered as a training organization, which led to it offering accredited training of Aboriginal health workers for the first time (Adams and Spratling 2001). A review of Aboriginal birthing services and birth outcomes was conducted, leading to the establishment of the Koori Maternity Services (KMS) Program, providing improved access to appropriate birthing services (Campbell 2000). A VACCHO and Cooperative Research Centre for Aboriginal Health (CRCAH) publication describes the KMS Program at the Victorian Aboriginal Health Service as having 'had lasting, ongoing, positive impacts in the Community' (VACCHO and CRCAH 2007: 21). The Health Service practice manager noted that 'we now have evidence that since the program has started, there has been an increase in the birth weights of babies born in the commu-nity despite all the media attention that has been given to Aboriginal Communities facing low birth weights' (VACCHO and CRCAH 2007: 21). The increase in birth weights, which is an early but important health status indicator, demonstrates the positive impact this programme has had and continues to have on the path towards a general improvement in health outcomes for the Aboriginal community. With improved programmes and partnerships has come improved VACCHO member support, Medicare and general practice accreditation, engagement with universities for ethical and community-led research, health promotion initiatives, and workforce training development and provision. These have also led to improved links with main-stream services such as hospitals, general practitioners (GPs) and community health centres.

In playing a leading role VACCHO has achieved some major outcomes for the Aboriginal health sector. In 1996 the Victorian Aboriginal Council on

Koori Health (VACKH) was established. VACKH provides a forum where the Australian federal government, the Victorian state government and the community-controlled health organization sector work collaboratively to improve the health and well-being of Aboriginal people. The members of VACKH are nominated representatives from the Australian government Department of Health and Ageing, the Victorian Department of Human Services, VACCHO, and its member organizations. VACCHO hosts the executive support for VACKH, which has several subcommittees, including those on oral health, mental health, health workforce issues and the implementation of Victorian Aboriginal health reforms under COAG. These subcommittees provide an opportunity for the development, implementation, monitoring and evaluation of specific Aboriginal health issues and COAG's Close the Gap health reform.

In 2008 VACKH initiated the development of the Victorian Aboriginal Health Plan (VACKH 2009) to provide a joint forum for planning across federal, state and Aboriginal community-controlled concerns. The idea was that the planning process would identify health priorities and strategies to close the gap between Aboriginal and non-Aboriginal people in Victoria. VACKH commissioned VACCHO to coordinate the development of the VACKH plan, with VACCHO undertaking extensive consultation with its member organizations and providing an analysis of existing programmes, policies and research evidence. This is in complete contrast to health policy development undertaken in the past. VACCHO member organizations were able to participate in meetings, discuss issues, voice their concerns and suggest ideas for programmes and strategies to address Aboriginal health and well-being issues. The Victorian Aboriginal Health Plan, through VACKH, aims to:

- coordinate action to improve outcomes across the social determinants that impact on health;
- strengthen health promotion and prevention responses;
- improve the provision of, and access to, culturally appropriate primary, secondary and specialist health care services;
- build health infrastructure and organizational capacity in Aboriginal Community Controlled Health Organisations;
- improve the cultural safety of mainstream services;
- build workforce capacity; and
- advance data collection, information management systems and research (VACKH 2009: 9).

The plan will be implemented through the development of a framework by VACKH and any further implementation will be monitored and evaluated to ensure that targets and performance indicators are achieved. The plan's implementation will also be integrated with Aboriginal health reforms under the COAG framework. This offers ACCHOs a great opportunity to ensure that future Victorian Aboriginal health-related programmes and policies are responsive, appropriate and meaningful for Aboriginal people.

The signing of the Close the Gap statement showed a commitment to a partnership with Aboriginal communities for health equality, both in Victoria and nationally. COAG underlined this commitment with AUS$1.6 billion of activities to address health inequities, while the Victorian state government committed a further AUS$47.4 million over 4 years (Mohamed in VACCHO 2009: 5). This is a substantial commitment from all governments to address the gap between the health of Aboriginal and non-Aboriginal Australians and Victorians, and will present VACCHO and its member organizations with many challenges (VACCHO 2009: 5).

The COAG initiatives combined with VACKH and the Victorian Aboriginal Health Plan provide a framework for change in Victoria, offering Aboriginal people the opportunity for real participation in processes that are about transformation across the state and in individual communities. Although decision-making power is still vested in governments, if there is to be meaningful, long-lasting change in the health status of Aboriginal people then continuing Aboriginal community participation in defining the problems and providing real community solutions is essential.

In the last 30 years governments have reconceptualized the role of Aboriginal people and communities in health policy decisions. In recent times governments have finally listened to these Aboriginal voices. Aboriginal people have known that there needed to be a variety of methods to address the gaps in Aboriginal health, along with appropriate funding and resourcing. It can be demonstrated that when Aboriginal people moved from being seen and treated as *objects* of policy to being *subjects* who themselves have a stake in policymaking, there was better control over health outcomes. This in turn has fostered partnerships and an equal stake in policymaking free from tokenism. It has also fostered sites of empowerment, self-determination and self-management (Wallerstein 1992; Freire 1970; Labonte 1986, 1989, 1991a, 1991b). Federal and state governments and Aboriginal people have come a long way since the first roundtable discussions under the National Aboriginal Health Strategy.

CONCLUSION

This chapter has explored both the changing health status of Victorian Aboriginal people as a result of colonization and the growth over time of Aboriginal health advocacy, empowerment, self-determination and self-management.

Aboriginal participation in the development of policy and in the planning, delivery, management and evaluation of health programmes enables policies and programmes to respond effectively to the needs of Aboriginal people and to change future health outcomes for them. Aboriginal involvement in decision-making has gone some way to decolonizing policymaking and has addressed the power imbalance – both of which have been critical in the improvement in Aboriginal health outcomes.

NOTES

1. In 2004 Michael Long, a well-known footballer, walked to Australia's national capital, Canberra, to draw attention to racism in Australian culture and Aboriginal disadvantage. At a reconciliation convention in Melbourne, Aboriginal people turned their backs on a hectoring Prime Minister John Howard who said that 'symbolic' reconciliation was useless and foreshadowed changes to Native Title legislation.

REFERENCES

Abbie, A.A. (1976), *The Original Australians*, Sydney. NSW: Rigby.

Adams, K. and M. Spratling (2001), 'Keepin ya mob healthy: Aboriginal community participation and Aboriginal health worker training in Victoria', *Journal of Primary Health*, **7** (1): 116–19.

Anderson, I. (1997), 'The National Aboriginal Health Strategy', in H. Gardner (ed.), *Health Policy in Australia*, Melbourne, VIC: Oxford University Press, pp. 119–35.

Australian Bureau of Statistics (ABS) (2007), *Number of Persons Usually Resident by Number of Bedrooms by Indigenous Status of Household – Victoria*, cat. no 2068.0–2006, Canberra: ABS.

ABS and Australian Institute of Health and Welfare (AIHW) (2008), *The Health and Welfare of Aboriginal and Torres Strait Islander Peoples*, cat. no 4704.0, Canberra: ABS and AIHW.

Australian Health Ministers' Advisory Council (AHMAC) (2006), *Aboriginal and Torres Strait Islander Health Performance Framework Report*, Canberra: AHMAC.

Australian House of Representatives Standing Committee on Family and Youth Affairs (2000), *Health is Life Report on the Inquiry into Indigenous Health*, Canberra: Australian Government Publishing Service.

Australian Human Rights Commission (2009), 'Will COAG deliver on indigenous health?', media release, 1 July, accessed 15 December at www.humanrights.gov.au/about/media/media_relases/2009/58_09.html.

Beresford, Q. and P. Omaji (1998), *Our State of Mind: Racial Planning and the Stolen Generations*, South Fremantle, WA: Fremantle Arts Centre Press.

Blainey, G. (1994), *Triumph of the Nomads: A History of Ancient Australia*, South Melbourne, VIC: Macmillan.

Calma, T. (2009), 'Little progress for indigenous people', media release, 2 July, accessed 15 December at www.unaa.org.au/pdf/Unity20601.pdf.

Campbell, S. (2000), *From Her to Maternity: A Report to the VACCHO Members and the Victorian Department of Human Services about Maternity Services for the Aboriginal Women of Victoria*, Melbourne, VIC: VACCHO.

Clark, M. (1966), *Sources of Australian History*, New York: Mentor.

Cleland, J.B. (1928), 'Disease amongst the Australian Aborigines', *Journal of Tropical Medicine and Hygiene*, 31: 53–70, 125–30, 141–5, 157–60, 173–7, 196–8, 202–6, 216–20, 232–5, 262–6, 281–2, 290–94, 307–13, 326–30 (a series of articles across the same volume, in different editions, available from the University of Queensland).

Elphinstone, J. (1971), 'The health of Australian Aborigines with no previous association with Europeans', *Medical Journal of Australia*, 2: 293–301.

Engels, F. (1892 [1976], *The Condition of the Working-Class in England in 1844*, reprinted in 1976, Moscow: Progress Publishers.

Evans, R., K. Saunders and K. Cronin (1988), *Race Relations in Colonial Queensland: A History of Exclusion, Exploitation and Extermination*, Brisbane QLD: University of Queensland Press.

Fredericks, B. (2007), 'Australian Aboriginal women's health: reflecting on the past and present', *Journal of Health and History*, 9 (2): 93–113.

Fredericks, B. (2008), 'Which way that empowerment?: Aboriginal women's narratives of empowerment', *Alter*Native: *An International Journal of Indigenous Scholarship*, 4 (2): 6–19.

Fredericks, B. (2009a), 'There is nothing that "identifies me to that place": Aboriginal women's perceptions of health spaces and places', *Cultural Studies Review*, 15 (2): 41–61.

Fredericks, B. (2009b), 'How the whiteness embedded in health services impacts on the health and well-being of Aboriginal peoples', in D. Riggs and B. Baird (eds), *The Racial Politics of Bodies, Nations and Knowledges*, Newcastle on Tyne: Cambridge Scholars Publishing, pp. 11–27.

Fredericks, B. (2010), 'Reempowering ourselves: Australian Aboriginal women', *SIGNS: Journal of Women in Culture and Society*, 35 (3): 546–50.

Freire, P. (1970), *Pedagogy of the Oppressed*, New York: Continuum Publishing Company.

Henderson, J.S.Y. (2000), 'Challenges of respecting indigenous world views in Eurocentric education', in R. Neil (ed.), *Voice of the Drum: Indigenous Education and Culture*, Brandon, MB: Kingfisher Publications, pp. 59–80.

Horton, D. (1999), *Aboriginal Australia*, Canberra: Australian Institute of Aboriginal and Torres Strait Islander Studies.

Hunter, P. (1998), 'Executive overview: chairperson's report', *NACCHO National Aboriginal Community Controlled Health Organisation Report 1997/98 Annual Report*, Canberra: NACCHO.

Kidd, R. (1997), *The Way We Civilise*, St Lucia, QLD: University of Queensland Press.

Koori Heritage Trust (2009), 'Oral history collection', accessed 23 December at www.koorieheritagetrust.com/collections/oral_history_collection.

Labonte, R. (1986), 'Social inequality and healthy public policy', *Health Promotion International*, 1 (13): 341–51.

Labonte, R. (1989), 'Community empowerment: the need for political analysis', *Canadian Journal of Public Health*, 80 (2) (March/April): 87–8.

Labonte, R. (1991a), 'Econology: integrating health and sustainable development, part one: theory and background', *Health Promotion International*, 6 (1): 49–65.

Labonte, R. (1991b), 'Econology; integrating health and sustainable development, part two: guiding principles for decision making', *Health Promotion International*, 6 (2): 147–56.

Lippmann, L. (1994), *Generations of Resistance: Mabo and Justice*, 3rd edn, Melbourne, VIC: Longman Cheshire.

Manne, R. (2001), 'In denial: the stolen generation and the right', *Quarterly Essay*, **1**: 1–113.

Mohamed, J. (2009), 'Chairperson's report', *Victorian Aboriginal Community Controlled Health Organisation Annual Report 2008–2009*, Melbourne, VIC: VACCHO.

Moodie, P. (1973), *Aboriginal Health*, Canberra: Australian National University Press.

National Aboriginal and Torres Strait Islander Health Council (NATSIC) (2001), *National Aboriginal and Torres Strait Islander Health Strategy, Consultation Draft*, Canberra: NATSIC.

National Aboriginal Community Controlled Organisation (NACCHO) and Oxfam Australia. (2007), *CLOSE THE GAP. Solutions to the Indigenous Health Crisis facing Australia*, Braddon, ACT: NACCHO and Oxfam Australia.

National Aboriginal Health Strategy (NAHS) Working Party (1989), *A National Aboriginal Health Strategy*, Canberra: Australian Government Publishing Service.

Nelson, E., S. Smith, and P. Grimshaw (eds) (2002), *Letters From Aboriginal Women of Victoria, 1867–1926*, Melbourne, VIC: The University of Melbourne.

Paradies, Y., R. Harris and I. Anderson (2008), *The Impact of Racism on Indigenous Health in Australia and Aotearoa: Towards a Research Agenda*, Casuarina, NT: Cooperative Research Centre for Aboriginal Health and Flinders University.

Phillips, G. (2003), *Addictions and Healing in Aboriginal Country*, Canberra: Aboriginal Studies Press.

Redbird, E. (1995), 'Honouring native women; the backbone of native sovereignty', in K. Hazlehurst (ed.), *Popular Justice and Community Regeneration: Pathways of Indigenous Reform*, London: Praeger, pp. 121–41.

Rintoul, S. (1993), *The Wailing: A National Black Oral History*, Port Melbourne, VIC: Heinemann.

Rintoul, S. (2002), 'A new age for Aboriginal issues', *The Australian*, 28 March.

Rosser, B. (1985), *Dreamtime Nightmares: Biographies of Aborigines under the Aborigines Act*, Canberra: Australian Institute of Aboriginal Studies.

Rudd, K. 2008, 'Apology to Australia's indigenous peoples', accessed 10 December at www.pm.gov.au/media/speech/2008/Speech_0073.cfm.

Saggers, S. and D. Gray (1991), *Aboriginal Health and Society: The Traditional and Contemporary Aboriginal Struggle for Better Health*, Sydney. NSW: Allen & Unwin.

Sanders, W.G. (2006), 'Indigenous affairs after the Howard decade: an administrative revolution while defying decolonisation', Centre for Aboriginal Economic Policy Research The Howard Decade Conference, 3–4 March, Canberra.

Schwartz, L. (2004), 'Tough journey ends, another begins', *The Age*, 1 December, accessed 23 December 2009 at www.theage.com.au/news/National/Tough-journey-ends-another-begins/2004/11/30/1101577485689.html.

Stone, S. (ed.) (1974), *Aborigines in White Australia: A Documentary History of the Attitudes Affecting Official Policy and the Australian Aborigine 1697–1973*, Melbourne. VIC: Heinemann Educational Books.

Thomson, N. (1984), 'Australian Aboriginal health and health-care', *Social Science & Medicine*, **18** (11): 939–48.

Vickery, J., A. Clarke and K. Adams (eds) (2005), *Nyernila Koories Kila Degaia: Listen to Koories Speak about Health*, Melbourne. VIC: Koori Heritage Trust and Onemda VicHealth Koori Health Unit.

Victorian Aboriginal Community Controlled Health Organisation (VACCHO) (2006), *VACCHO: About Us*, Melbourne. VIC: VACCHO.

VACCHO (2009), *Victorian Aboriginal Community Controlled Health Organisation Annual Report 2008–2009*, Melbourne, VIC: VACCHO.

VACCHO and Cooperative Research Centre for Aboriginal Health (CRCAH) (2007), *Communities Working for Health and Wellbeing: Success Stories from the Aboriginal Community Controlled Health Sector in Victoria*, Fitzroy, VIC: VACCHO and CRCAH.

Victorian Aboriginal Council on Koori Health (VACKH) (2009), *Victorian Aboriginal Health Plan*, Melbourne, VIC: VACKH.

Wallerstein, N. (1992), 'Powerlessness, empowerment and health: implementation for health promotion programs', *American Journal of Health Promotion*, **6**: 197–205.

Wallerstein, N. and Bernstein, E. (1988), 'Empowerment and education: Freire's ideas adapted to health education', *Health Education Quarterly,* **15** (4): 379–94.

7. The Irish Health Service's Expert Advisory Groups: spaces for advancing epistemological justice?

Orla O'Donovan

In February 2006 the Irish Health Services Executive (HSE) placed notices in national newspapers seeking expressions of interest for membership of its proposed Expert Advisory Groups (EAGs). Replacing 11 regional health boards with a single centralized apparatus, the HSE had been established a year earlier and was heralded in official discourses as signifying the beginning of not just major reform of the Irish health care system but its transformation. Acknowledging the dysfunctional and expensive character of the existing system, in his opening comments in the HSE's *Transformation Programme 2007–2010* (2007: 5), HSE CEO Brendan Drumm stated that he deliberately used the term 'transformation' to describe the radical changes underway because 'reform' had come to refer to the modest project of organizational and administrative change: 'Our transformation must extend much further and touch almost every aspect of our work; the way we work, the way we relate to each other, our culture and our ambitions.' In contrast to this official celebration of the HSE, critics, including some senior bureaucrats, argued that the health service would not be better governed by further centralizing responsibility for service delivery or by reducing the role of elected representatives who served on the regional health boards (Donnellan 2003). For others the new division of labour – the Department of Health and Children would be responsible for health care legislation, policy and financial accountability, and the HSE in charge of management and delivery of health care – constituted an outsourcing of government, reducing the government department to a small policymaking unit and undermining democratic involvement in day-to-day decision-making (Allen 2007).

Shortly after the expression-of-interest notices were published, Drumm described the EAGs as a pioneering mechanism of participatory governance:

> We are inviting people such as members of the public, front line physicians, paramedics and therapists to join a forum that will act as a driving force for the development of policies for the provision of health services and will be responsible for

monitoring the implementation of the policies. This is the first time for any health organisation in the world that front line service providers and the people who use our services will be made central when deciding policy implementation plans. (Joint Committee on Health and Children 2006)

However, just three years later the EAGs featured in the *Irish Medical News'* 'Whatever Happened?' series devoted to 'high profile health-related projects, reports, and schemes which have stalled or been abandoned' (Lynch 2009).

In this chapter, I tell the story of this short-lived institutional mechanism by way of elucidating a significant aspect of the bio-political landscape in which Irish health advocacy organizations are embedded. The historical narrative I offer is recounted with a view to revealing the prevailing systems of thought and action, or governmental rationality and technologies (Rose and Miller 1992), through which the HSE sought to give effect to health advocacy organization involvement in the health policy process. 'Governmental rationality' refers to a collective mentality, way of thinking or complex of justifications and meanings 'capable of making some form of activity thinkable and practicable both to its practitioners and to those upon whom it is practiced' (Gordon 1991: 5). 'Governmental technologies' are the complex of programmes, procedures, structures and documents through which the HSE sought to operationalize health advocacy organization involvement. The story is pieced together using publicly available documentation, and information provided to me through a series of conversations and email communications with HSE personnel, and conversations with two members of an EAG.

STRUGGLES FOR EPISTEMOLOGICAL JUSTICE

HSE governmental rationalities and technologies form a significant aspect of the 'field of contention' in which Irish health advocacy organizations are embedded, the web of 'interactions, relationships, and interdependencies in which agents and particularly organizations who elect to contest an area of life ... find themselves enmeshed' (Crossley 2006: 562). As in other countries, Irish health advocacy organizations are highly diverse in disposition, culture of action and scale (O'Donovan 2007), and the existence of a distinct patients' movement is questionable. However, many organizations converge around broadly similar contentious concerns, among which are struggles for recognition of the experiential knowledge they can bring to the health policy process. Boaventura de Sousa Santos and colleagues (2007) conceive of these struggles for epistemological justice as efforts to replace the existing 'monoculture of scientific knowledge' with a multicultural 'ecology of knowledges'. They argue that this ambitious project, already significantly underway globally, can avoid the much-discussed pitfalls of collapsing knowledge into belief resulting in 'new ways of knowing nothing' (Collins and Yearly 1992: 310), and of romanticizing experiential knowledge in a manner that ignores its limitations (Prior 2003). The validity of experiential knowledge claims does not escape scrutiny; rather, the ecology of knowledges allows for 'a pragmatic discussion of alternative criteria of validity, which does not straightforwardly disqualify whatever does not fit the epistemological canon of modern science' (de Sousa Santos et al. 2007: xlix). Furthermore, in this understanding of democracy, embracing the principle of the incompleteness of all knowledges is a precondition for dialogue between people drawing upon different ways of knowing.

The struggle for epistemological justice is evident, for example, in the claim made by the Irish National Council of AD/HD Support Groups (INCADDS) that its members 'are ideally placed to have a major input into the development of policies in relation to AD/HD as they are the people who live with the condition and its consequences every day' (INCADDS 2003: 14). Similarly, mental health activists involved with the Irish Advocacy Network position themselves as 'experts by experience' who can 'speak authoritatively and humanely from the inside out' (Dublin City University 2007). In many instances of health advocacy organizations' demands for formal inclusion in the policy process and recognition of the distinctive knowledge of their members, new patient identities are in the making as people once deemed incapable of self-advocacy are recast as knowing and able policy actors. As the Chairperson of the Alzheimer Society of Ireland in a letter to *The Irish Times* (Tierney 2007) put it, people diagnosed with the disease 'must be heard, understood and responded to' in policy processes concerning nursing home care and more generally. It is important to recognize that these epistemological struggles are nested within 'environing fields' (Crossley 2006) that make up the bio-political landscape in which health advocacy organizations operate and that many seek to transform. In this discussion, I approach the HSE as a significant environing field impinging upon Irish health advocacy organizations and their struggles for recognition of the distinctive knowledge that they bring to the health policy process. Health advocacy organizations are not just situated in fields of contention; they also help constitute them through generative interactions with each other, state institutions, the mass media and a variety of other actors. However, the analysis in this chapter focuses mainly on HSE discourses about health advocacy organization involvement, leaving consideration of the dynamic interplay between them and health advocacy organization discourses for another day. I also limit my analysis to official activities and pronouncements made between 2006 and 2010, the period when the EAGs were both introduced and abandoned. The problems associated with participatory governance mechanisms are by now well understood (Clarke 2005); my purpose here is to elucidate those problems as they were played out in the specific context of the Irish health services.

SHORT-LIVED NEW GOVERNANCE SPACES – EXPERT ADVISORY GROUPS

Official talk in Ireland about health service public involvement long predates the establishment of the HSE. 'New managerialism', embodying the neo-liberal economic decision-making calculus and aimed at making public services more 'business like' (Clarke 2004) was evident in Irish health care discourses by the mid-1980s. For example the 1986 policy document *Health – The Wider Dimensions* addressed the importance of mechanisms for active 'consumer' feedback and input. Since then a series of managerialist governmental technologies have been introduced (and subsequently abandoned), including the 1992 'Charter of Rights for Hospital Patients' that conferred non-legally-binding 'rights' to information and redress (O'Donovan and Casey 1995). Before the new millennium Irish state institutions were also experimenting with new health 'governance spaces' (Taylor 2007) in which civil society organizations and actors were invited to engage in the policy process. One senior Department of Health figure championed the regional women's health advisory committees established in the 1990s as the best example of state efforts to promote democratic dialogue with women's organizations (Barrington 1998). These committees were among the profusion of 'partnership' forums formed at this time which came to be seen by many civil society organizations as the primary arena, if not the only one in which they might shape state policy. This hegemony of state corporatism in Ireland has been the focus of extensive critical commentaries (Ó Cinnéide 1999; Allen 2000; Meade and O'Donovan 2002). Among them are assessments of civil society organization participation in governance spaces and processes despite ambivalence about the implications of this for their autonomy and influence – a conflicted sentiment expressed by Rosie Meade (2005) as: 'We hate it here, please let us stay!'

The legislation underpinning the establishment of the HSE provided for '[m]echanisms (including advisory panels) to enable [the] Executive to consult with local communities and others' (Government of Ireland 2004). Blending managerialist with partnership speak, according to the initial HSE Corporate Plan one objective was to develop as a 'dynamic, effective and learning organisation in partnership with service users, patients, staff, not-for-profit/Voluntary/Community sector and other stakeholders'. The Plan went on to state that this 'means we are committed to listening to and learning from the experience of our service users ... and other stakeholders' (HSE 2005: 18). It was in the context of these provisions and commitments that the EAGs were established. The HSE CEO made many pronouncements about the significance of their establishment, echoed by government ministers. Speaking in the Seanad (the Irish parliament's upper house) in 2006, the Minister of State at the Department of Health and Children declared that the establishment of the EAGs represented 'a major step in the [health services] reform programme' and that they would enable 'patients, clients and service users' and other 'stakeholders' to play 'an influential role in service development' (Seanad Éireann 2006). Similarly, HSE documentation explained that the EAGs 'will formalise meaningful engagement with the clinical and professional community and with patient, client and user representatives so that they can influence the strategic direction of the relevant area' (HSE 2006: 7).

In a further explanation of the official rationale for the EAGs, the HSE's CEO argued that frontline staff, patients and service users have insights and can identify practical solutions to problems that evade health service managers: 'They often have a level of clarity and see solutions that we managers in the wider context of managing overall services and having to make compromises do not see' (in Hunter 2006a). On this occasion Brendan Drumm differentiated HSE managers from EAG members on the basis of their knowledge, with EAG members recognized as possessing insightful, if particularistic, knowledge that contrasted with managers' transcendent, pragmatic but occasionally blinkered and thus incomplete knowledge. But as will be shown, in other contexts EAG members' particularistic knowledge was constructed as potentially flawed and serving narrow sectional interests. Indeed, as experienced in other countries, hand in hand with the rise of managerialism came the depoliticizing commitment to 'evidence-based' policy-making (Clarke 2004) which elevated managers' allegedly transcendent and pragmatic knowledge over the knowledge of other policy actors.

Here, it is worthwhile noting that the managers mentioned by Drumm are a class of well-paid state actors which grew significantly once the HSE was established. Critics on the left pointed to the 'bloated, over-paid managerial layer' that appeared in the era of neo-liberalism, during which time Irish public services followed the model of the corporate sector (Allen 2009: 39). Some senior medical professionals also accused the HSE of cultivating an 'opaque and labyrinthine bureaucracy' that excluded senior doctors, not to mention patients, from the management process (Hardiman 2007). In addition to the spawning of HSE managers, when Drumm became CEO he brought with him a handpicked 'reform team', referred to in the media as his 'kitchen cabinet' (Donnellan 2009). Drumm negotiated a salary for himself of 400 000 – significantly above that of the Taoiseach (head of government) – together with substantial bonuses, and 1 million annually to spend on his team of advisers (Burke 2008). Embedding managerialist ideology and processes, the brief of these advisers included providing guidance on performance management and value for money.

The HSE's call for membership of the EAGs unambiguously defined the terms of engagement of the new governance spaces. The number of EAGs to be established was already decided, as was their focus. The notice indicated that five EAGs were to be set up: one each for older people, children, mental health, diabetes, and accident and emergency services. The last was never appointed, possibly because accident and emergency services became extremely contentious as hospital services were centralized and belief in 'bigger is better' ideology was instantiated (O'Connor 2007). Despite use of the term 'representatives' to refer to some EAG members, the notice seeking expressions of interest specified that 'Members will be appointed on a personal basis and not as a representative of a group or professional body', thus avoiding processes of democratic mandating and accountability between the members of the group and the various organizations and constituencies they ostensibly represented. The HSE equated such democratic processes with partisan parochialism; a spokesperson explained that their preferred model of representation 'removes any obligation members may feel to put forward the views of peer groups and interest groups with specific local and regional agendas'; that it enabled them to 'retain their impartiality and apply a national perspective' (not unlike the supposedly transcendent perspective of managers, discussed above) (Hunter 2006b). In other words, in a measure that suppressed the particularistic knowledge that the HSE CEO specified elsewhere as underpinning the rationale for the new governance spaces, EAG members were officially envisioned as individuals rather than as members of collectivities or publics. The 'rules of the game' for EAGs were further elaborated in an information pack which stated that members and chairs would be appointed by the CEO, that chairs would report to the CEO via the national director (a member of his kitchen cabinet), that group reports would be submitted to the HSE Strategic Planning, Reform and Implementation division, and that members would be required to sign a declaration of confidentiality prior to appointment. In sum, from the outset the EAGs had all the hallmarks of 'invited spaces', 'into which communities/citizens are invited by the state and which are created and defined by the state' (Taylor 2007: 300).

Despite the constraints imposed, the HSE received over 600 expressions of interest (Hunter 2006a) and in October 2006 the membership of the first four EAGs was announced, with final selections made by the HSE CEO. Upholding the hierarchies and expert culture typical of the Irish health service, the chair of each group was a medical consultant, and the majority of members were health professionals. At most there were two members who could be regarded as patient representatives and most of these were professional advocates. For example, a consultant geriatrician chaired the EAG on services for older people and the only civil society actors were the CEO of the Alzheimer Society of Ireland, a highly professionalized patient organization, and the CEO of the smaller Senior Help Line. The predominance of professionals was also a feature of the mental health EAG. It was chaired by a consultant psychiatrist, and among its 20 members were four other consultant psychiatrists, three senior nurses and a psychologist, general practitioner, occupational therapist and social worker. The two service user representatives were professionalized peer advocates associated with the Irish Advocacy Network. The appointment of group members was met with public criticism due to the virtual absence of 'ordinary patients', prompting one medical journalist to ask 'Where are the patients?' (Hunter 2006a). Significantly, in many later official pronouncements reference to the inclusion of patients or their representatives was omitted. For example, in 2008 in Dáil Éireann (the Irish parliament's lower house), the Minister for Health and Children stated that EAGs 'are made up of a wide range of health professionals' (Dáil Éireann 2008a). Similarly, according to an article in the *Irish Medical News*, the EAG on diabetes was established to give 'the medical profession a voice to talk to HSE management on policy matters' (Mulholland 2008). According to the HSE's 2008–11 corporate plan EAGs were 'providing a central platform within the HSE for the front line professionals and leaders to contribute to operational policy' (HSE 2008: 44). A possible explanation for this repeated omission is that behind the managerialist mythology of 'stakeholder involvement' the actual purpose of EAGs was to incorporate, through a combination of flattery and semblance of inclusion, senior health professionals who were critical of and marginalized by the centralized system of managerial authority and the CEO's personally appointed kitchen cabinet. As will be shown, this erasure of patient representatives is consistent with their exclusion from the category 'experts' employed by the HSE in relation to the EAGs.

In contrast to the identification of citizens as 'consumers' that by 2006 was widespread in Irish health service discourses, the EAG newspaper notice invited expressions of interest from 'patients', 'clients' and 'service users', as well as clinicians and professionals. Mention of these three distinct identities suggests an official awareness of the significance of words as carriers of meanings, and of the heterogeneous identities assumed by and ascribed to members of the public in their interaction with health services. The decision not to use 'consumer' may have stemmed from an awareness that this term is tainted in the context of participatory initiatives or, as suggested by an EAG member, recognition of the absence of choice of services available to Irish public patients. A further significant lexical choice was the inclusion of 'Expert' in the title of the Advisory Groups. This could be interpreted as conferring on patient, client and service user representatives the status of experts, possibly on the basis of claims about experiential knowledge (as made by members of INCADDS and the Irish Advocacy Network noted above). However closer inspection of the notice reveals that from the outset this was not part of the governmental rationality behind these new governance spaces. Indeed, the EAGs' purpose was 'to bring the *expertise* of the clinical and health community and the *voice* of patients/clients and service users to a more influential role within the HSE' (my emphasis). In other words, a boundary was set up between clinicians/professionals and patients/clients/service users, with *expertise* the property only of the first and *voice* a property of the second. Even though differences between 'patients', 'clients' and 'service users' seem to have been acknowledged, they collapsed when the character of the knowledge these actors possessed was a consideration. *Expertise* was used only with reference to credentialized experts. The distinction drawn between professional and clinical actors was also noteworthy, as expressions of interest were sought from 'persons with professional/clinical expertise in the specified areas of focus' – presumably an encouragement to medical and 'allied' health professionals to nominate for membership of the groups. However, the appointment of senior clinicians as the EAG chairs restated the status distinction between these two groups.

The vocabulary, distinctions, and identities evident in the initial public notice became stock phrases used repeatedly in official pronouncements about the allegedly pioneering governance spaces. In 2007 when the Minister of State at the Department of Health and Children spoke about the EAGs in Dáil Éireann he too subscribed to the distinction between 'expertise' and 'voice' (Dáil Éireann 2007). Moreover members of EAGs who were health professionals were constructed not just as experts but as 'esteemed' ones: the 'presence of esteemed doctors, nurses and other practitioners in the structure should help to influence change reform and the development of best practice in a more consistent way throughout the system' (HSE 2006: 7). No reference was made to esteemed patient representatives.

In May 2007 the HSE called for expressions of interest from groups that might offer advice about maternity services, oral health, and health and personal social services for people with a disability. By then the four original groups were meeting on a regular basis and the EAG on diabetes had submitted a report and series of recommendations to the HSE. As late as June 2008 senior political actors were continuing to talk up the significance of the new health governance spaces and processes. Speaking in the national parliament, the Minister for Health and Children noted that the HSE was also establishing an EAG on maternity services which would 'provide a central platform for clinical and health communities, patients, clients and managers to become actively involved in the development and transformation of maternity services' (Dáil Éireann 2008c).

However, second-round EAGs were never appointed. In November 2008 the Irish medical press noted that the HSE had revealed that their establishment had been 'delayed as a result of the review of the Executive's organisational structure and associated plans for restructuring' (Mulholland 2008). By then, members of the EAG on diabetes were publicly criticizing the HSE for its slow response to their recommendations, which became the focus of a number of parliamentary questions in 2008, while some members of the EAG on mental health had stopped attending meetings or had formally resigned because they felt the group to be a mere talk-shop dominated by senior clinicians. The decision to apply an HSE embargo on travel expenses (due to the crash in the so-called 'Celtic Tiger' economy) and resort to teleconferencing were interpreted by some members as a convenient way of undermining the troubled structures of participatory governance. In 2009 there was evidence that the HSE experiment in what the Minister for Health and Children referred to as 're-engineer[ing] how it gathers views and opinions from patients and staff' (Dáil Éireann 2008b) was over. When I enquired of the HSE why the EAGs were no longer functioning I was told that: 'in 2008, Prof. Drumm, CEO, decided to pause the EAGs to allow a period of reflection on the first 2-year term and also to understand how EAG type structures might contribute to policy development in the context of the significant structural re-organisation of the HSE which was under consideration at the time' (HSE 2010). In the same communication I was also informed that a 'qualitative review/evaluation of the EAG process was undertaken; however a report has not been published'. The 'pause' was really the abandonment of the participatory governance mechanism, as signalled by the inclusion of the EAGs in the *Irish Medical News*' 'Whatever Happened?' series.

Contradictory Governmental Rationalities

Clues that help explain the fate of these short-lived health governance spaces can be found in official pronouncements about another participatory institutional mechanism introduced just as the EAGs went into abeyance: the National Strategy for Service User Involvement in the Irish Health Service 2008–2013. This was launched in June 2008, apparently with renewed enthusiasm for participatory governance, CEO Drumm declaring that this mechanism represented 'a significant step forward in actively involving the public in this [transformation] programme of change' (HSE and Department of Health and Children 2008: 5).

Alongside the National Strategy the HSE published a literature review titled *Service User Involvement in the Irish Health Service: A Review of the Evidence* (McEvoy et al. 2008). As explained in the Executive Summary, the *Review* formed 'part of the foundations' on which the National Strategy was built. The review and the strategy, however, revealed profound contradictions in HSE governmental rationalities as it tried to reconcile commitments to participatory governance and evidence-based policy. Not only were the shaky foundations of the HSE's governmental rationality around service user involvement revealed, it being concluded that an 'evidence base' for this did not exist; so too was the shaky nature of its commitment to evidence-based policy as, despite the lack of evidence, it proceeded with its National Strategy.

The review considered research addressing the benefits of service user involvement in health service decision-making. Significantly, such benefits were never discussed in relation to democracy, or to democratizing health service decision-making, rather only in respect to effects on quality of care, patient satisfaction levels and health outcomes. It highlighted gaps in the literature documenting the outcomes and effectiveness of service user involvement. Demonstrating the HSE's increasingly scientistic rationality – that justifications for participatory governance have to be founded on or filtered through scientific evidence – the review bemoaned the fact that 'service user involvement is rarely amenable to the "gold standard" of evaluation: the randomised control trial' (McEvoy et al. 2008: 27). Reinforcing the epistemic authority of the new 'gold standard' of evaluation which emerged in the 1980s, they emphasized the conclusion of a systematic review that found: 'An evidence base for the effects [of involving patients in the planning and development of health care] on use of services, quality of care, satisfaction, or health of patients does not exist' (Crawford et al. 2002). Just as participatory governance was officially constructed as a technical challenge, something to be engineered, so too were its effects viewed in technical, calculative terms. Furthermore, knowledge attributed with the status of 'gold standard' was that generated through scientific methods. Drawing directly on the work of Nina Fudge and colleagues (2008) and upholding the bottom line of value for money, the HSE review concluded that 'given the resource implications of undertaking user involvement in service development there is a need for critical debate on the purpose of such involvement as well as better evidence of the benefits claimed for it' (McEvoy et al. 2008: 37). Nonetheless, in the absence of any such critical debate or evidence, the HSE, together with the Department of Health and Children, proceeded to launch the National Strategy for Service User Involvement in the Irish Health Service 2008–2013. In direct contradiction of the conclusions of the literature review, the National Strategy declared that service user involvement 'promotes health and personal social services that are safer, more accessible and of a higher quality' and even directed readers to the website where they could find the 'review of the literature supporting this strategy' (HSE and Department of Health and Children 2008: 19). In a further display of the HSE's capacity for cognitive dissonance, the then faltering EAGs were first on the list of HSE 'initiatives promoting service user involvement' in the 2008 literature review.

CONCLUSION

The story of Ireland's EAGs reveals the highly controlling and contradictory systems of thought and action through which the HSE experimented with participatory governance. It is a tale of the HSE's grappling with and eventual failure to make participatory governance either 'thinkable' or 'practicable' using the device of the EAG; and it is a story that provides no evidence of self-reflection on this failure and its introduction of yet another 'new' participatory device. What emerges is an image of a new state agency not only with a penchant for experimenting with and reconfiguring its participatory governance structures, but also with institutional amnesia about its failed experiments.

Despite official claims about transformation and culture change there is little evidence of any dismantling of the epistemological privilege granted to credentialized experts and scientific knowledge, nor of any emergent epistemological justice, which for some is essential to democratizing health. Even if we set questions of epistemological justice aside and lower the bar significantly, official recognition of plural systems of expertise and even the hybrid 'expert patients' who feature prominently in health policy discourses in other countries (Taylor and Bury 2007) were absent from the HSE's discursive repertoire. What we see is this state agency's commitment to 'boundary work': its unrelenting demarcation of the boundaries between credentialized expertise and other modes of knowing, combined with a constant reinforcing of the epistemic authority of the former and marginalizing of service users' experiential knowledge. Emerging from the story is evidence of severe constraints on the democratic potential of EAGs, which functioned within a hypermanagerialist agency with an intensely centralized system of authority. However, in keeping with John Clarke's (2004) argument that public sector managerialism, and more generally the logics of neo-liberalism, have not been wholly hegemonized and still have their troubles, the EAG experience shows a profound dissonance between the HSE's systems of thought and action regarding participatory governance and evidence-based policy. Dissonance such as this can potentially be used by those struggling for recognition for non-credentialized ways of knowing. This has been done by Irish mental health activists who have pointed to the incompleteness of medical knowledge and the absence of an evidence base for practices such as electroconvulsive therapy (ECT) and the prescribing of selective serotonin reuptake inhibitor antidepressants when there is no system for measuring serotonin levels (Lynch 2008). Troubles in the HSE's rationalities also raise questions about the distinctiveness of new public sector managerialism vis-à-vis the original private sector variety, as even in the context of this participatory governance mechanism 'the public' and commitments to democracy were dissolved.

   Clearly this account raises yet again the question of whether 'to participate or not' for Irish health advocacy organizations. The significant response to the HSE's latest invitation to 'service users and community group representatives' to submit their details to a database of parties 'interested in participating in local or national events relating to the design, development and-or delivery of Irish health and social services', as reported by the Minister of State at the Department of Health and Children in July 2009 (Dáil Éireann 2009) suggests an enduring willingness to become involved in 'invited' participatory governance processes, even when such processes are forever changing and very troubled. But this should not be read as evidence that participating organizations have been enrolled into the HSE's governmental rationality. As one service user representative on an EAG explained, he used the governance space as a 'training ground' that afforded him opportunities to learn how clinicians think, especially those he identified as opponents of his movement's cause. Additionally, significant recent victories by the Irish psychiatric survivor movement in generating debate in parliamentary and media arenas about the coercive administration of ECT, and calling for recognition of the agency of the 'psychiatric patient', show that in Irish mental health politics the invited spaces of partnership governance are not 'the only game in town' (Murphy 2002). Perhaps most significantly, this recent battle has also been fought in popular spaces created and defined by citizens, such as Mad Pride Days (McCarthy 2010), where the abnormality of madness has been contested, and alternative criteria of validity of knowledge that would value the experiential knowledge of the mad have been mooted.

REFERENCES

Allen, K. (2000), *The Celtic Tiger: The Myth of Social Partnership in Ireland*, Manchester: Manchester University Press.
Allen, K. (2007), *The Corporate Takeover of Ireland*, Dublin: Irish Academic Press.
Allen, K. (2009), *Ireland's Economic Crash: A Radical Agenda for Change*, Dublin: Liffey Press.
Barrington, R. (1998), 'The future political, legislative and social framework of the health services', in A. Leahy and M. Wiley (eds), *The Irish Health System in the 21st Century*, Dublin: Oak Tree Press, pp. 83–101.
Burke, S. (2008), 'A house built on shaky ground', *The Irish Times*, 8 March.
Clarke, J. (2004), 'Dissolving the public realm? The logics and limits of neo-liberalism', *Journal of Social Policy*, **33** (1): 27–48.
Clarke, J. (2005), 'New Labour's citizens: activated, empowered, responsibilized, abandoned?', *Critical Social Policy*, **25** (4): 447–63.
Collins, H. and S. Yearly (1992), 'Epistemological chicken', in A. Pickering (ed.), *Science as Practice and Culture*, Chicago, IL: Chicago University Press, pp. 301–26.
Crawford, M., D. Rutter, C. Manley, T. Weaver, K. Bhui, N. Fulop and P. Tyrer (2002),

'Systematic review of involving patients in the planning and development of health-care', *British Medical Journal*, **325** (7375): 1263–5.

Crossley, N. (2006). 'The field of psychiatric contention in the UK, 1960–2000', *Social Science & Medicine*, **62** (3): 552–63.

Dáil Éireann (2007), vol. 630, 31 January.

Dáil Éireann (2008a), vol. 645, 31 January.

Dáil Éireann (2008b), vol. 653, 29 April.

Dáil Éireann (2008c), vol. 657, 24 June.

Dáil Éireann (2009), vol. 687, 8 July.

de Sousa Santos, B., J.A. Nunes and M.P. Meneses (2007), 'Introduction: opening up the canon of knowledge and recognition of difference', in B. de Sousa Santos (ed.), *Another Knowledge is Possible. Beyond Northern Epistemologies*, London: Verso, pp. xviii–lxii.

Donnellan, E. (2003), '"Not enough credit" given to health boards' work', *The Irish Times*, 18 June.

Donnellan, E. (2009), 'Drumm loses his dream team', *The Irish Times*, 10 November.

Dublin City University (2007), 'Thinking, Feeling, Being. Critical Perspectives and Creative Engagement in Psychosocial Health, 10–12 September 2007', conference programme, Dublin: Dublin City University.

Fudge, N., C. Wolfe and C. McKevitt (2008), 'Assessing the promise of user involvement in health service development: ethnographic study', *British Medical Journal*, doi: 10.1136/bmj.39456.552257.BE.

Gordon, C. (1991), 'Governmental rationality: an introduction', in G. Burchell, C. Gordon and P. Miller (eds), *The Foucault Effect. Studies in Governmentality*, London: Harvester Wheatsheaf, pp. 1–48.

Government of Ireland (2004), *Health Act 2004*, section 43.

Hardiman, O. (2007), 'Whose health service is it anyway?', address given to the McGill Summer School, Glenties, Co. Donegal, 18 July.

Health Services Executive (HSE) (2005), *Corporate Plan 2005–2008*, Naas, Ireland: Health Services Executive.

Health Services Executive, (2006), *Information Pack Re: Expert Advisory Groups*, Naas, Ireland: Health Services Executive.

Health Services Executive (2007), *Transformation Programme 2007–2010*, Naas, Ireland: Health Services Executive.

Health Services Executive (2008), *Corporate Plan 2008–2011*, Naas, Ireland: Health Services Executive.

Health Services Executive (2010), E-mail from the business manager, leadership, education and development, 12 February.

Health Services Executive and Department of Health and Children (2008), *National Strategy for Service User Involvement in the Irish Health Service 2008–2013*, Dublin: Department of Health and Children and the Health Services Executive.

Hunter, N. (2006a), 'Expert groups – where are the patients?', accessed 2 February at www.irishhealth.com/article.html?id=10468.

Hunter, N. (2006b), 'HSE defends expert group membership', accessed 2 February at www.irishhealth.com/article.html?id=10475.

Irish National Council of AD/HD Support Groups (INCADDS) (2003), *INCADDS Strategic Plan*, Galway, Ireland: The Irish National Council of AD/HD Support Groups.

Joint Committee on Health and Children (2006), vol. 85, 30 March.

Lynch, P. (2009), 'Whatever happened to the EAGs?', *Irish Medical News*, 28 July.

Lynch, T. (2008), 'The dominance of drug-based mental health care in Ireland: a personal account of a general practitioner turned psychotherapist', in O. O'Donovan and K. Glavanis-Grantham (eds), *Power, Politics and Pharmaceuticals*, Cork, Ireland: Cork University Press, pp. 135–50.

McCarthy, J. (2010), 'What a day', *Cork Independent*, 10 June.

McEvoy, R., C. Keenaghan and A. Murray (2008), *Service User Involvement in the Irish Health Service. A Review of the Evidence*, Dublin: Department of Health and Children and the Health Services Executive.

Meade, R. (2005), 'We hate it here, please let us stay! Irish social partnership and the community/voluntary sector's conflicted experiences of recognition', *Critical Social Policy*, **25** (3): 349–73.

Meade, R. and O. O'Donovan (2002), 'Editorial introduction. Corporatism and the ongoing debate about the relationship between the state and community development', *Community Development Journal*, **37** (1): 1–9.

Mulholland, P. (2008), 'Establishment of EAGs delayed', *Irish Medical News*, accessed 14 June 2010 at www.irishmedicalnews.ie/index.php/current-issue/news/392-establishment-of-eags-delayed.

Murphy, M. (2002), 'Social partnership – is it the 'only game in town?', *Community Development Journal*, **37** (1): 80–90.

Ó Cinnéide, S. (1999), 'Democracy and the Constitution', *Administration*, **46** (4): 41–58.

O'Connor, M. (2007), *Emergency. Irish Hospitals in Crisis*, Dublin: Gill & Macmillan.

O'Donovan, O. (2007), 'Corporate colonization of health activism? Irish health advocacy organizations' modes of engagement with pharmaceutical corporations', *International Journal of Health Services*, **37** (4): 711–33.

O'Donovan, O. and D. Casey (1995), 'Converting patients into consumers: consumerism and the Charter Rights for Hospital Patients', *Irish Journal of Sociology*, **5**: 43–66.

Prior, L. (2003), 'Belief, knowledge and expertise: the emergence of the lay expert in medical sociology', *Sociology of Health & Illness*, **25**: 41–57.

Rose, N. and P. Miller (1992), 'Political power beyond the state: problematics of government', *British Journal of Sociology*, **43** (2): 173–205.

Seanad Éireann (2006), vol. 183, no. 7, 5 Apri.

Taylor, D. and M. Bury (2007), 'Chronic illness, expert patients and care transition', *Sociology of Health & Illness*, **29** (1): 27–45.

Taylor, M. (2007), 'Community participation in the real world: opportunities and pitfalls in new governance spaces', *Urban Studies*, **44** (2), 297–317.

Tierney, N. (2007), *The Irish Times*, 7 December.

8. Patient empowerment in the Netherlands

Atie Schipaanboord, Diana Delnoij and Roland Bal

INTRODUCTION

Regulated competition was introduced into the Dutch health care system in 2006. Although this was regarded as a radical break with the past, some elements of the reform, such as competition between social health insurers, had been implemented from the 1990s onwards (Helderman et al. 2005). What was new was the introduction of an obligatory basic package of health insurance for all citizens, with health insurers obliged to accept all enrolees and compensated for 'bad risks' through a risk equalization fund and introduction of competition between health care providers over price and quality.[1] Increased transparency of costs and quality were also part of the shift, with the introduction of a diagnosis-related group system for financing health care and the publication of performance indicators measuring quality.

As a result of these changes, government involvement in the health care sector was minimized and replaced by additional audit procedures. The 'triangle' of insurers, providers and patients became the main regulating and coordinating mechanism in three interdependent markets, namely the health insurance market, in which health care users have a free choice of health plans and insurance companies; the provider market, where health care users can choose between providers, such as hospitals, nursing homes, and family practices; and the health care purchasing market, where health insurance companies contract health care providers (see Figure 8.1).

Voice and Choice in Health Care

As patients have traditionally been a weak force in the health care sector much effort has been put into empowering them, both individually and collectively. Since the mid-1990s legal measures to strengthen patients at the micro, meso and macro levels have been introduced and continue to expand. Increasing the transparency of the health care sector is also aimed at empowering patients.

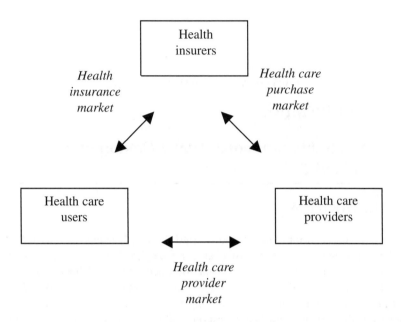

Figure 8.1   Markets in the Dutch health care system

Arguments put forward in favour of patient empowerment see patient involvement as a 'counterbalancing power' or as upholding traditional democratic ideals, as well as helping to improve the quality of care. Health is clearly a public good of concern to us all. Deliberations on the functioning of health care are regarded as a normal part of democracy and – together with the input of the state, health care organizations, professionals and insurers – patients and patient organizations have come to be recognized as legitimate voices in the process. Patients' experiential knowledge is increasingly seen as a crucial factor in the advancement of quality care. Patients not only know what it is to live with a specific disease; they also have extensive experience of health care organizations and specific treatments. Patient participation and feedback is therefore sought after in almost all aspects of health care: in setting national policies (van der Kraan 2006); in decisions about the basic insurance package (Bal and van de Lindeloof 2006); in scientific research and advice (Bal et al. 2004; Epstein 2008); in guideline development (Moreira 2005; van de Bovenkamp and Trappenburg 2009); in quality improvement (Bate and Robert 2007); and, not least, in the consulting room itself.[2]

In the context of health care reforms occurring across the industrialized world, arguments for increased patient 'voice' are accompanied by pleas for 'choice' (Le Grand 2007). Working from the opposition between 'voice' and 'exit' (the right to opt out and choose a different provider) as introduced by Hirschman (Hirschman 1970), authors like Le Grand have argued that only if there are channels for 'exit' are service providers made aware it is in *their* interest to listen to clients.[3] Patient choice induces competition between providers and between insurers who have to 'win' clients by offering high-quality services at the best price. Choice is thus thought to advance both the quality and cost containment of health care. For exit to function in this context a number of assumptions must hold true. Alternatives must be available, together with information about the relative quality of these options, and consumers must actually be able to exercise choice.[4] Theoretical assumptions about how choice impacts on achieving policy objectives in health care depend on how choice is exercised, including the way choice is mediated by social and technical agents (Dixon et al. 2010). Of course whether choice has an impact is an empirical question, one that will be addressed below.

Efforts to increase choice have been accompanied by pleas for a more transparent system. Performance indicators are a key instrument in this regard. Following countries like the United Kingdom, in 2003 the Healthcare Inspectorate of the Netherlands published a 'basic set' of performance indicators (Berg et al. 2005). The Inspectorate's major goal was priority-setting, but since then furthering patient choice has become part of the discourse around performance indicators.[5] However, given the different goals attached to performance indicators the question remains whether they can indeed be used to enhance patient choice. The question is, what kind of transparency is being created in health care and for whom? Patient voice seems crucial in ensuring that choice is exercised, for example by developing relevant indicators for patients. In the Netherlands patient and consumer organizations have therefore become involved in developing indicators, sometimes putting forward their own indicator sets.

A Collective Voice?

In a way, one could argue that *the* patient movement does not exist, either in the Netherlands or elsewhere. Or, to put it differently, organizing patients into one collective voice should be seen as an achievement rather than a given. There are at least three reasons for this. First, patient organizations have traditionally been formed around specific diseases for the purpose of sharing experiences, organizing contact with professionals and scientists, and drawing attention to policy issues. As a result they have competed for scarce resources (funding, research and so on). Second, subsequent generations of patient organizations have adopted different ways of expressing patient voice, particularly in relation to research and policy. Whereas traditional patient organizations have generally followed scientific agendas as set by experts, newer organizations have set their own research agendas, some even placing themselves outside the world of experts (Barbot 2006). This trend is an expression of the further politicization of the body, resulting in patient organizations embracing kinds of expertise different from those offered by the traditional biomedical model. Similarly, patient organizations use different strategies in relation to governmental policies, sometimes perceiving the state as a means of furthering patients' interests, but at times seeking policy alternatives outside the state. Third, since the introduction of market mechanisms, being a patient is no longer the only mobilizing factor; consumer organizations are now more active and pursue strategies less connected to the medical world of doctors, operating on the basis of something more like a 'business' model. As a result of the above, in most countries the patient movement is rather fragmented. What are the driving forces behind attempts to create a single patient voice and what issues are they focused on? What are the pros and cons of a fragmented patient movement?

Patients and the organizations representing them are increasingly asked to participate in policymaking, guideline development, research funding and more, requiring them to have professional expertise, to the extent that the term 'professional patient' has been coined. Not all patient organizations are able to professionalize to the same degree, which means that some are less able to make their voices heard (van de Bovenkamp et al. 2010). Moreover, professionalization of patient organizations limits their ability to voice experiential knowledge, which is a core factor legitimizing patient participation. Whether and in what way patient organizations individually and collectively are able to deal with this dilemma is an issue gaining in importance.

In this chapter we analyse and evaluate the changing position of Dutch patients, focusing initially on *voice* and the role of patient organizations and subsequently on *choice* in relation to individual patients or their representatives. Several key questions guide our analysis. Can patients actually function as a 'third partner' vis-à-vis providers/professionals and insurers in the health care system? What legal tools, support systems and resources are provided for choice and voice? How are patients being represented? Are patients well enough organized to protect their own interests against those of suppliers and insurers in a market-oriented environment? Are patients willing and able to make choices and is consumer choice effective in a climate where mergers frequently occur? How is patient empowerment translated into voice and choice options? What prevents patients being involved and what changes could make them more active in the system? Can patients make a difference and how could they become a counterbalancing power?

PATIENT PARTICIPATION: THE ORGANIZED VOICE

Over 400 patient organizations exist in the Netherlands. For each disease there is some way for patients to find information and other people with whom to share their experiences. Patient organizations provide patients with information, answer their questions and facilitate opportunities for individuals to meet others in the same situation. In the case of rare diseases they know where specialist doctors work and have regular contact with them. Some organizations also work on public interest issues by influencing government and health supplier policies.

But patient organizations vary greatly in their scope, financing and activities, with some run mainly by volunteers while others are large and serviced by a professional staff. In a society where people are more educated and financially better off, citizens behave more assertively to achieve equal opportunities in relation to their rights. Patients want to be treated equally and receive better services, and patient organizations campaign to achieve these outcomes. New possibilities for patient empowerment exist because changes in the health care system have put the position of patients increasingly to the fore.

Activities of Patient Organizations

Most patient organizations are associations representing people who have a specific disease (for example diabetes, Parkinson's, epilepsy) while others are foundations, for example for people with lung cancer. Regardless of their legal structure they organize meetings, establish local working groups and usually rely on a large number of volunteers to carry out their various functions. Patient organizations also participate in research funding; devise clinical guidelines and standards; and help develop patient-oriented health indicators.

Patient groups cooperate in alliances or in federated structures, for example, the Dutch Federation of Cancer Patient Organizations, uniting all kinds of cancer groups, the Group for Heart and Artery Diseases, the Union for Rheumatic Diseases and the Dutch Association for Muscle Diseases. Nationally, there are umbrella organizations, such as the National Patient and Consumer Federation (NPCF), the Council for Chronically Ill and Disabled People, the Coordinating Group for the Elderly, the Platform for Psychiatric Diseases and the Platform for Parents of Disabled Children. Umbrella organizations provide support activities and consolidate the strength of their member groups around common problems. Alliances across organizations are especially important for campaigning around common problems, for example, the NPCF's successful campaign for a new law on patient rights.

Patient organizations are funded through membership fees and receive grants from charities and government. Sometimes they also receive money from the pharmaceutical industry, but this is heavily criticized because of possible conflicts of interest and loss of independence.

Patient organizations function at all levels of the health care system, from patient involvement in the client councils of health care organizations to patient organizations working at local, regional and national levels (see Figure 8.2).

At the *national* level, alliances and national federations organize campaigns, monitor policy implications and are involved in policymaking and lobbying legislators. They also carry out support activities for the movement as a whole. The Dutch government has been supportive of their role, making an annual budgetary allocation of 32 million euros (about 2 per capita annually) for patient organizations. When health care reform was introduced in 2006, the government provided 10 million euros to help patient organizations adjust to their new roles.

At the *regional* level, so-called *Zorgbelang* (literally meaning 'interest in care') organizations have direct contact with regional and local hospitals, long-term care institutions like nursing homes, and primary care centres. Their activities also include handling complaints and providing information. Regional patient organizations are funded by provincial governments.

At the *local provider* level, hospitals and institutions for disabled people, nursing homes and homes for the elderly each have a statutory client council to advise their boards of directors. The councils form part of the internal governance structure of health care organizations and comprise volunteers who usually serve four-year terms. Their influence and performance vary greatly, depending on the scope of their operations and the professionalism and expertise of their members (van der Kraan et al. 2008).

A Changing Health Care System

Changes in the health care system have meant that the role of patient organizations has also had to change (Grit et al. 2008). But are they equipped to take up their new role? Currently the interests of suppliers and health insurance companies tend to dominate, and patients are not in a position to know whether or not they are receiving value for money. They lack proper information to make informed choices and cannot influence the purchasing policies of health insurance companies, many of which exercise control rather than allowing people to make their own decisions.

Also, patients' needs are changing, with more people suffering from one or more chronic illnesses (co-morbidity and multi-morbidity) and needing greater support to properly manage their health. In order to continue working and living as normal a life as possible they need to have more control over and be involved in decisions regarding their treatment, lifestyle adjustment and

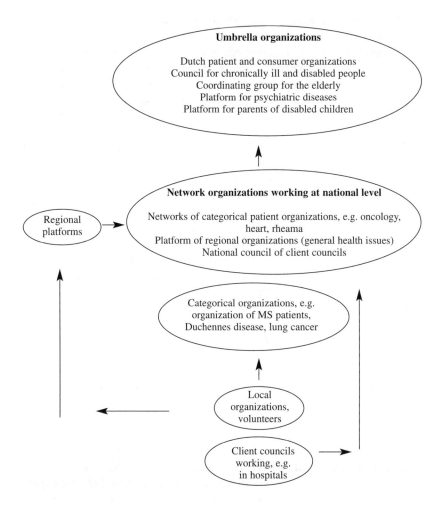

Figure 8.2   Patient organizations in the Netherlands

medication. Although patient organizations are valued for the information they provide and their promotion of patients' interests, their membership is far from representative of those suffering from chronic illnesses.

Although the internet is an important instrument for patient empowerment it also partly undermines the traditional position of patient organizations because it provides patients with new ways of searching for information and meeting others through electronic communities, weblogs, Twitter and so on. Patients increasingly want individualized support tailored to fit their specific situation. The internet enables patients to search for relevant expertise world-wide and to organize themselves in new ways, for example for peer support via internet fora. Although little research has been done on the role of internet fora in relation to how patients organize or relate to policy and expertise, there is some evidence that the internet is becoming a means of developing new political agendas (Akrich et al. 2009). It can also, however, reinforce the traditional lay–expert divide, which is the case with most patient portals set up to 'prevent health illiteracy' (Adams and Bal 2009).

Stakeholders value the work of patient organizations (Berk et al. 2008). There is a need to embed the patient perspective in health protocols, quality and safety policies, and government policies generally. Policymakers need patient organizations to legitimize their policies and as a source of experiential knowledge. There are now many examples of their influence. For example:

- The breast cancer foundation and prostate cancer organizations have negotiated with health insurance companies to include patient-oriented quality criteria in their purchasing policy.
- The diabetes association offers diabetes products through a membership benefit programme.
- Patient organizations for people with rheumatoid diseases have actively participated in a project of the Utrecht Academic Medical Centre to design a portal where patients can not only find but also add information about the disease. The portal offers discussions on sport, sex, study and work; videos; and the opportunity to read one's health records and lab results and request e-consultations.

But many patient organizations find it difficult to keep up with the demands for participation imposed on them. Organizations meeting these demands have become increasingly professionalized, which distances them from the experiential 'patient perspective' (van de Bovenkamp et al. 2010). If this patient perspective lies in the unique expertise that patients have from 'living a disease', including treatment and the ways they organize their own patient-hood in relation to other social roles (school, work, family, and so on), then one might wonder whether participating at all levels of health care is always necessary.

PATIENT EMPOWERMENT AND CHOICE

Patient choice is an important element of the health care reforms. However, patient choice is not in itself a new feature of the system. As Dixon et al.

(2010) point out, patients have always been free to choose a hospital after referral, although choice was not on the policy agenda and was not actively supported. This changed in the 1990s when the individual's choice of hospital was promoted as a way to reduce growing waiting times for hospital care. Today patient choice is higher on the political agenda.

Patient choice contributes to a more demand-driven system, and accordingly greater emphasis is being placed on transparency and providing information to patients. The Medical Treatment Act requires providers to inform patients about alternative treatment options and their respective side effects, while under the Healthcare Market Regulation Act providers are obliged to inform the public, among other things, about price and quality of services to promote transparency in the system.

Public Reporting and Patient Choice

Patients/consumers are encouraged to exercise choice in both the provider and health insurance markets. For regulated competition to work, consumers and their representatives need comparable information about providers' performance (Williamson 2008). The Netherlands is not unique in this respect. Public reporting about health care performance is important in other countries too, notably in the United States and the United Kingdom, where it was introduced in the late 1980s (Marshall et al. 2000).

It is now common in many countries for comparative information about services to be made public, for instance information about waiting times, products and quality, as well as some general background about providers (Lugtenberg and Westert 2007). Quality can be measured by different indicators and from different perspectives, for example from the professional's perspective and from the service user's. Therefore comparative information is usually drawn from a variety of data sources, including clinical and administrative records and surveys of patients' care experiences (Zaslavsky 2001; Brien et al. 2009; Delnoij 2009).

Although publication of comparative information for consumers is vital to the functioning of the market, the Ministry of Health, Welfare and Sports has delegated decision-making on health care to the main actors. However the Ministry did initiate the website www.kiesBeter.nl ('choose better') through the National Institute of Public Health and the Environment. This site aims to provide both health information (disease description and treatment options) and comparative service information (location, opening hours and so on), as well as information about product quality.

Other sites have been developed by the commercial sector (www.independer.nl) and not-for-profit organizations (www.consumentendezorg.nl), the latter being an initiative of the NPCF providing comparative information

about cataract surgery and total hip and knee replacements. On
www.kiesBeter.nl there is comparative information about health plans, nursing
homes, home care and care for the disabled. The Dutch Consumer Association
(the Consumentenbond) presents comparative information for its members
about health plans on www.consumentenbond.nl. Several health insurance
companies also publish comparative health care information on their websites.

Defining Quality of Care

Steering committees made up of national representatives of patient/consumer
organizations, health care providers and health insurers negotiate and implement national indicator sets for each health sector and decide on their publication. Indicators include effectiveness and safety (in the Dutch context these
are called 'professional indicators') and patient experiences of the quality of
services, such as access, timeliness, information, communication, respectful
treatment and so on.

Steering committees define quality of care for the disabled, long-term nursing (nursing homes, homes for the elderly, home care), mental health, hospital
care, general practice, physiotherapy and pharmaceutical care. They can
commission and use research to develop indicators and surveys; decide what
indicators are to be measured, which measuring instruments are to be used and
the frequency of measurement; and also decide which indicators are to be
made public.

Use of Comparative Health Care Information

International research has provided mixed results concerning patients' interest
in and use of comparative information. When asked about their preferences,
patients/consumers generally say they want free choice in health care and that
they are interested in comparative quality information (Edgman-Levitan and
Cleary 1996; Robinson and Brodie 1997; van Rijen 2003; Nelson et al. 2005;
O'Meara et al. 2005). In the United States this kind of information has been
published for nearly two decades, but it is not widely used by consumers
(Schneider and Epstein 1998; Marshall et al. 2000; Fung et al. 2008; Castle
2009). A review conducted by Faber et al. (2008) found that when individuals
were choosing a new health care plan, fewer than 5 per cent said that quality
information had influenced their choice of provider. However, having seen
quality information was a strong determinant for choosing higher-quality-
rated health plans (Faber et al. 2008).

In the Netherlands little empirical research has been conducted into the
actual use of websites or the degree to which patients base their choices on
comparative information. The degree to which people exercise choice in the

insurance market is monitored by the Dutch Consumer Panel in Health Care. In 2009, overall only 3 per cent of the population switched to another health plan, while 8 per cent of people aged under 40 switched (Vos and de Jong 2009). To what extent 'switchers' based their choice on comparative information about a health plan performance (available on www.kiesBeter.nl) is unclear. This site is accessed by more than 10 000 people daily and in December 2008, 19 per cent of the population were familiar with the name 'kiesBeter' (Colijn and van der Graaf 2008). The usability of the website is regularly investigated but it remains unclear as to how visitors use the information provided.

CONCLUSION

In Western societies people are encouraged to choose healthy lifestyles and when they fall ill they are expected to act as rational consumers who search for information about their disease, question their doctors about expected benefits and possible side effects of treatment, compare the performance of health care providers, and find the doctor or hospital that best suits their needs. Market mechanisms have been introduced into a system that was built on trust: societal trust in professionals as a group and interpersonal trust in the provider–patient relationship. This shift reflects a libertarian view of society, with a strong emphasis on individual responsibility, autonomy and self-determination (Maarse and ter Meulen 2006; Pratt et al. 2006). We agree with Milewa (this volume) that today there is more emphasis on the 'governmentality' (Foucault 1991) of patients through which they are made into self-managing subjects responsible for their own health care: responsible both for the various aspects of their illnesses and their own integration into society. In this discourse the traditional Parsonian patient (Parsons 1975), dependent on their environment – on the expertise of health professionals and the support of government structures – no longer exists. Instead patients have become agents of their own health care. In this chapter we have critically engaged with this view in relation to patient voice, patient choice and the role of patient organizations.

According to the findings reported in the review by Faber et al. (2008), expectations should be modest about patient choice based on comparative information. Apart from using websites to facilitate patient choice, other direct forms of stimulating choice should be investigated. The possibility of stimulating choice through 'surrogate consumers', such as health insurers, or referring general practitioners (GPs), should be explored. In the Dutch system GPs have always functioned as gatekeepers to specialist and hospital care and are therefore in an excellent position to advise their patients. They have engaged in mediating activities, for example providing documentation to support patients' choices at the point of referral (Dixon et al. 2010). Currently an experiment is taking place where comparative information about hospital performance is being made available to GPs for use in consultations with patients being referred to a hospital. The role of health insurers as advisers guiding their customers through the system is not new either. Since the mid-1990s health insurers have established 'waiting time mediation' services. In 2000 some 6000 patients accessed this service and between 70 and 80 per cent were directed to health organizations with shorter waiting times (Knippers et al. 2001).

Obviously professionals find it difficult to cope with consumerism and a demanding society forcing them to disclose information about quality. Governments too struggle to determine what their role should be in empowering patients and protecting the public from misleading information. Patient and consumer organizations also have difficulty keeping abreast of new developments to help their members find relevant information to assist them in finding caregivers.

Internationally the Netherlands is seen as a leader with regard to its well-organized system of patient organizations. Although they are funded by government and are part of policy negotiating fora there are so many organizations that it is often difficult for them to cooperate or to centralize their activities. In general, patient organizations are small-scale and are not highly professionalized. Their activities fail to achieve the necessary scale and level of expertise to make them serious players alongside providers and insurers or for them to be a real counterbalancing power in the health care system. As a result they run the risk of legitimizing other parties' agendas instead of proactively setting their own.

Whether participation per se is a good thing is debatable. One can argue that the only way to gauge the success of participation is the extent to which the patient voice is heard. Much of this 'the more the better' kind of discourse is based on Arnstein's 'ladder of participation' (Arnstein 1969). While it furthered the participatory agenda it was put forward at a time when participation was the exception rather than the rule. In recent years this approach has been criticized for neglecting the complex issues involved in effective participation and for assuming a 'zero sum game' regarding the division of power between patients, professionals and health care organizations (Tritter 2009). It also neglects the negative impacts participation can have on patient movements – which indicates that more is not always better (Trappenburg 2008). This is not an argument against participation but rather a call for finding new ways to further the participatory agenda. Defining new choice mechanisms in which the patient perspective is fully embedded could be one way. Using ethnographic techniques for expressing the patient perspective could be another.

Given the range and diversity of patient and consumer organizations, most people can find a body to identify with, but diversity also results in significant disadvantages, namely lack of cohesion and competition. Patient organizations rarely articulate a united point of view, thus inhibiting their capacity to act as a counterbalancing power. Major challenges require new and innovative approaches. If patients are asked to exercise more influence in a demand-oriented system then they have to manoeuvre themselves into a position to fulfil that promise. This requires a strong, coherent patient movement that is able to centralize patients' experiences and use them to set the policy agenda for evaluating services and advocacy, but for this to occur long-term structural funding programmes are required.

Patient organizations are the experts in the domain of customers' or patients' needs in the health market and without them the health care system would not be demand-oriented. They should capitalize on their knowledge and exercise their potential influence by supporting patients in making choices and by guiding people towards the right doctor and hospital. Rather than seeing them as opposites (Tritter 2009), *choice* can then become an important factor in strengthening *voice*.

NOTES

1. Regulated competition has also introduced new terminology, so health care organizations are 'providers of care' and patients are 'consumers'. We will use these terms interchangeably.
2. Doubtless instrumental reasons are important as well: 'playing the patient card' is an important legitimizing strategy in discussions on health care (Harrison and Mort 1998).
3. Interestingly, Hirschman's third concept (loyalty) has barely been explored in these debates, despite the dependent position in which many patients find themselves. See Benschop et al. (2003) for their discussion of loyalty in relation to patient participation in the development and use of genetics in health care.
4. Although economists say that the actual number of people who exit need not be high and high exit would even be detrimental to the functioning of the system, the mere possibility of exit and the use of this route by a limited number of clients would be sufficient.
5. This 'logic of escalation' is evident in other indicator systems (Pollitt et al. 2010) and has huge consequences for the governance of health care in a broader sense.

REFERENCES

Adams, S. and R. Bal (2009), 'Practicing reliability: reconstructing traditional boundaries in the gray areas of health information review on the web', *Science, Technology & Human Values*, **34** (1): 34–54.
Akrich, M., C. Meadel and V. Rabeharisoa (2009), *Se mobiliser pour la santé*, Paris: Presses de l'Ecole des Mines.
Arnstein, S.R. (1969), 'A ladder of citizen participation', *Journal of the American Institute of Planners*, **35** (4): 216–23.

Bal, R., W.E. Bijker and R. Hendriks (2004), 'Democratisation of scientific advice', *British Medical Journal*, **329** (7478): 1339–441.

Bal, R. and A. van de Lindeloof (2006), 'Publieksparticipatie bij pakketbeslissingen. Leren van buitenlandse ervaringen', in Raad voor de Volksgezondheid en Zorg (ed.), *Zicht op zinnige en duurzame zorg*, Zoetermeer, Netherlands: RVZ.

Barbot, J. (2006), 'How to build an "active" patient? The work of AIDS associations in France', *Social Science & Medicine*, **62** (3): 538–51.

Bate, P. and G. Robert (2007), *Experience-Based Design: From Redesigning the System around the Patient to Co-designing Services with the Patient*, Abingdon: Radcliffe Publishing.

Benschop, R., K. Horstman, and R. Vos (2003), 'Voice beyond choice: hesitant voice in public debates about genetics in health care', *Health Care Analysis*, **11** (2): 141–50.

Berg, M., Y. Meijerink, M. Gras, A. Goossensen, W. Schellekens, J. Haeck, M. Kallewaard and H. Kingma (2005), 'Feasibility first: developing public performance indicators on patient safety and clinical effectiveness for Dutch hospitals', *Health Policy*, **75** (1): 59–73.

Berk, M., H. van der Steeg and G. Schrijvers (2008), *Stille Kennis. Patienten-en gehandicaptenorganisaties: waardevolle bronnen van informatie*, Utrecht, Netherlands: Universiteit van Utrecht.

Brien, S.E., E. Dixon and W.A. Ghali (2009), 'Measuring and reporting on quality in health care: a framework and road map for improving care', *Journal of Surgical Oncology*, **99** (8): 462–6.

Castle, N.G. (2009), 'The nursing home compare report card: consumers' use and understanding', *Journal of Aging and Social Policy*, **21** (2): 187–208.

Colijn, J.J. and M.L. van der Graaf (2008), *Gebruik en waardering van kiesBeter.nl in 2008*, Bilthoven, Netherlands: RIVM.

Delnoij, D. (2009), *Zicht op kwaliteit. Transparantie in de zorg vanuit patientenperspectief*, Tilburg, Netherlands: Tranzo, Universiteit van Tilburg.

Dixon, A., R. Robertson and R. Bal (2010), 'The experience of implementing choice at point of referral: a comparison of the Netherlands and England', *Health Economics, Policy and Law*, **5** (3): 295–317.

Edgman-Levitan, S. and P.D. Cleary (1996), 'What information do consumers want and need?', *Health Affairs*, **14** (4): 42–56.

Epstein, S. (2008), 'Patient groups and health movements', in E. J. Hackett, O. Amsterdamska, M. Lynch and J. Wajcman (eds), *The Handbook of Science and Technology Studies*, 3rd edn, Cambridge, MA: MIT Press, pp. 499–539.

Faber, M., M. Bosch, H. Wollersheim, S. Leatherman and R. Grol (2008), 'Public reporting in health care: how do consumers use quality-of-care information?' *Medical Care*, **47** (1): 1–8.

Foucault, M. (1991), 'Governmentality', in G. Burchell, C. Gordon and P. Miller (eds), *The Foucault Effect: Studies in Governmentality*, London: Harvester Wheatsheaf, pp. 87–104.

Fung, C.H., Y-W. Lim, S. Mattke, C. Damberg and P.G. Shelleke (2008), 'Systematic review: the evidence that publishing patient care performance data improves quality of care', *Annals of Internal Medicine*, **148** (2): 111–23.

Grit, K., H. van den Bovenkamp and R. Bal (2008), *Positie van zorggebruiker in veranderend stelsel. Een quick scan van aandachtspunten en wetenschappelijke inzichten*, Rotterdam, Netherlands: iBMG, Erasmus Universiteit Rotterdam.

Harrison, S. and M. Mort (1998), 'Which champions, which people? Public and user involvement in health care as a technology of legitimation', *Social Policy & Administration*, **32** (1): 60–70.

Helderman, J-K., F.T. Schut, T.E.D. van der Grinten and W.P.M.M. van de Ven (2005), 'Market-oriented health care reforms and policy learning in the Netherlands', *Journal of Health Politics, Policy and Law*, **30** (1–2): 189–210.

Hirschman, A.O. (1970), *Exit, Voice, and Loyalty. Responses to Decline in Firms, Organizations, and States*, Cambridge, MA and London: Harvard University Press.

Knippers, E.W.A., E.J. Breedveld, M.G. Andela and S. Lambeck (2001), *Wachtlijstbemiddeling in de curatieve zorg. Het aanbod in beeld; eindrapport*, the Hague: ZonMw.

Le Grand, J. (2007), *The Other Invisible Hand. Delivering Public Services through Choice and Competition*, Princeton, NJ and Oxford: Princeton University Press.

Lugtenberg, M. and G.P. Westert (2007), *Kwaliteit van de gezondheidszorg en keuze-informatie voor burgers*, Tilburg, Netherlands: Tranzo.

Maarse, H. and R. ter Meulen (2006), 'Consumer choice in Dutch health insurance after reform', *Health Care Analysis*, **14** (1): 37–49.

Marshall, M.N., P.G. Schekelle, S. Leatherman and R.H. Brook (2000), 'The public release of performance data: what do we expect to gain? A review of the literature', *Journal of the American Medical Association*, **283** (14): 1866–74.

Moreira, T. (2005), 'Diversity in clinical guidelines: the role of repertoires of evaluation', *Social Science & Medicine*, **60** (9): 1975–85.

Nelson, E.C., K. Homa, M.P. Mastanduno, E.S. Fisher, P.B. Batalden, E.F. Malcolm, T.C. Foster, D.S. Likosky, J.A. Guth and P.B. Gardent (2005), 'Publicly reporting comprehensive quality and cost data: a health care system's transparency initiative', *Joint Commission Journal on Quality and Patient Safety*, **31** (10): 573–84.

O'Meara, J., M. Kitchener, E. Collier, M. Lyons, A. De Billwiller-Kiss, L.P. Simon, and C. Harrington. 2005. 'Case study: development of and stakeholder responses to a nursing home consumer information system', *American Journal of Medical Quality*, **20** (1): 40–50.

Parsons, T. (1975), 'The sick role and the role of the physician reconsidered', *The Milbank Memorial Fund Quarterly*, **53** (3): 257–78.

Pollitt, C., S. Harrison, G. Dowswell, S. Jerak-Zuiderent and R. Bal (2010), 'Performance regimes in health care: institutions, critical junctures and the logic of escalation in England and the Netherlands', *Evaluation*, **16** (1): 13–29.

Pratt, W., K. Unruh, A. Civan, and M. Skeels (2006), 'Personal health information management', *Communications of the ACM*, **49** (1): 51–5.

Robinson, S. and M. Brodie (1997), 'Understanding the quality challenge for health consumers: the Kaiser/AHCPR Survey', *Joint Commission Journal on Quality Improvement*, **23** (5): 239–44.

Schneider, E.C. and A.M. Epstein (1998), 'Use of public performance reports. A survey of patients undergoing cardiac surgery', *Journal of the American Medical Association*, **279** (20): 1638–42.

Trappenburg, M. (2008), *Genoeg is genoeg. Over gezondheidszorg en democratie*, Amsterdam, Netherlands: Amsterdam University Press.

Tritter, J.Q. (2009), 'Revolution or evolution: the challenges of conceptualizing patient and public involvement in a consumerist world', *Health Expectations*, **12** (3): 275–87.

van de Bovenkamp, H.M. and M.J. Trappenburg (2009), 'Reconsidering patient participation in guideline development', *Health Care Analysis*, **17** (3): 198–216.

van de Bovenkamp, H.M., M.J. Trappenburg and K. Grit (2010), 'Patient participation in collective healthcare decision making: the Dutch model', *Health Expectations*, **13** (1): 7–85.

van der Kraan, W.G.M. (2006), *Vraag naar vraagsturing. Een verkennend onderzoek naar de betekenis van vraagsturing in de Nederlandse gezondheidszorg*, Rotterdam, Netherlands: iBMG, Erasmus Universiteit Rotterdam.

van der Kraan, W.G.M., P. Meurs and S. Adams (2008), *Effectieve medezeggenschap. Een verkennend onderzoek naar effectieve vormgeving van medezeggenschap van clienten in algemene ziekenhuizen*, Rotterdam, Netherlands: iBMG, Erasmus Universiteit Rotterdam.

van Rijen, A.J.G. (2003), *Internetgebruiker en kiezen van zorg* [*Internet users and demand-driven care*], Zoetermeer, Netherlands: Raad voor de Volksgezondheid en Zorg.

Vos, L. and J. de Jong (2009), *Percentage overstappers van zorgverzekeraar 3%. Ouderen wisselen nauwelijks van zorgverzekeraars*, Utrecht, Netherlands: Nivel.

Williamson, C. (2008), 'The patient movement as an emancipation movement', *Health Expectations*, **11** (2): 102–12.

Zaslavsky, A.M. (2001), 'Statistical issues in reporting quality data: small samples and casemix variation', *International Journal for Quality in Health Care*, **13** (6): 481–8.

9. Health policy in Germany: consumer groups in a corporatist polity

Jens Geissler

The making of German health policy is characterized by a corporatist 'division of labour' between, on the one hand, parliament, government and the Ministry of Health and, on the other, numerous self-governing bodies (especially insurance funds and doctors' associations) to which considerable responsibilities have been delegated.

In this arena there is no individual organization that can claim to speak for 'the patient'. However there is a highly differentiated scene of patient organizations, with a large number of organizations targeting different groups, especially the chronically ill. These organizations have developed structures adjusted to the complexity of the German health care system with its large number of decision-making bodies.

Patient organizations act as advocacy organizations when interacting with the political sphere. Umbrella organizations and senior citizens' organizations are especially involved in debates about the general structure of the health care system and its funding arrangements. The patterns of interaction have long remained essentially unchanged. However patient organizations have recently been given a larger role in the self-governing bodies of the health insurance system. In particular, in 2004, health consumer groups were granted observer status on the Federal Joint Committee (Gemeinsamer Bundesausschuss) which makes final decisions about health insurance benefits.

Since 2000 health insurance funds have been required to spend 0.56 per year per insuree to support patient organizations. After initial difficulties and a simplification of funding procedures, insurance funds are starting to reach this amount, which supports patient organizations' self-help, information and lobbying activities. Organizations applying for funding have to fulfil certain formal criteria and confirm their independence from industry interests. Generally the transparency of funding for patient organizations in Germany has improved, but balance sheets detailing income and expenditure are, in the main, still not published.

In the first section of this chapter I explain the political significance of insurance funds being self-governing. In the second I provide a brief overview of the German health care system, especially social health insurance, which covers about 90 per cent of the population. The mechanics of German policy-making and self-governance of health insurance funds are then outlined. An overview of patient organizations introduces those organizations that can legitimately claim to represent the interests of patients and health care users. Some speak for specific groups of chronically ill people, others are umbrella organizations or speak for large sections of the general population, like senior citizens or consumers. The funding mechanisms of these organizations are then analysed. In the final section I elaborate on patient organizations' political influence on health policy and on health insurance self-governance.

THE POLITICAL DIMENSION OF SELF-GOVERNANCE[1]

In a context of neo-pluralism, interest groups voice their concerns but elected politicians make the final decisions. Under neo-corporatism, interest groups find a consensus which is then implemented by the decision-makers. This reduces the autonomy of the political sphere, but formally the government still has the final say. What happens though when competencies are fully delegated to autonomous bodies? This is the case in the German social security and health insurance system where far-reaching administrative responsibilities have been delegated to health insurance funds. One could say that these responsibilities are only of an administrative nature and thus not of political interest or relevance. I would argue however that in times of increasing financial pressure on the health insurance system these powers are no longer merely administrative but also political.

The first reason for this system being self-governed is historical. The roots of Germany's health insurance system lie first in the cooperative or guild insurance schemes that covered basic risks like death (funeral expenses) and illness, and second in company-based schemes for workers. Schemes of both kinds are much older than Bismarck's social security legislation of the 1880s, and neither type was a government initiative (Tennstedt 1981). Bismarck's reforms provided a legal framework for these and all new funds, but allowed their independence from direct government interference. Since then, the health insurance funds have been self-governing bodies carrying out legally mandated tasks under government supervision but otherwise organizationally and financially independent.

The second reason for this system of self-governance is what I call its 'depoliticization'. The medical system was taken out of the political sphere and handed over to specialists who had to tackle the numerous day-to-day technical questions of running a highly complex system. This delegation of competencies to self-governing health insurance bodies and health care providers worked well as long as these decisions were indeed administrative and *not* political in character. I argue that this has changed over recent decades, with increasing financial pressure on the health care system. In the context of increasing scarcity of resources, decisions about health insurance benefits are not merely administrative but also political, and thus require political legitimacy. With health insurers and providers making decisions without political scrutiny, political legitimacy appears to be lacking. One solution would have been to restore power to the political decision-makers. But this would have forced government to make difficult, detailed and contentious choices about the allocation of resources. Consequently, an alternative was adopted that sought to restore political legitimacy to policy decisions by giving health care users a stronger voice in decision-making (see also Etgeton 2009). This chapter will show how and to what extent health care user representatives are now included in decisions and how the financing of patient groups has been changed to reflect their new role.

THE GERMAN HEALTH CARE SYSTEM

Insurance Coverage and Benefit Package

About 90 per cent of the German population[2] is covered by mandatory social health insurance, which provides a comprehensive benefit package (preventive medicine, outpatient and inpatient care, rehabilitation, medicines) and is funded by member and employer contributions.

The scheme is currently organized into about 170 health insurance funds. Insurees are free to choose a fund. Before the reforms of January 2009, the main factor influencing decisions to join an insurance fund was the premium, since all funds offered much the same package of benefits (and still do). Now all funds charge the same premium, currently 14.9 per cent of gross income, so the benefit package and the premium are not criteria people use to choose a fund.

Provision of Health Care Services

In Germany, primary health care (general practitioners (GPs) and specialist care) is provided by physicians operating private practices. Family GPs (about half of all physicians providing care outside the hospital system) are not gatekeepers for referral to specialists, although their role as coordinators of care has been strengthened in recent years. Hospitals are owned by local government, by charitable organizations (for example, the churches) or else privately. Note that there is no central unit responsible for the delivery of health care.

There are regional planning committees that determine the number of both social health insurance-accredited primary care practices and hospital beds. Otherwise, the relation between physicians and insurance funds is based primarily on collective contracts between funds and physician organizations (Busse and Riesberg 2004). This means patient and consumer organizations can influence the provision of GP and hospital care only through the insurance funds.

HEALTH CARE POLICY AND HEALTH INSURANCE SELF-GOVERNANCE

Policymaking for health care is characterized by a 'division of labour' between parliament, government and the Ministry of Health, on the one hand, and a large number of self-governing bodies (especially insurance funds and doctors' associations), on the other. The latter have been delegated considerable responsibilities.

Nationally, the Federal Assembly (parliament), the Federal Council (the lower chamber representing the Länder, or states) and the Federal Ministry of Health are the key actors. It is here that the regulatory framework (*Sozialgesetzbuch* or social code) for health insurance is set: guidelines about benefits and contributions, organizational arrangements and, since 2009, the contribution rate.

The government does not get involved in questions related to specific diseases, except for issues that have a special relevance for public health, like HIV/AIDS and, to give a recent example, 'swine flu'. For patient organizations this means that the government only becomes a lobbying target when fundamental and systemic questions are concerned.

Below the federal level, Germany is divided into 16 Länder with their own ministries of health. Länder health care responsibilities include hospital planning, disease prevention, vaccination and prevention of drug abuse.

Health insurers act as intermediaries between providers and patients. The funds' formal self-governance organs are their administrative councils and executive boards. Insurees and employers are usually represented equally on a fund's administrative council. Representatives on the administrative council are elected by secret ballot every 6 years by insurees and employers. The administrative council sets the budget and the articles of the health insurance fund, and elects and monitors the executive board.

These elections, commonly called 'social elections', are at the democratic heart of this system of health insurance, but most people take a very limited interest in the elections, and participation is quite low (Braun et al. 2008; Gesellschaft für Versicherungswissenschaft und -gestaltung 2007). Theoretically, these social elections could provide an opportunity to make consumers' voices heard within the funds. But the large number of funds – 170 over all of Germany – is prohibitive. Consumer groups cannot possibly participate in all the elections that take place, let alone the demanding work of governance after elections. Thus, there are no indications that elections so far have played any role in representing specific patient-group interests in health insurance matters.

Benefit Package Decisions

The key player determining the benefit package offered by the German insurance system is the Gemeinsamer Bundesausschuss (Federal Joint Committee). With equal representation from insurance funds and doctors' associations, this committee determines spending limits for the services offered by physicians in private practice; the inclusion of new medical procedures and preventive services and medicines; and guidelines for the distribution and joint use of sophisticated medical technology and equipment for ambulatory (or out-patient) care and hospital services (Geissler 2004).

Until 2004 the committee was a closed shop of insurance fund and doctor association representatives, with little public interest shown and no outside scrutiny of decisions. Since 2004, patient organizations have enjoyed observer status on all of the committee's working groups. This must be considered an important step in giving consumers a stronger voice at a crucial point in health care decision-making. It enables patient organizations to make their concerns known and it increases the pressure on insurance fund and doctor representatives to justify their decisions (Meinhard et al. 2009). Recently consumer representatives have been advocating – with little prospect of early success – for increased rights in procedural matters, for example, setting the committee's agenda.

Legal Basis for Patient Organization Participation in Policymaking

Self-governance in the German health insurance system has roots going back almost 130 years. Giving patient organizations an officially recognized (though still limited) role in this corporatist system has made it necessary to set clear standards about who may legitimately speak in the patient's name and receive government funding to support their activities.

There is no official government-run organization representing patients. Instead, existing organizations have been offered representation and funding if they fulfil certain criteria and are willing to play by certain rules.

There are two levels of criteria. One applies to organizations playing an official part in health policymaking, for instance, on the Federal Joint Committee; the second defines criteria for receiving public funding. Of course the criteria for the former are more demanding than for the latter.

OVERVIEW OF GERMAN PATIENT ORGANIZATIONS

Disease-specific Organizations

The health care scene in Germany is highly differentiated. Organizations exist for all major chronic diseases as well as for many rare conditions. There are no comprehensive evaluations of the sector, but estimates are of about 50 000 regional or local self-help groups, about 800 Länder-level organizations and 300 organizations at the national level. The membership lists of one of the major umbrella organizations shows a total of 107 disease-specific organizations active at the federal level. One can safely assume that these organizations not only undertake self-help activities but also have a health policy agenda. Here I will present only the Deutscher Diabetiker Bund (DDB, the German Diabetics Association) as one example. (See Engelhardt (1989) for an interesting account of the founding of diabetes organizations in Germany, Britain and the United States.)

Since diabetes is one of the most common chronic diseases it is not surprising that the DDB is one of the largest patient organizations in Germany. Structurally DDB is typical of many of the larger patient organizations. DDB members are not patients or carers, but 16 diabetes organizations at the Länder level. Patients and carers are members of these Länder organizations, which undertake information and prevention activities and support the work of self-help groups.

DDB's political focus is on issues with direct relevance to people living with diabetes, like instituting the disease management programme in 2003, the funding of rapid-acting insulin analogues, and the vaccination of diabetics against swine flu.

DDB membership excludes medical doctors and other diabetes-related professionals. This is quite typical of Germany, where medical professionals are usually organized in their own associations, and not together with the patients.

Membership seems to have reached a high point around 2001, with 40 000 members, compared with 29 500 members in 1997 and 34 000 in 2009. This makes the DDB considerably smaller than diabetes organizations in the United States and United Kingdom.

There is no obvious indication why the DDB has not managed to mobilize people living with diabetes in numbers as large as those of US and UK diabetes associations. It is clear however that the increased availability of public funding via health insurance funds since 2000, discussed below, has not resulted in an increase or even a stabilization of the membership.

The DDB is an example of the difficult relation between professionals and patients. As mentioned, traditionally there were separate organizations for

Table 9.1   Membership of diabetes organizations in Germany, the United States and the United Kingdom

	DDB	American Diabetes Association	Diabetes UK
Total patient/carer membership	34 000	407 655	170 000
Total number of diabetics	8 million	23.6 million	3 million
Percentage of membership	0.4	1.7	5.7

Source: www.ddb.de, www.diabetes.org.uk and www.diabetes.org
The total number of diabetics is estimated according to the following prevalence rates: United Kingdom, 4 per cent; United States, 7.8 per cent; Germany, 9.7 per cent.

patients and carers (DDB), medical doctors specializing in the treatment of diabetes (Deutsche Diabetes Gesellschaft) and other diabetes-related professionals (Verband der Diabetesberatungs und Schulungsberufe Deutschland) (Geissler 2004). Since 1990, these organizations have worked together in the umbrella organization, the Deutsche Diabetes Union (DDU). The DDU dissolved when the medical professionals decided to leave the organization to found a new, more centralized structure. This new organization, which came into being in October 2008 under the name diabetesDE, operates on a model based on Diabetes UK and the American Diabetes Association, bringing professionals and patients together in one organization (see www.diabetesde.org).

The DDB was invited to participate in the new organization but declined as it was felt the organization would be dominated by professionals. As a result, there are now two organizations, both of which claim to advocate in the interest of, and both of which offer membership to, people living with diabetes. It remains to be seen how this relationship will develop.

Umbrella Organizations

Disease-specific patient organizations offer self-help groups and specific information to members. But this specialization means many groups are quite small, which in turn means they have limited scope for employing professionals to undertake marketing and lobbying activities. As well, many share similar political aims. This has led to the forming of two umbrella patient organizations. Both provide organizational support to their members (for example, seminars) and act as political voices for their member organizations on decision-making bodies.

The Bundesarbeitsgemeinschaft Selbsthilfe (BAG Selbsthilfe, the Federal Working Group of Self-Help Organizations) was founded in 1967 as an umbrella structure for self-help organizations focused on the needs of children with disabilities. This focus started to shift when the children grew up and it became clear that there was a continuing need for support and advocacy. There are two types of membership of the BAG Selbsthilfe. First, 107 disease-specific organizations active at the federal level (like the DDB) are direct, individual members. Second, there are 15 Länder-level organizations (for example, the Landesarbeitsgemeinschaft Selbsthilfe Baden-Württemberg). They in return offer membership to organizations that are active mainly at the regional or local level. Federal-level patient organizations are thus represented directly in the BAG Selbsthilfe, while regional or local organizations are represented indirectly via the Länder organizations.

The second umbrella organization is the Deutscher Paritätischer Wohlfahrtsverband (DPWV). Initially a provider of social services for disabled, elderly and disadvantaged groups independent of religious or political affiliations, the DPWV is now also notable for its 'Working Group of Self-Help Organizations'. It represents 100 federal-level patient organizations and more than 3000 self-help groups. Many of these are simultaneously members of the BAG Selbsthilfe. The DPWV has a broader agenda than the latter, including migration issues, family policy, unemployment, and income generation (Geissler 2004).

Senior Citizens' Organizations

The two world wars saw the founding of two organizations to support and lobby for invalid soldiers and civilians. The organisation known today as Sozialverband Deutschland (SoVD) was founded in 1917, the VdK in 1950. Today, both have very similar membership profiles, mainly senior citizens and people with disabilities.

Both are large organizations, with 525 000 and 1.4 million members respectively. Members receive legal advice in dealing with the health and social security systems. Both have a broad political agenda, including any topic relevant to senior citizens, with health policy an important focus.

Consumer Protection Societies

The *Verbaucherzentralen* (consumer protection societies) are organizations *for* consumers, but not organizations *of* consumers. They provide advice and information about topics relevant to consumers. They also act as advocates and lobbying organizations to protect consumer interests against those of 'big business'. Like many of the organizations mentioned above, consumer organizations are structured within one federal level umbrella organization, with 16 Länder-level organizations. Even though their most important source of funding is the German government, they are generally regarded as independent and highly trustworthy. An important source of this trust is the day-to-day advice they provide to consumers. This also makes it possible for them to speak for the health care consumer in general. While self-help and senior citizens' organizations each speak for a specific segment of health care users, consumer organizations can claim to give voice to the interests of the general public in health care. Like the senior citizens' organizations, consumer organizations have a broad agenda. The issues addressed are not only in the interest of current health care users but also of many potential ones, for example around topics like pharmaceutical legislation, genetic testing for diseases and bacterial resistance to antibiotics. Another important issue is the quality of medical care.

The German Society for Insurees and Patients and the Union of German Health Insurees

The other organizations described in this chapter can legitimately claim to speak in the interest of patients. There are, however, two organizations that claim to represent the interests of patients without having a legitimate basis to do so: the Deutsche Gesellschaft für Versicherte und Patienten (DGVP, the German Society for Insurees and Patients) and the Verband der Krankenversicherten Deutschlands (VKVD, the Union of German Health Insurees). The most striking feature of both organizations is their lack of transparency. Their websites offer only vague or misleading information about the size of their membership, and there is no information at all about their finances. There are ongoing rumours that both are funded largely by the pharmaceutical industry, but this is difficult to substantiate. Their political influence seems to be limited, but they do appear regularly in television discussions as patient representatives. These organizations are a good illustration of how having a catchy name will get you a certain level of public recognition (see Geissler 2004; also www.dgvp.de and www.vkvd.de).

FUNDING OF PATIENT ORGANIZATIONS

In Germany there is very limited information about patient organization funding. Even analysis at the level of individual organizations is difficult because they are not required to publish balance sheets. A review of the websites of the diabetes organization DDB shows that out of the one federal and 16 Länder organizations only one (DDB Hamburg) publishes comprehensive, detailed information about its membership and financial situation. (See www.ddb.de and the websites of the Länder-level diabetes organizations.) In one 2006 study, the participating organizations reported that 42 per cent of their income came from membership fees, 25 per cent from health insurance funds and 5 per cent from sponsoring activities, including but not restricted to the pharmaceutical industry (Klemperer 2009: 75).

Patient organizations are repeatedly criticized for accepting funds from the pharmaceutical industry. There are allegations that the industry even 'buys' the support of individual groups which then lobby to promote the funding of specific drugs under the social health insurance. But it is hard to prove how prevalent any such influence over consumer groups might be, or if it exists at all (Geissler 2004; Klemperer 2009).

Since 2000 the health insurance funds have gained in importance as sources of funding for patient organizations undertaking self-help activities.[3] Health insurers are required to spend 0.56 per year per insuree on funding patient organizations (SGB [Sozialgesetzbuch] V §20c, 'Förderung der Selbsthilfe').

Table 9.2 provides an overview of the development of the total funding and the funding per insuree since 2000 (Gesundheit und Gesellschaft Spezial 2008: 4).

Initially it was difficult for the health insurance funds to find enough projects to support. Legal changes in 2007 made it mandatory for health insurance bodies to carry over funds they did not spend in one year to following years. Previously it had been in the financial interest of insurance funds not to spend the total amount because any leftover monies could be used for other purposes.

The changes in 2007 also aimed at simplifying disbursement procedures for the funds. Previously all money had to be disbursed through individual projects initiated by each individual insurance fund, of which there were, at that time, more than 300. Since 2008, 50 per cent of this funding goes into a pool which is administered jointly by all funds. This reduces the administrative burden on patient organizations in making applications.

Table 9.2 *Funding from German health insurance funds to support the work of patient organizations*

	2000	2002	2004	2006	2008
Total annual funding (m.)	9.5	21.5	26.4	27.5	39.9
Annual funding per insuree ( )	0.13	0.30	0.38	0.39	0.56

Source: Laaff (2008).

The conditions for the disbursement of the funds are set by the federal umbrella organization of the German social health insurance (Spitzenverband Bund der Krankenkassen) together with the federal-level self-help umbrella organizations (see above). Money goes to (umbrella) organizations at the federal level, organizations at the Länder level, and self-help groups at the community level.

To receive funding, all groups have to sign a 'declaration of neutrality and independence'. Patient organizations signing this declaration confirm that they will make public any event financially supported by, for example, the pharmaceutical industry, to ensure that no undue outside influence is being exerted on the organization. Additionally, organizations commit to publishing their income from industry sponsorship annually.

Increasing Funding Transparency

In the period 2002 to 2003, both the BAG Selbsthilfe and the DPWV independently published guidelines concerning acceptance by their members of funding from the pharmaceutical industry. Since 2005 both organizations have worked together in formulating joint criteria. Initially there was only a non-binding set of suggestions, but now there is a trend towards stricter enforcement of these conditions. Funded by the health insurers, a project has been initiated to strengthen monitoring and enforcement capacities. Member organizations can now submit a request to check if ongoing or planned activities are in line with the regulations. A monitoring commission has been established which can act upon its own initiative, but which can also be called upon by anyone to review an organization's activities. The commission publishes annual reports about its activities. The 2008 report gives concrete examples of what constitutes a legitimate activity and what is considered a breach of funding guidelines, but it does not disclose the names of organizations whose activities were critically reviewed (Danner 2008; BAG Selbsthilfe and Paritätischer 2008).[4]

Surprisingly, an increase of transparency in the funding of patient organizations comes from the pharmaceutical industry. The major companies have developed their own standards for cooperating with patient organizations and are publishing quite detailed information about the amounts donated to different groups. Considering this new source of information, it is even less understandable that patient organizations do not themselves systematically make public their sources of income.

THE POLITICAL INFLUENCE OF PATIENT ORGANIZATIONS

Influencing Politics at the Federal Level

The voice of patient organizations in German health care policymaking is probably not as strong as that of doctors, pharmacists and insurance funds, and, realistically, it will never be so (Offe 1974; Geissler 2004). But Mancur Olson's assessment that consumers (including patients) are 'suffering in silence' (Olson 1968) clearly does not hold true for Germany.

In the political sphere, German patient organizations are similar to any other advocacy or lobbying organization. They are, however, especially like consumer and environmental lobbying organizations in that they have less funding and often less direct political influence than industry organizations. But organizations like BAG Selbsthilfe or the disease-specific groups can claim a high degree of legitimacy as authentic representatives of patients' interests. I argue that this authenticity, and the often passionate support of organizations' members and leadership, can to a large extent replace traditional (that is, mostly financial) resources.

Again, it is difficult to assess and quantify the political impact of lobbying activity in a general sense. But German patient organizations have managed to develop individual mechanisms that allow them to make the best use of their specific situation and resources. (For a more detailed analysis see Geissler 2004.) The BAG Selbsthilfe holds regular information meetings for journalists and members of parliament, submits written statements on legislative proposals and testifies before parliamentary committees. Many patient organizations develop questionnaires (*Wahlprüfsteine*) for political parties during elections. The responses to the questions are then circulated to members. Many organizations have developed individual personal contacts with decision-makers. It often helps to work together with well-known public figures to increase their visibility.

It is difficult to judge to what extent this lobbying is successful, but the same would be the case for the lobbying of doctors or any other health-related interest group. Yet German patient organizations are clearly in a position to get their messages across to political decision makers in the right form and at the right time. At the end of the day, they possess a high degree of professionalism in the lobbying methods and tools employed, which determines their often significant political influence as patient organizations (Geissler 2004). It remains to be seen if increased public funding will be the basis of a sustainable improvement in the lobbying capacities of German patient organizations.

Länder-level Policies

In order to be successful, consumer groups have to lobby at the Länder level as well. To take the city-state of Hamburg as an example, patient representatives sit on committees determining the number of doctors who can register in a certain area, on ethics committees making decisions about medical research projects, and on hospital planning committees deliberating on investments in hospital infrastructure (Verbraucherzentrale Hamburg 2008). Again, since they are not the only ones on the committees, it is hard to determine if or to what extent health consumer groups influence decision-making. But at least they are represented at the place of decision-making, and they act as watchdogs to ensure decisions are not made in a closed shop of health insurance fund and provider representatives.

Influencing Social Health Insurance Decisions

Health consumer representation on the Federal Joint Committee certainly represents an important step towards making the social health insurance scheme more responsive to consumer interests. The committee still attracts little public attention. But patient representatives are now present at a crucial decision-making point, and insurance fund and doctor representatives at least have to justify their decisions if they do not follow consumer representative opinion (Etgeton 2009).

Legal changes in 2007 further strengthened the role of patient representatives on the Federal Joint Committee. A support unit (*Stabsstelle Patientenbeteiligung*), established within the Federal Joint Committee, provides training and information to patient representatives and makes relevant documents available. These measures are intended to reduce the knowledge gap between patient representatives and insurance fund and doctor association representatives (Meinhardt et al. 2009). The findings of Meinhardt et al. suggest that patient representatives on the Federal Joint Committee do feel that they can influence decisions. The sample size of eight patient representatives out of a total of 182 is too small to allow statistical evaluations. But it is still relevant to note that seven out of eight people participating in the study said that they were able to influence decisions and were generally able to support decisions reached by the committee (Meinhardt et al. 2009: 100).

CONCLUSION

Germany has a vibrant patient organization scene consisting, especially, of disease-specific organizations, which in turn are members of two umbrella organizations. Senior citizens' health-related interests are also advocated by two organizations, and consumer protection societies lobby on behalf of 'health care users' in general. I still consider funding transparency to require further practical improvement. The umbrella organizations BAG Selbsthilfe and DPWV have certainly improved the situation by setting up a committee to scrutinize the activities of their members and to publish its findings. But there is no reason why patient organizations should not be required to publish their balance sheets, as they are in other countries.

Two events in recent years have considerably strengthened the position of patient organizations in German health care policymaking. In 2004, consumer groups were given observer status on all the working groups of the Federal Joint Committee, which is the decision-making body for the social health insurance benefits package. This decision put patient organizations in a position to scrutinize decisions taken by this important self-governing body. Since 2000 the insurance funds have been required to provide direct funding to patient organizations. The impact of this is still difficult to judge, in part because the stipulated funding level of 0.56 per insuree was only achieved in 2008. There is no analysis showing whether the additional funding has resulted in an increase in membership or professionalization of lobbying activities. I would expect this to happen over time, though the example of the DDB suggests that it will not be automatic.

The lobbying activities of patient organizations in Germany are essentially the same as those of other lobbying organizations. Their targets are policymakers at the federal and Länder level. In the sphere of social security self-governance, the only indication of patient organization activities relates to the Federal Joint Committee. There is no indication that patient organizations are participating in the social elections for the governing councils of insurance funds, and there is no indication that this will change in the future. But despite this, patient organizations have gained a firm position as lobbying organizations. They may not be in a position to veto parliamentary decisions or the insurance funds, but they are certainly able to make their positions known.

NOTES

1. I am using the term 'self-governance' as a translation of the German *Selbstverwaltung*, which literally translates as 'self-administration'. However, 'self-governance' puts a stronger emphasis on the fact that the activities in question are not of a purely administrative nature. Self-governance here refers to the *concept* or *principle* of delegating competencies from government to independent bodies. At the same time, the term is used to denote the *organs* or *organizations* of self-governance (also called self-governance bodies).
2. The remaining 10 per cent use private health insurance. Private health insurees are primarily civil servants and the self-employed, who are not covered by social health insurance. Additionally, people earning above 4000 a month can voluntarily leave the social health

insurance system to join private health insurance. As private health insurance covers only a small portion of insurees, it is not considered further in this chapter. Henceforth, 'health insurance' refers only to social health insurance.

3. Only organizations undertaking self-help activities are eligible for this kind of funding. Others, like senior citizens organizations, consumer protection societies and trade unions, are not eligible.

4. Martin Danner in GG Spezial 12/08, S. 14; Gemeinsamer Bericht zum Monitoring-Verfahren von BAG Selbsthilfe von Menschen mit Behinderung und chronischer Erkrankung und ihren Angehörigen e.V. und FORUM chronisch kranker und behinderter Menschen im Paritätischen Gesamtverband e.V. (2008)

REFERENCES

BAG Selbsthilfe and Paritätischer (2008), Gemeinsamer Bericht zum Monitoring-Verfahren, accessed at www.bag-selbsthilfe.de.

Braun, B. and T. Klenk, W. Kluth, F. Nullmeier and F. Welti (2008), 'Gutachten zur Geschichte und Modernisierung der Sozialversicherungswahlen', expert report on behalf of the Federal Ministry for Labour and Social Security.

Busse, R. and A. Riesberg (2004), *Healthcare Systems in Transition: Germany*, Copenhagen: WHO Regional Office for Europe on behalf of the European Observatory on Health Systems and Policies.

Danner, M. (2008), 'Prüfung fragwürdiger Praktiken', in *Gesundheit und Gesellschaft Spezial, Gemeinsam stark: Die Selbsthilfeförderung der AOK. Ziele, Konzepte, Hintergründe*, December, Berlin: KomPart-Verlag, p. 14.

Engelhardt, D. von (1989), *Diabetes in Medizin und Kulturgeschichte. Grundzüge – Texte – Bibliographie*, Berlin: Springer.

Etgeton, S. (2009),Patientenbeteiligung in den Strukturen des Gemeinsamen Bundesausschusses', *Bundesgesundheitsblatt – Gesundheitsforschung – Gesundheitsschutz*, **52** (1): 104–10.

Geissler, J. (2004), *Organisierte Vertretung von Patienteninteressen: Patienten-Organisationen als gesundheitspolitische Akteure in Deutschland, Großbritannien und den USA*, Hamburg, Germany: Verlag Dr Kovac.

Gesellschaft für Vesicherungswissenschaft und -gestaltung (2007), *Zur Bedeutung der Selbstverwaltung in der deutschen Sozialen Sicherung. Formen, Aufgaben, Entwicklungsperspektiven*, Bonn: Nanos Verlag.

Gesundheit und Gesellschaft Spezial (12/2008), *Gemeinsam stark: Die Selbsthilfeförderung der AOK. Ziele, Konzepte, Hintergründe*, Berlin: KomPart-Verlag.

Klemperer, D. (2009), 'Interessenkonflikte der Selbsthilfe durch Pharma-Sponsoring', *Bundesgesundheitsblatt – Gesundheitsforschung – Gesundheitsschutz*, **52** (1): 71–6.

Laaff, H. (2008), 'Hilfe für die Selbsthilfe', in *Gesundheit und Gesellschaft Spezial, Gemeinsam stark: Die Selbsthilfeförderung der AOK. Ziele, Konzepte, Hintergründe*, December, Berlin: KomPart-Verlag, p. 4.

Meinhardt, M., E. Plamper and H. Brunner (2009), 'Beteiligung von Patientenvertretern im Gemeinsamen Bundesausschuss. Ergebnisse einer qualitativen Befragung', *Bundesgesundheitsblatt – Gesundheitsforschung – Gesundheitsschutz*, **52** (1): 96–103.

Offe, C. (1974), 'Politische Herrschaft und Klassenstrukturen – Zur Analyse spätkapitalistischer Gesellschaftssysteme', in H.P. Widmaier (ed.), *Politische Ökonomie des*

Wohlfahrtsstaates. Eine kritische Darstellung der Neuen Politischen Ökonomie, Frankfurt am Main, Germany: Fischer, pp. 264–93.

Olson, M. Jr (1968), *Die Logik des kollektiven Handelns. Kollektivgütern und die Theorie der Gruppen*, Tübingen, Germany: Mohr.

Tennstedt, F. (1981), *Sozialgeschichte der Sozialpolitik in Deutschland*, Göttingen, Germany: Vandenhoek & Ruprecht.

Verbraucherzentrale Hamburg (2008), '20 Jahre Gesundheit und Patientenschutz in der Verbraucherzentrale Hamburg', accessed at www.vzhh.de.

10. Austrian health consumer groups: voices gaining strength?

Rudolf Forster, Gudrun Braunegger-Kallinger and Karl Krajic

It will be argued in this chapter that Austria's dominant political culture does not encourage the emergence of social movements in general, and that political activism is even more unlikely in health care. While Austria has not seen the rise of a broad health consumer or patient movement so far, it has seen the emergence of self-help groups seeking to complement professional care and to compensate for its deficiencies. Based on our own recent research it will be shown that the self-help field offers potential for mobilizing the collective interests of members and others. Empirical evidence will be provided to show how this potential is currently realized, drawing on a theoretical framework that stresses the capacity of health care consumers to organize interests and become relevant to established stakeholders.

POLITICAL SYSTEM, POLITICAL CULTURE AND POLITICAL PARTICIPATION

Austria is a 'late democracy' by Western European standards and has followed a non-linear path to its present situation as a basically representative democracy with few options for direct democratic participation. Its political culture after the Second World War stressed political collaboration between the formerly highly antagonistic parties of the right and left. In light of this the relationship between the political class and citizens has been characterized by paternalism and clientelism, generating a citizen mentality of high expectations and dependence (Gerlich and Pfefferle 2006).

Since the Second World War, then, the Austrian political system has experienced 'hyperstability'. This was further consolidated by its particular 'social partnership' model, in which corporations of employers and employees negotiate economic and social policies beyond and before parliamentary procedures, striving for compromise (Talos 2006). Massive, consensus-based welfare state expansion after 1945 contributed to political stability and Austria's identity as a viable democratic state (Talos 2005).

A traditional element of Austria's political system is federalism. Despite a relatively small population base of 8.3 million inhabitants, Austria's nine Länder (autonomous provinces constituting the federal state) enjoy considerable political autonomy, based less on the constitution than on tradition and culture and successful identity politics (Pelinka 2009).

However the past 25 years have seen a gradual erosion of this political culture. Austria's democracy has changed from a 'consociation' type to a more 'competitive' one (Pelinka 2009). In the perception of many, the 'Golden Age' of welfare state expansion has ended, revealing structural problems typical of conservative-corporatist type regimes (Esping-Andersen 1990).

The extent and modes of political participation are also changing. Turnout at general elections has decreased but options for direct democracy and readiness to participate have increased, as have unconventional styles of political activity. Additionally some have noted a gradual transition from corporatist to more pluralist modes of interest aggregation (Karlhofer 2007). Some new initiatives have claimed the status of new social movements. Especially in the areas of women's rights and ecology, permanent and professional structures have been developed that have achieved specific successes as well as better access to the policy process (Gottweis 1997).

Civil society – understood as a sector of organizations and networks independent of established political bodies or churches – is underdeveloped in Austria. Nevertheless, recent decades have seen the rise of more independent associations and a move towards greater autonomy of a voluntary third sector alongside the state and market (Brix 2003).

HEALTH POLICY AND THE ROLE OF HEALTH CONSUMERS

In comparative health systems analysis, Austria has been categorized as a social health insurance system (Saltman et al. 2004), displaying some elements of all Saltman's structural characteristics (Saltman 2004: 6):

- Risk-independent, transparent contributions.
- Health insurance funds acting as payers/purchasers. (In Austria there are several funds – mainly regionally organized, with some professional groups like farmers, small businessmen and public employees organized in separate funds at the national level.)
- Near universality in population coverage (99 per cent) and funding, and nearly uniform benefits.

- Pluralism in actors/organizational structure.
- A corporatist model of negotiation.
- Shared governance arrangements.
- Individual choice of provider (but not of health insurance fund).

But the Austrian social health insurance system manifests also several of the paradoxes of this type of system identified by Marc Danzon (Foreword in Saltman et al. 2004). It is formally 'self-governed' by contributors, who are represented on the governing bodies by the 'social partners' (employer corporations and trade unions). Self-government is limited however, as social health insurance is regulated and supervised by the federal government. Only 45 per cent of health care costs (including those of long-term care) are financed by social health insurance funds. Taxes cover another 25 per cent, users another 25 per cent, but the system is considered a social health insurance system. Austria is proud of the 'solidarity'/(near) universality of its system, yet socio-economic status and region still influence contributions and benefits and private contributions are high and growing. A final, important point is that although the health care system is considered in expert and public discussions to be expensive, requiring higher funding levels than tax-funded systems, it is very popular with Austrians.

Social health insurance funds play a central role in corporatist-style governance of public ambulatory (or out-patient) care, but in the hospital and long-term care sectors it is the nine Länder that play the main role in governance, as well as being deeply involved in service provision (social health insurance funds have little say in the hospital sector, despite spending half of their resources on hospitals). The 2004 health care reform modified this imbalance by involving social health insurance in provincial governance structures ('Health Platforms') in the nine Länder, but these seem a rather weak coordinating mechanism (Hofmarcher and Rack 2006: 209). The Austrian federal government has a primarily supervising, coordinating and mediating role. However, its constitutional responsibilities for health, social insurance and especially public finance ensure that health care reform remains a national concern. Recent decades have seen some experimentation in federal interventions (legal, financial, organizational), but success has been limited.

There are major imbalances in service provision. The large hospital sector is expanding (staff, technology, services) and is heavily used (the inpatient admission rate of 28 per 100 population is 65 per cent above the EU average: Hofmarcher and Rack 2006: 133). In contrast, there is stagnation in public primary care – only 43 per cent of all doctors in private practice have contracts with social health insurance funds (Hofmarcher and Rack 2006). Solo practice is the dominant form – and there are few more complex organizational models. General practitioners are in an especially unenviable position. They are expected to fulfil their traditional role of providing primary diagnoses, acting as family doctors and coordinators of personal care in a complex system, as well as having many administrative duties. Their ability to do all this, however, is limited by their lack of prestige and formal power, and their weak gatekeeper function. In addition to this *public* system, a medical market of doctors in *private* practice has evolved, offering a lot of consumer choice but creating questions concerning the impact of social inequality and increasing fragmentation of services, especially for the chronically ill. Integration/coordination and continuity between hospitals and primary care, generalists and specialists is an area of special concern (Eichwalder and Hofmarcher 2008). Long-term care is understood as social welfare rather than health care, causing problems at the interface (see Peinhaupt et al. 2004). Long-term care services are also provided by less-qualified staff, and patients with income and assets pay a large proportion of care costs out of their own pockets.

The high level of consumer satisfaction with Austrian health policy bodes well for the government's re-election chances. The Eurobarometer of 2001 found Austria the leader in patient satisfaction (Leopold et al. 2008), and Health Consumer Powerhouse (2007) awarded it number-one position for 'consumer friendliness'. Debates around service oversupply have led several experts to demand a re-engineering of the whole system, but resistance from local government and citizens has usually constrained policy actors.

In health policymaking, user/patient perspectives are not represented directly. Austria has not so far embraced the patient involvement initiatives launched by WHO Europe and the European Council. Various stakeholders claim to speak for patients. The national and Länder parliaments generally represent citizen concerns, including those about health care. Social health insurance funds are supposed to be self-governing bodies, but in practice are controlled by actors with a primarily economic perspective (cost containment) acting within a tight framework of federal laws and state supervision. The medical profession traditionally claims to represent the best interests of patients and refers to surveys showing high levels of patient trust to support its claim. In Austria, so-called patient advocates are generally considered the institution closest to patient interests. National legislation has been passed requiring Länder to establish these ombudsman-like institutions. Their legal remit is to represent patients vis-à-vis hospitals, nursing homes and primary care services (Bachinger 2008). This legislation was prompted by public concern about the vulnerability of patients in general, but particularly in geriatric care (after the killing of numerous patients by nurses in a Viennese hospital) and psychiatric care (where a special kind of patient advocacy has been operating since 1991: Forster and Vyslouzil 1991). Another aim of patient advocacy has been to facilitate extrajudicial handling of complaints to forestall a culture of damages litigation. As patient advocacy has to be provided by the nine Länder, there has been a diversity of solutions, for example concerning the resource base. Patient advocacy across the Länder is independent of political control and accessible free of charge. The mandate includes information about rights, take-up of complaints, support in extrajudicial conflict resolution and facilitation of out-of-court settlement of compensation cases for treatment errors. Service providers are legally obliged to cooperate. Most patient advocates also consider themselves mouthpieces for general patient concerns and as contributors to quality and error management and to higher awareness of patient rights. This extended role is supported by their membership of central health care governance bodies. Their position is further strengthened by general improvements in patient rights and protection over the past 20 years, although these are criticized for their tendency towards placatory symbolic politics (Kopetzki 2006). Some patient advocates have become strong supporters of direct patient representation by formally authorized spokespersons.

Health activism has never developed into a broad social movement in Austria. Health issues have however been central to the concerns of some new social movements, and some protest groups have gained a profile, for example in psychiatry. The campaign to legalize abortion in the 1970s – primarily stressing health risks – was formative for the women's movement (Groth 1999). Resistance to nuclear power plants and their health risks helped establish the ecology movement. And engagement in HIV/AIDS prevention strengthened the emancipatory claims of the gay movement.

Austria shares many of the problems described by Saltman et al. (2004) for social health insurance systems in general in relation to prevention and public health, with the weak role of national government in health care also extending to prevention. There are no explicit national health targets as responsibilities are devolved to the Länder and even to the local level, while health reporting, monitoring and research is erratic. Expenditure on prevention and health promotion is low (only 0.9 per cent of public health expenditure; Hofmarcher and Rack 2006: 68). Adequate funding is limited to those programmes that are closely linked to curative health care and its stakeholders: screening and early detection of disease and rehabilitation after surgery or other major interventions. Thus Austria may face the same difficulties in restraining future costs in an ageing society as other social health insurance systems.

HEALTH CONSUMER GROUPS IN AUSTRIA

As in many other developed countries (Baggott and Forster 2008) the number and societal relevance of self-organized health- and illness-related groups in Austria is increasing. Based on our recent research (Box 10.1), it will be argued that these groups have become an important basis for the mobilization of the collective interests of condition-specific groups, as well as patients in general. As political activism remains closely related to other activities we will first characterize the whole field.[1]

Self-definition as well as public perception of such groups in Austria has mainly evolved around the term 'self-help group', which emphasizes members' personal affliction, voluntary engagement, informal communication and independence from professional and commercial interests (Robinson and Henry 1977). The main distinguishing characteristic of self-help groups in both the self-definition of their members and in public perception has been their difference from professional medical care and the complementary and/or compensatory function of self-help. Self-help groups are considered *complementary*, offering mutual psycho-social support to their members that is usually not, or is no longer, provided by professionals, who have become increasingly specialized and bureaucratized. Though not professional themselves, these groups are also often expected to *compensate* for typical deficiencies in professional care in information provision, patient-oriented communication, management of everyday life, discrimination and stigmatization – thus reflecting the general growth of critical attitudes towards professional expertise (Kelleher 2006).

BOX 10.1   KEY FEATURES OF THE STUDY 'PATIENTS AND CARER ORGANIZATIONS IN AUSTRIA'

Target group: groups/organizations which by self-definition:

- constitute themselves around problems of (somato-psycho-social) health and illness;
- are organized or controlled by patients/users/health consumers or carers themselves;
- have no commercial interests;
- perform regular activities for a long period of time in Austria, independently of their formal status and geographical reach.

In total 1654 groups/organizations were identified, mostly via directories made available by self-help support institutions. Only a small segment of disability groups define themselves as patient and carer organizations according to these criteria.

Data collection: accomplished in three phases and by different methods:

- Phase 1 (2008): Questionnaire based on instruments from the studies of Baggott et al. (2005) in the United Kingdom, Trojan (2006) in Germany and Stremlow et al. (2004) in Switzerland; sent to 1550 groups/organizations; a return rate 40.3 per cent (*N* = 625); the sample generally reproduces key characteristics of the total target group quite well, but more highly organized groups seem to be slightly overrepresented.
- Phase 2 (2008–9): Interview study with self-help groups/organizations (seven focus group interviews and seven single interviews).
- Phase 3 (2009): Interview study with stakeholders of the political and administrative system, the health system (professionals and social health insurance), the pharmaceutical industry and patient advocacy (17 expert interviews).

Source: Forster et al. (2009)[2]

In Austria, around 1700 groups (20 per 100 000 inhabitants) define themselves as health-related self-help groups (Box 10.1). About half of the groups active in 2008 were founded within the previous decade. Yet it is not only numbers but also social visibility that has grown.

Of the various, partly competing, typologies canvassed in the literature (Epstein 2008), we have chosen for the purpose of this chapter those that focus on self-help groups' main activities and functions. Our data contain information on the frequency of a broad spectrum of activities. Two of the dimensions identified correspond to what has been portrayed in the literature as the distinction between 'inner- and outer-focused' functions (Katz and Bender 1976; Kelleher 2006). What we call 'mutual-support' activities are considered to be inner-oriented, as they relate to sharing experiences and feelings in a reciprocal way and individuals supporting each other in processes of identity reconstruction, management of everyday life, and adjustment to treatment. What we call 'collective-advocacy' activities correspond to the characteristics of 'outer-focused groups' that represent and advocate their collective interests to other stakeholders and the public to challenge features of service provision and adverse social structures and cultural concepts.

A third group which we call 'individual-support' activities expands this dual conception. On the basis of their accumulated expertise some groups offer advice and support not only in a reciprocal way and not only to members. Such activities partly blur the boundaries between professional and self-help approaches (McCormick et al. 2003) and could become the object of systematic efforts to include 'expert patients' in welfare service provision (Lindsay and Vrijhoef 2009).

Most groups included in our study could be classified as 'cumulative' in type. A first type of group engages primarily in activities of mutual support. A second combines mutual-support and individual-support activities. A third engages in collective advocacy as well. That means, on the one hand, that genuine 'self-help' was the common attribute of nearly all groups studied while on the other hand collective advocacy was nearly always performed in combination with both mutual and individual support. The fact that the 'organizational age' of groups with more complex patterns of activity is higher on average might result from a process of internal development. It might also indicate that the ability to adopt such outward-oriented goals increases longevity.

Further analysis showed characteristic differences between these three types of group. 'Mutual-support groups' are small, mostly informally organized, and locally oriented. They rely on personal communication and common decision-making. Voluntary engagement of members is their main resource, and this is mostly considered to be sufficient. About half these groups have relations with other groups dealing with the same health problem as themselves, as well as health care professionals. These groups see their main impact as being in improving coping abilities, social integration and problem- or illness-related knowledge.

'Individual-support groups' are larger in membership, more formalized and cover a larger area. They use external advice and information more often, and are less content with the resources at their disposal. Frequency and intensity of relations with health care professionals is higher and relations with pharmaceutical companies are more important. Self-assessment of impacts asserts effectiveness in the same areas as mutual support groups, but at a higher level; in addition, these groups see themselves as effective in promoting autonomous health behaviour.

'Collective-advocacy groups' differ significantly from the two other types. They are larger, include an extended range and scope of activities, and structures become more formalized, including decision-making being moved to central executive bodies. They also have more resources and their external relations are more complex. These groups are analysed in more detail in the next section.

The self-help group field in Austria has two general features. First, most groups try to combine experiential knowledge built up by themselves with formal knowledge 'imported' from experts. Interestingly, leaders of Austrian groups assessed the improvement of (formal) knowledge about the identifying problem (illness) as the highest single effect their groups have had. This might indicate ineffective patient information in professional health care. Access to (professional) knowledge is also a main reason for the close cooperation with medical specialists.

Second, self-help support institutions have been established at Länder level since the 1990s. Groups consider them to be their most important resource besides their own members' voluntary work. They provide assistance in founding and organizing groups, developing infrastructure, training and information. As most of these institutions are provided by regional cross-condition self-help group alliances, there are good reasons to understand them as being controlled by the groups themselves (self-government). But financial support comes mainly from the Länder governments, so these institutions are also an object of state governance.

POLITICAL ACTIVISM FOR HEALTH CONSUMER INTERESTS

Self-help groups are mostly 'condition-based groups' (Baggott et al. 2005: 21) whose collective interests relate first of all to the availability and quality of services for their members and fellow sufferers, services that are controlled by professional experts and welfare state bureaucracies. As well, they sometimes advocate for their specific needs in areas of possible discrimination such as employment, housing and transport. Their shared experience of what it means to live with a specific problem legitimizes them as advocates for their interests. On the other hand they are in competition for attention, resources and influence with other condition-based groups similarly entitled to press their own specific needs.

A way out of this potentially problematic situation is to build alliances within and across conditions – a trend noted by some observers but one scantily researched so far (Epstein 2008). In a study on alliance formation in the United Kingdom, Jones (2007) shows that the expectation of gaining political strength by pooling limited resources was the main driver of alliance formation. But she also refers to changes in the policy environment and new opportunity structures as potential factors encouraging cooperation. The study points out that building and maintaining alliances also carries high opportunity costs and the risk of groups losing their identity, so alliance-building remains fragile and is vulnerable to a fluctuating policy context and associated pressures.

What preconditions are necessary for organizing collective interests? Offe (1974) suggested the concepts of 'organizational capacity' and 'conflict capacity'. Geissler (2004) has proposed the use of these concepts for analysing patient organizations. He specifies the sources of 'organizational capacity' as strong common concerns, adequate resources, definable group identity, special incentives for membership and participation, and good prospects of success. The capacity to advocate condition-specific or cross-condition collective interests can be analysed using these criteria. In addition, claiming an advocacy role for collective interests raises issues of legitimacy such as the authorization of spokespersons (Contradiopoulus 2004).

'Conflict capacity' is defined by Offe (1974) as the power of a collective to deny a performance or benefit, which includes control over something that others urgently need. What are the assets controlled by people organized around health problems? Usually it is they who are dependent on specialized services and experts. Alternative options or complaints mechanisms can be used individually but cannot easily become instruments of collective activism. Voting in general elections as an aggregated way to voice needs and preferences is not well suited to expressing complex and specific concerns around health problems. Yet as Hirschman (1970) and Stichweh (2005) have argued, professional expert systems are to some degree dependent on their clients. They are based on 'loyalty', that is, trust in the competence and disinterestedness of professionals. Partnerships between self-help groups can thus become an asset in the symbolic struggles (Contradiopoulos 2004) of various stakeholders who legitimize their positions by referring to the true interests of patients. And vice versa: public critique by such groups can undermine their public standing.

The three main stakeholders in social health insurance systems like Austria's – state authorities, social health insurance institutions and professionals – relate differently to the main interests of self-help groups. Our assumptions are as follows:

- Self-help groups are of interest to all stakeholders for the complementary role they play to professional service provision. For the state, self-help groups offer the prospect of financial relief as challenges in health care are increasing faster than budgets. For the social health insurance institutions which are required to provide 'necessary care', self-help groups can help restrict expanding demand and supply of professional services (medicalization). Self-help groups are of interest to specialized health professionals not only because they complement and improve their work but also because they expand their field of influence.
- Lobbying by condition-specific groups is more ambiguous. For governments and social health insurance institutions it may convey important information about service gaps but it might also question the established

balance between different needs. For professionals, lobbying might support expansion and sub-specialization but also present the risk of clashes between different perspectives.

- Political activism referring to the health and health care concerns of (chronically ill) patients in general clashes with the established balance of stakeholders and their claims to represent collective health needs. Democratically legitimized political bodies and social health insurance institutions are especially challenged.

In the following section, based on our study (see Box 10.1), we analyse the organizational and conflict capacities of both condition-specific groups and cross-condition alliances, and their role in policy processes in Austria.

Condition-specific Groups and Their Collective Advocacy Role

Of the Austrian self-help groups represented in our study, 29 per cent are 'collective advocacy' type groups as characterized above. All of these groups are also engaged in 'inner-oriented' activities, which they generally consider to be the most important. As this subgroup of 'collective advocacy groups' is still heterogeneous we will focus on those groups which combine their claim of 'collective advocacy' with a formal status and which also operate beyond the local level (representing 15 per cent of the whole sample).

In analysing the organizational capacity of these groups, a first issue is the membership base. Quantitatively, collective advocacy groups have the biggest membership of all self-help groups. It is usually assumed that condition-specific groups are bound together by strong common concerns. It is not self-evident that outer-oriented activities enjoy the same support from members as inner-oriented ones since they entail the risk of shifting priorities and causing cleavages between ordinary members and leaders or expert members (that is, between 'lay-lay' and 'lay-expert' members: Epstein 2008). Interview data from leaders of condition-specific alliances indicate that there are different group identities and that a balance of interests has to be found. Coordination must be undertaken with care. The dominance of leaders or (non-afflicted) professional staff is often viewed sceptically and can provoke internal conflicts and resistance. What might also complicate collective interest formation is the remarkably diverse membership base even of condition-specific groups. Asked who belongs to the groups, not only did most groups include relatives, but often also medical doctors and other (health) professionals.

Resources are seen by most as the crucial measure of organizational capacity. Different sorts of resources are important: money, voluntary engagement, availability of professional staff, organizational know-how and infrastructure,

as well as supportive relationships. For self-help groups, voluntary engagement of members is usually the central resource. This holds true also for
collective advocacy groups. Yet about half of these assess members' voluntary
engagement as not being sufficient to accomplish their complex aims.
Although annual budgets far exceed those of the majority of self-help groups,
nearly half of them have less than 5000 annually at their disposal, and only
about a fifth command a budget of more than 20 000 – so not surprisingly
most of the groups consider money to be scarce. This holds also for the availability of professional staff. More than half of collective advocacy groups have
no paid staff at all; those that do have it have to make do, on average, with one
full-time employee. Thus it is not surprising that group leaders assess their
effectiveness in advocating collective interests as low compared with claimed
achievements in knowledge, management of everyday life, and autonomous
health behaviour.

Concerning 'external support', collective advocacy groups consider public
authorities, private sponsors, medical professionals and, to a lesser extent,
social health insurance funds and pharmaceutical companies to be very important. But medical professionals, health care organizations, public authorities
and funds are both principal sources of support and addressees of demands.
Thus collective advocacy groups have to find a balance between self-mainte-
nance and political activism. As the 'conflict capacity' of collective advocacy
groups is embedded in such ambiguous relations to main stakeholders these
relations need more detailed exploration.

Various indicators suggest that by far the most important 'external' relationships are with health professionals, especially experienced specialists in the
condition of concern to the group. More than half of the groups analysed here
report 'close relations' with physicians. Medical professionals participate in the
foundation of groups and remain members. Groups value access to medical
knowledge and information about services, as well as doctors informing
patients about the groups. They also emphasize opportunities for promoting
improvement of service provision and raising their public profile. And more
than 80 per cent of collective advocacy groups consider (selected) health
professionals as their partners in the common representation of the groups'
concerns. Various concepts in the literature have tried to capture the essence of
such relations, some stressing symmetry as in Epstein's concept of 'interpene-
tration' (2008) or Rabeharisoa's concept of 'partnership' (2003); others suggest
asymmetry, for example Kelleher's notion of 'colonization' (2006). The strong
inclination of Austrian groups towards 'sympathetic' health professionals, especially when it comes to advocating interests, indicates a rather dependent position. Nevertheless the great majority of groups analysed assess themselves as
being able to achieve their goals vis-à-vis health care stakeholders, and most
intend to increase their involvement in reshaping the health care system.

Health policy stakeholders seem to be less accessible and relevant to collective advocacy groups. Most claim to have relationships with actors in the political system, especially at the Länder level, but these are mostly considered to be 'loose'. Maintenance of self-organization and improvement of care are central issues. In interest advocacy, these groups assess themselves as much less assertive vis-à-vis health policy than health care. But variation between groups concerning intensity of relations and assertiveness is high – and this might depend on the strategic and social skills of particular group members, as well as on opportunities to develop stable, trusting personal relationships. This interpretation is supported by what have been observed as the main reasons for failed political activism by such groups: lack of knowledge of political processes, poor access to and interest on the part of decision-makers, and lack of support from the media and health professionals.

Relationships between collective advocacy groups and social health insurance funds are the most diverse, consultative relations around issues like self-help support, service provision and quality having been built up in only half the Länder. This also reflects insurance institutions' lack of a common policy towards self-help groups.

Cross-condition Self-help Alliances and their Collective Advocacy Role

Cross-condition alliances have emerged in eight of the nine Länder, reflecting their common interest in establishing self-help support institutions. Alliances are organized formally and their members are various condition-specific groups. Some of these regional alliances have started to include collective advocacy for general patient interests. The organizational capacity for this stems from their professional competence as well as from organizational know-how gained in self-help support work. Alliances gain legitimacy by having a broad membership base. Yet the main incentive for membership seems to be access to support and resources rather than identification with common concerns.

As far as the capacity to manage conflict is concerned, the situation is diverse. For example, access of regional alliances to various governance bodies varies considerably between Länder. While some have gained access to ethics committees, bodies for compensation claims, or even the above-mentioned Health Platforms, others remain outside these structures. It is not clear whether access has been denied, not offered or not even requested by the alliances concerned. Alliance representatives on these bodies consider the main benefit of participation to be proximity to ongoing developments. They complain that decision-making seems opaque and that important decisions are predetermined by traditional stakeholders (in the corporatist tradition of Austrian health policy), thus sometimes making official deliberations merely tokenistic.

In 2000, regional alliances and self-help support institutions established an informal national alliance, which also cooperates with (some) condition-specific groups at the national level. Originally focused on improving self-help support quality and promoting public acceptance of self-help groups, the national alliance now seeks to represent general patient interests. This has so far proved difficult. Interview data indicate disagreements about common concerns and priorities, lack of a clear mandate for spokespersons and a severe lack of resources. So far the national alliance has established only a few, weakly structured relationships with the main stakeholders. National government authorities have so far ignored the national alliance, neither offering support nor providing access to governance bodies.

Perspectives of Main Stakeholders

Representatives of the relevant stakeholders in our study generally welcomed the inner-oriented functions of self-help groups. All stakeholders vaguely endorse a stronger patient voice. Yet expectations and preconditions formulated by other stakeholders seem incompatible with the current organizational characteristics of the self-help field in Austria, and, potentially, also with the autonomy of their work in general. The vision of the main actors in health care governance is to gather all groups into a single alliance. This alliance would have to accept the rules of the political game and eschew financial support from commercial companies, especially pharmaceutical ones. The alliance would have to be strong enough to give a clear mandate to representatives who are competent and not motivated by self-interest, and whose continuity in office is secure.

SUMMARY AND CONCLUSIONS

We began by pointing to the macro context of political culture in Austria. For a long time it was strongly moulded by a tradition of party dominance, corporatism, clientelism and paternalism, as well as weak development of political self-organization and civil society institutions. But as the established modes of interest articulation have grown weaker more pluralistic modes have developed and new kinds of political activism and lobbying have begun to emerge.

At least in the perspective of many political actors, health care is a field where it is easy to lose voter support when problems emerge. Specialized acute care is highly developed, consumer satisfaction is the highest in Europe and expectation of continuous improvement of services is widespread. Many options for consumer choice in the public and the private sector, and extrajudicial mechanisms for complaint and redress, contribute to individualistic strategies of health consumer involvement. As challenges increase, more conflicts and struggles are likely to arise. The decentralized and fragmented system certainly offers opportunities for influencing health policies by well-organized interest groups, including health consumer groups.

Health consumer activism in Austria is connected mainly to the growing field of self-help groups. Their prevailing function is mutual exchange and support, offering a complementary role to professional care. This function is central for inner-focused legitimacy (meeting member expectations), as well as outer-focused legitimacy (recognition and support from key external stakeholders), and also constitutive for building cross-condition alliances. Yet many self-help groups and organizations, as well as some cross-condition alliances, have also developed ambitions to advocate collectively, thus complementing their inner-oriented activities with outer-oriented ones, articulating interests vis-à-vis health care providers, health policy, the media and the public. In this their overall impact so far has been modest.

Organizational capacity implies strong common concerns, availability of knowledge and resources, and the ability to reconcile diverging expectations, various interests and identities. The organizational capacity of condition-specific self-help groups was assessed generally as being low on average but highly variable. While cross-condition alliances have a fairly stable organizational basis as a result of running publicly subsidized support institutions, only some of them use this for political representation, depending on their overall priorities and different regional opportunity structures.

A second crucial prerequisite is conflict capacity in politically relevant matters. We understand this as the capacity to hold or command resources that established health care stakeholders consider relevant for their public standing and in the political struggles in which they are engaged. A first overall indicator of low general conflict capacity is the fact that Austrian health consumer and patient groups have so far been denied formal participation in most health care governance. Health policy stakeholders get away with paying lip-service to the desirability of better health consumer representation while simultaneously referring to a lack of necessary preconditions in the self-help field. Thus groups and alliances usually have to use informal means to gain access to and influence health care governance.

For many groups a main strategy to overcome lack of organizational and conflict capacity seems to be intense partnership with medical specialists, including common representation of interests. This strategy suggests itself as particular doctors not only seem to be prepared to cooperate but also hold highly influential positions in Austrian health policy. The price that self-help groups presumably pay for such partnership is a bias towards interests that are compatible with doctors' interests, in so far as they increase doctors' legitimacy and 'territory'. Furthermore, the apparent identity of consumer and provider interests might make the other relevant stakeholders reluctant to engage with these groups.

In the climate of uncertainty created by the global economic crisis, tighter budgets and increasing challenges for health policy, future development is difficult to predict. It can, however, be assumed that the conflicts in health policy which were on the rise in recent years will become aggravated and that more lobbying activism will undermine the prevailing corporatist governance style of Austrian health policy. This will provide new opportunities but also new risks. From our analysis, it seems questionable whether many self-help groups – including their alliances – have developed their capacities sufficiently to make the voice of patients and health consumers more audible in an increasingly complex political environment.

NOTES

1. The results of this first comprehensive study are in obvious disagreement with a recently published report, 'The Patient Movement in Austria' (*HCSNews International* 2009). This report is based on a very sketchy understanding of the situation, and also on misleading and partly wrong data, and should not be regarded as a reliable source.
2. The study was conducted at the Institute of Sociology, University of Vienna, in collaboration with Ludwig Boltzmann Institute Health Promotion Research and funded by the Austrian Health Promotion Agency (FGÖ), the Federation of Austrian Social Security Institutions, Vienna Health Promotion, and the Länder Kärnten and Vorarlberg.

REFERENCES

Bachinger, G. (2008), 'Außergerichtliche Streitbeilegung', in G. Aigner, A. Kletecka, M. Klectecka-Pulker and M. Memmer (eds), *Handbuch Medizinrecht für die Praxis*, Vienna: Manz, pp. II/51–II/81.

Baggott, R., J. Allsop and K. Jones (2005), *Speaking for Patients and Carers. Health Consumer Groups and the Policy Process*, Basingstoke: Palgrave Macmillan.

Baggott, R. and R. Forster (2008), 'Health consumer and patients' organizations in Europe: towards a comparative analysis', *Health Expectations*, **11** (1): 85–94.

Brix, E. (2003), 'Liberales und Kommunitaristisches in der österreichischen Gesellschaft', in E. Brix and P. Kampits (eds), *Zivilgesellschaft zwischen Liberalismus und Kommunitarismus*, Vienna: Passagen Verlag, pp. 219–26.

Contradiopoulos, D. (2004), 'A sociological perspective on public participation in health care', *Social Science & Medicine*, **58** (2): 321–30.

Eichwalder, S. and M.M. Hofmarcher (2008), 'Failure to improve care outside hospitals', *Health Policy Monitor*, in S. Schlette, K. Blum and R. Busse (eds), *Health Policy Developments 11: Focus on Primary Care. Appropriateness, Transparency, National Strategies*, Verlag Bertelsmann Stiftun, accessed at www.hpm.org/survey/at/a11/2.

Epstein, S. (2008), 'Patient group and health movements', in E.J. Hackett, O.

Amsterdamska, M. Lynch and J. Wajcman (eds), *The Handbook of Science and Technology Studies*, 3rd edn, Cambridge, MA: MIT Press, pp. 499–539.

Esping-Andersen, G. (1990), *The Three Worlds of Welfare Capitalism*, Cambridge: Polity Press and Princeton University Press.

Forster, R. and M. Vyslouzil (1991), 'Patient advocacy in Austria', *Medicine and Law*, **10** (4): 335–40.

Forster, R., G. Braunegger-Kallinger, P. Nowak and S. Österreicher (2009), 'Funktionen gesundheitsbezogener Selbstorganisation – eine Analyse am Beispiel einer österreichischen Untersuchung', *SWS-Rundschau*, **49** (4): 468–90.

Geissler, J. (2004), *Organisierte Vertretung von Patienteninteressen. Patienten-Organisationen als gesundheitspolitische Akteure in Deutschland, Großbritannien und den USA*, Hamburg, Germany: Verlag Dr. Kovaĉ.

Gerlich, P. and R. Pfefferle (2006), 'Tradition und Wandel', in H. Dachs, P. Gerlich, H. Gottweis, H. Kramer, V. Lauber, W.C. Müller and E. Tálos (eds), *Politik in Österreich. Das Handbuch*, Vienna: Manz Verlag, pp. 501–11.

Gottweis, H. (1997), 'Neue soziale Bewegungen in Österreich', in H. Dachs, P. Gerlich, H. Gottweis, F. Horner, H. Kramer, V. Lauber, W.C. Müller and E. Tálos (eds), *Handbuch des politischen Systems Österreichs. Die zweite Republik*, 3rd edn, Vienna: Manz Verlag, pp. 342–58.

Groth, S. (1999), 'Bewegte Frauengesundheit', in S. Groth and E. Rasky (eds), *Frauengesundheiten*, Innsbruck, Austria: Studienverlag, pp. 84–97.

Health Consumer Powerhouse (2007), *Euro Health Consumer Index 2007*, Brussels, Stockholm, Winnipeg.

Hirschman, A.O. (1970), *Exit, Voice and Loyalty: Response to Decline in Firms, Organisations, and States*, Cambridge, MA: Harvard University Press.

Hofmarcher, M. and H. Rack (2006), *Health Systems in Transition: Austria – Health System Review*, European Observatory of Health Systems and Health Policy, Vienna: Medizinisch Wissenschaftliche Verlagsgesellschaft.

Jones, K. (2007), 'Building alliances: incentives and impediments in the UK health consumer group sector', *Social Policy and Society*, **6** (4): 515–28.

Karlhofer, F. (2007), 'Filling the gap? Korporatismus und neue Akteure in der Politikgestaltung', *Österreichische Zeitschrift für Politikwissenschaft*, **36** (4): 389–403.

Katz, A.H. and E.I. Bender (1976), *The Strength in Us. Self-Help Groups in the Modern World*, New York: New Viewpoints.

Kelleher, D. (2006), 'Self-help groups and their relationship to medicine', in J. Gabe, D. Kelleher and G. Williams (eds), *Challenging Medicine*, 2nd edn, London and New York: Routledge, pp. 104–21.

Kopetzki, C. (2006), 'Patientenrechte in Österreich – Entwicklungen und Fehlentwicklungen', in G. Kern and C. Kopetzki (eds), *Patientenrechte und ihre Handhabung*, Vienna: Verlag Österreich, pp. 13–32.

Leopold, C., C. Habl, S. Morak, I. Rosian and S. Vogler (2008), *Leistungsfähigkeit des österreichischen Gesundheitssystems im internationalen Vergleich*, Vienna: Gesundheit Österreich GmbH.

Lindsay, S. and H.J.M. Vrijhoef (2009), 'Introduction: a sociological focus on "expert patients"', *Health Sociology Review*, **18** (2): 139–44.

McCormick, S., P. Brown and S. Zavestoski (2003), 'The personal is scientific, the scientific is political: the public paradigm of the environmental breast cancer movement', *Sociological Forum*, **18** (4): 545–76.

Offe, C. (1974), 'Politische Herrschaft und Klassenstrukturen – Zur Analyse spätkapitalistischer Gesellschaftssysteme', in H.P. Wiedmaier (ed.), *Politische Ökonomie des Wohlfahrtsstaates. Eine kritische Darstellung der Neuen Politischen Ökonomie*, Frankfurt am Main, Germany: Fischer, pp. 264–93.

Peinhaupt, C., A. Keclik, B. Greiner, P. Nowak and J.M. Pelikan (2004), 'Patient role in integrated care: concepts, experiences and challenges in Austria', *Integrated Care Digital Library*, Article 54: 1–21, International Network of Integrated Care: accessed 27 May 2010 at www.integratedcarenetwork.org/publish/articles/000054/article_print.html.

Pelinka, A. (2009), 'Das politische System Österreichs', in W. Ismayr (ed.), *Die politischen Systeme Westeuropas*, Wiesbaden, Germany: Verlag für Sozialwissenschaften, pp. 607–41.

Rabeharisoa, V. (2003), 'The struggle against neuromuscular diseases in France and the emergence of the "Partnership Model" of patient organisation', *Social Science & Medicine*, **57** (11): 2127–36.

Robinson, D. and S. Henry (1977), *Self-Help and Health: Mutual Aid for Modern Problems*, London: Martin Robertson.

Saltman, R., R. Busse and J. Figueras (2004), *Social Health Insurance Systems in Western Europe*, Maidenhead: Open University Press.

Saltman, R. (2004), 'Social health insurance in perspective: the challenge of sustaining stability', in R. Saltman, R. Busse and J. Figueras (eds), *Social Health Insurance Systems in Western Europe*, Maidenhead: Open University Press, pp. 3–20.

Stichweh, R. (2005), *Inklusion und Exklusion. Studien zur Gesellschaftstheorie*, Bielefeld, Germany: Transcript-Verlag.

Stremlow, J., S. Gysel, and E. Mey (2004), *'Es gibt Leute, die das Gleiche haben ...'. Selbsthilfe und Gesundheitsförderung in der deutschen Schweiz*, Lucerne, Switzerland: Hochschule für soziale Arbeit.

Tálos, E. (2005), *Vom Siegeszug zum Rückzug. Sozialstaat Österreich 1945–2005*, Innsbruck, Austria: Studien Verlag.

Tálos, E. (2006), ´Sozialpartnerschaft. Austrokorporatismus am Ende?', in H. Dachs, P. Gerlich, H. Gottweis, H. Kramer, V. Lauber, W.C. Müller and E. Tálos (eds), *Politik in Österreich. Das Handbuch*, Vienna: Manz Verlag, pp. 425–42.

Trojan, A. (2006), 'Selbsthilfezusammenschlüsse als vierte Säule des Gesundheitswesens?', *Jahrbuch für Kritische Medizin*, 43: 86–104.

11. Malaysia: the consumer voice in the policy process

Simon Barraclough and Phua Kai Lit

In seeking to theorize the role of social movements in health, Brown and Zavestoski suggest three 'ideal types' (Brown and Zavestoski 2005: 7–8). Health access movements seek equity and improvements in health care, while embodied health movements approach 'disease, disability or illness experience by challenging science on aetiology, diagnosis, treatment and prevention' (Brown and Zavestoski 2005: 7). The third type, constituency-based movements, target health inequalities proceeding from factors such as race, ethnicity, gender, class and sexual preference. Overlapping concerns are possible in this typology, but it serves to alert the analyst to the social factors influencing health consumer movements.

In Malaysia, health access groups have been the most significant, although they can hardly be described as movements with a mass membership. A number of illness-related organizations have lobbied the government on specific issues (for example, HIV/AIDS, mental health, heart disease and cancer). Constituency groups have not been significant; despite the country's ethnically plural population, there have not been notable demands for health care based upon ethnic considerations, with the exception of advocacy for the *Orang Asli* (Aborigines of Peninsular Malaysia). However, consumer bodies claiming a population-wide constituency have been active for 40 years, arguing for equitable access to health care for all Malaysians and improvements in the health system. They have challenged the commodification of heath care by the medical profession, asserting the need for preventive care and recognition of the social determinants of illness.

Two major consumer organizations have been conspicuous in their efforts to influence national health care policy: the Consumers' Association of Penang (CAP) and the Federation of Malaysian Consumers Associations (FOMCA). To explain their role in seeking to 'democratize health' it is necessary to understand the dynamics of both the political system and the formulation of health care policy.

THE MALAYSIAN POLITICAL SYSTEM

Malaysia is a federation, but the central government controls almost all policy areas, including health services. The country has enjoyed impressive rates of long-term economic growth and is now a middle-income nation aspiring to achieve developed status by the year 2020.

Malaysia's political system is substantially different from the liberal democratic polities described in other chapters of this book. Crouch has characterized Malaysia as having a 'repressive-responsive regime' that remains in power through a combination of repression, manipulation and responsiveness (Crouch 1996: 240–47). The political system has three major features: the primacy of ethnic factors, the close management of civil society participation by the regime, and the continuity of governance by various compositions of the original coalition party that negotiated Malayan independence from Britain in 1957 and the subsequent formation of Malaysia in 1963.

Malaysia's political parties are for the most part ethnically based, some more substantially than others. In the 2000 Census, Malays (with the smaller populations of other so-called indigenous groups) were the largest ethnic group, comprising approximately 66 per cent of the population, compared with 25 per cent Chinese and 7.5 per cent Indians (Department of Statistics Malaysia 2008). The government is formed by a multi-ethnic coalition – the Barisan Nasional (National Front) – dominated by the United Malays National Organization (UMNO). The National Front claims that this coalition provides national cohesion through the representation in government of all the major ethnic groups.

Ethnic factors have often divided Malaysians. Ramasamy avers that

> the state, by a combination of coercive and non-coercive measures, has succeeded in imposing a particular kind of ethnic ideology in the society as a whole. Non-ethnic contestations have been raised from time to time, but they fall short of seriously challenging the ideological basis of the state. (Ramasamy 2004: 214)

Another significant feature of the political system for civil society is that Malaysia's version of democracy has historically been closely managed by the regime. Opposition political parties have been permitted and have even won office in several states, although never at the federal level. Interest groups have been accorded limited access to the policy process. However, political participation has always been subject to limitations, controlled coverage by the mass media, and legislation restricting the political agenda. Most major television and radio stations are operated by the national government. Malaysia's major newspapers and some electronic media are dominated by owners close to the ruling coalition. Self-censorship is widely practised, leading many Malaysians to turn to the internet for political information and opinions.

Almost three decades ago, the National Front government attempted closer regulation of the activities and affiliations of interest groups. Under amendments to the Societies Act an organization could be designated a 'political society' and closely controlled if it sought 'in any manner' to influence public policy or the operations of government at national or state level (quoted in Barraclough 1984: 451–2). Facing concerted opposition to these amendments from several Malaysian civil society groups, including CAP, the government offered a partial compromise, revising the legislation to remove the category 'political society' and the need for official approval of international affiliations (Barraclough 1984: 459). This episode set the tone for closely managed 'rules of engagement' for civil society groups in the policy process for the following two decades. During the prime ministership of Dr Mahathir bin Mohamed political participation was tightly controlled. In 1987 more than 100 civil society activists were detained without trial under the Internal Security Act.

The departure of Mahathir in 2004 was followed by a more accepting attitude to the role of interest groups. The new leader, Abdullah Badawi, observed that 'NGOs function as a check and balance to inform the Government about its shortcomings ... They also help ensure that the government's programmes are implemented effectively' (*New Straits Times* 2004). The administration of Najib Abdul Razak, Badawi's successor in 2009, has maintained a similar position in relation to civil society.

A further problem for civil society groups seeking to engage in the political process, as well as for researchers of their role and influence, is a long-standing culture of secrecy in governance. Few detailed policy documents are made public and the flow of information is closely managed. Individuals from consumer groups participating in policy consultations face the paradox of being given access to the policy process by dint of representing their group, yet being denied permission to report on the proceedings to their organization or to use information gained through these consultations. Even development of one of Malaysia's most important health care policies – the National Health Financing Scheme – has been subject to almost total secrecy, leading FOMCA to lament that the policy 'is set to bring about a total restructuring and reform of the national healthcare system but as of yet, details of it are vague and the development progress [sic] lacks transparency and civil society participation' (FOMCA 2008: 3).

THE MALAYSIAN HEALTH CARE SYSTEM: FROM WELFARISM TO PLURALISM

In the past 25 years, the Malaysian health care system has undergone substantial change. In 1991, Roemer considered Malaysia to have an essentially welfare-based health system in which the government ensured subsidized direct provision of curative care (Roemer 1991: 129). As well as government hospitals, there were some charitable hospitals cross-subsidizing poorer patients with revenue from richer patients. In parallel with government services, the private sector offered specialist, general practice and dental services. However, private hospitals operated by profit-seeking corporations gradually became part of the Malaysian health care system, encouraged by the government and responding to rising levels of wealth (Barraclough 1997). Approximately 25 per cent of hospital beds are now in the private sector.

The ascent of Mahathir to the prime ministership in 1981, in the wake of Margaret Thatcher's new market-oriented and anti-welfarist Conservative government in the United Kingdom, was followed quickly by his adoption of neo-liberal ideology and policies, including privatization (Phua 2001). The mobilization of CAP, FOMCA and other groups in the debate over neo-liberal policies in the health services sector and the privatization of public hospitals can be considered a reaction to this change in the government's formerly welfarist approach to health care policy. The government privatized the hospital pharmaceutical drug supply system, corporatized some hospitals and privatized hospital maintenance and waste disposal services (Barraclough 1999). In introducing the Seventh Malaysia Plan (the official economic blueprint) in 1996, Prime Minister Mahathir stated that the government intended 'to privatize many health facilities, including hospitals and specialist units' (quoted in Barraclough 1999: 60).

The growth of the private sector, moves away from a universal welfare model and increasing privatization posed new challenges for consumer representatives in Malaysia. Their role in monitoring 'value for money' and quality of care was intensified by the rapid growth of private hospitals and the more intensive use of medical technology. Many Malaysians were increasingly becoming customers in a health care market driven by the profit motive, rather than citizens exercising their civic rights to public care. There were concerns that overcharging and overtreatment were occurring. Quality of care and patients' rights had previously been largely the preserve of the Ministry of Health since the overwhelming majority of Malaysians were treated in government hospitals. But who would now press for the rights of the increasing number of Malaysians using the private sector?

Alongside the traditional functional concern of consumer organizations was an ideological challenge to the government's stated goals of reducing the public financing of health care and privatizing the public agencies responsible for its delivery. This was a particularly political challenge since opposition to such policies brought consumer organizations into fundamental conflict with the governments. Such a challenge would inevitably be used by political parties contesting the electoral process as evidence of opposition to the government policy and support for the opposition policy.

Health Care as a Public Policy Issue

Historically, most medical services were provided in government hospitals and health centres, and public policy for health care was largely a matter for the health minister and civil servants, with occasional consultations with representatives of medical bodies. Health care policy was rarely on the political agenda. As Snodgrass observed in his 1980 study of equity in Malaysia's economic development, in comparison with education policy 'health has been relatively neglected by citizens, politicians and analysts alike' (Snodgrass 1980: 260).

In terms of the role of consumer groups in the Malaysian democratic process, health care serves a unifying purpose and also gives these groups potential political influence since access to health care is a sensitive political issue for the ruling coalition. Health care is a basic necessity for all, regardless of ethnicity or social class. Those Malaysians dependent upon public care – especially in rural and remote areas – fear privatization policies. Many middle-class Malaysians are sympathetic towards state-subsidized health care and do not want to see the dismantling of welfare provisions. These sentiments stem from both altruism and self-interest since in times of economic recession they might lose their jobs and hence also employer-funded health care insurance and the income to pay for out-of-pocket costs. Most significantly, from a political perspective, health care, unlike policy issues such as education, culture and religion, is not ethnically divisive. Nonetheless, it is clear that any reduction in the public provision of health care is especially sensitive in predominantly Malay rural constituencies and is therefore of particular concern to UMNO.

The Rationale for Consumer Group Participation in the Policy Process

Consumer group participation in policy development can serve several functions for a political system, such as alerting the government to the interests of lower socio-economic sections of the population and to particular problems with health care. Consumer groups can articulate citizen interests to decision-makers and assert societal values. Sometimes they also develop new policy ideas through their own research and networks. By aggregating interests, consumer groups contribute to a more manageable policy process, allowing decision-makers to consult with key representatives, thereby saving time and human resources. Consumer participation and consultation are important elements in legitimizing policy in democratic political systems. Finally, consumer groups can assist in disseminating information from policymakers to those affected by the policy.

In Malaysia, the potential for interest groups to contribute to policymaking in the field of health care has received only limited official endorsement. For example, writing in 2002 about future needs, Ministry of Health officials identified a need to establish a 'National Health Advisory Council' to represent stakeholders and offer advice to the Ministry (Merican and Rohaizat 2002: 21). But the Ministry's strategic plan for 2006–8 listed no concrete strategies to achieve these ends (Ministry of Health 2008). To date, no advisory council has been convened.

MALAYSIAN CONSUMER GROUPS

A problem for health consumer groups in any political system concerns their fundamental role. Should they restrict their public policy activities to seeking the best value for customers within a health care market and watching over the quality and safety of goods and services, or should they articulate broader societal values such as equity of access?

Many Malaysian consumers of health care – most notably those unable to pay for private care, and civil servants who are entitled to heavily subsidized public care – do not operate in a market: care is provided by the government for free or for a nominal sum and there are limited opportunities to seek alternative government services, especially in rural areas. Yet alongside government services is an ever-growing array of commercial, for-profit providers, operating in a competitive environment and providing goods and services for those able to pay. Malaysia's major consumer groups are mindful of both an operational role representing consumer interests and a wider role promoting equity within the health care system. FOMCA has summarized its work in stating that 'it goes beyond the traditional role of consumer protection in the marketplaces, which has been called the "value for money" approach. Instead FOMCA advocates the "value for people", "value for the environment" and "value for money" paradigm' (FOMCA 2009b: 3).

Malaysian health consumer organizations perform some of the functions of equal health advocates, identified in the United States by Alford (1975). Many consumers, particularly those of lower socio-economic status, are unable to articulate their interests against dominant structural interests, especially professional monopolists (the medical and dental professions), who are 'served by the structure of social, economic and political institutions' (Alford 1975: 14). In Alford's discussion of interests in the US health care system, equal health care advocates and professional monopolists are not always opposed. This phenomenon is also evident in Malaysia where health consumer groups have joined the Malaysian Medical Association (MMA) in criticizing moves towards privatization, yet on other issues have endorsed government policy opposed by the MMA.

Another difficulty for Malaysian consumer groups involved in health policy derives from their status as generic consumer organizations. Both FOMCA and CAP represent consumers in a wide range of fields of which health is but one and health care a subset of that field. Lacking the expertise required for analysis of more technical health care issues, they risk being disadvantaged when participating in policy deliberations.

Both FOMCA and CAP seek to influence policy by several means. Both submit annual memoranda to the government at national budget time. Lobbying and written communications are used in response to particular issues. Regular use is made of the mass media and the CAP publishes its own periodical, *Utusan Konsumer*. It also publishes booklets on specific health-related issues. FOMCA publishes *Consumer Digest* twice yearly. Both bodies hold public seminars and events devoted to raising public awareness of health issues. Finally, in varying degrees, they participate in permanent and ad-hoc official bodies and in dialogue sessions to offer policy advice.

The Federation of Malaysian Consumer Associations

FOMCA is Malaysia's principal national consumer organization and is composed of 16 affiliated consumer groups in various states. It is affiliated with Consumers International, a global coalition of consumer organizations, and is regarded favourably by the government as the voice of Malaysian consumers.

FOMCA performs a significant operational role in the health sector since health services are included in the brief of the National Consumer Complaints Centre (NCCC). Established by FOMCA in collaboration with and financially supported by the Ministry of Domestic Trade, Co-operatives and Consumerism, this service deals with all kinds of consumer complaints. FOMCA is regarded by the Ministry as playing 'a positive role in complementing the government's effort to protect, promote and safeguard the consumers' (NCCC 2008: 3). Given the size of Malaysia's population, the number of health care complaints processed has been modest; in 2008, a total of 208 health service complaints were received (NCCC 2008: 83). Despite this small number, FOMCA has succeeded in gaining recognition for a direct consumer complaints mechanism at arm's length from the government and the medical establishment.

FOMCA is also included on a number of government committees and bodies concerned with industrial standards, including medical devices, food, agriculture and beverages. Food is the policy area in which FOMCA has enjoyed the highest degree of official recognition and involvement with the Ministry of Health. It also serves on various national technical and advisory bodies, and is represented on the National Codex Alimentarius Committee and its subcommittees. However this substantial engagement with food policy bodies is not matched in health care. Although FOMCA is a member of the Ministry of Health Technical Advisory Committee on Continuous Medical Education and Consumer Education, no permanent consultative body on health care has been established.

An examination of FOMCA's annual memoranda to the government reveals aspects of both its operational role and its engagement with fundamental societal values. FOMCA articulates a discourse strongly counter to that of neo-liberal elements seeking to change the shape of Malaysia's health care system.

FOMCA presents some of the changes in public policy on health care as a problem, arguing that past achievements are threatened by moves to reduce real levels of public expenditure on health care. According to FOMCA, the 'government's health financing through taxes and other public revenues have [*sic*] achieved laudable coverage for primary health care' (FOMCA 2009a: 2). However, the Malaysian government's expenditure on health care still falls short of the 5 per cent of the budget recommended by the World Health Organization and in recent years the growth of private health care has reflected a 'slowdown in public healthcare expenditure' (FOMCA 2007: 3). FOMCA's equal health advocacy role is manifest in its demands that any national health financing scheme should be universal to ensure fairness and equity (FOMCA 2007: 3) and that the government should 'minimise the quality disparity' between the public and private sectors (FOMCA 2007: 4).

According to FOMCA, the growing private sector is so denuding the public sector of staff that there is risk of the 'eventual collapse of the public health-care sector'. The government therefore needs to protect and sustain public health care (FOMCA 2009a: 3). FOMCA is particularly concerned that medical tourism will divert scarce resources from the public health care system.

FOMCA is also strongly opposed to 'fee-for-service' payment, arguing that it tends to cause overtreatment, thus contributing to cost escalation. It rejects any further moves to privatize the public health care system, asserting that previous privatizations have resulted in higher costs without much improvement in quality and efficiency (FOMCA 2007: 4).

The threat of privatization to equity is emphasized in reference to the private sector:

> A look at our private health sector and how it operates and [is] motivated solely by profit should be able to give us an insight into the repercussions of the move to encourage privatisation in parts of the public health sector. While the rich in Malaysia may have healthcare services at luxury private hospitals, the poor have to wait in long queues at the government hospitals. (FOMCA 2008: 5–6)

In order to 'educate and empower the people' on health care issues, FOMCA argues that the government should provide more grants to non-government organizations (FOMCA 2007: 4).

At a functional level, FOMCA has encouraged the government to provide improved technical, communications and ethics training for health professionals, and higher levels of remuneration for public sector health workers (FOMCA 2007: 4; FOMCA 2009a: 3).

The Consumers' Association of Penang

Operating from Penang, and closely identified with the leadership of its long-standing president, Haji S.M. Mohamed Idris, CAP has always presented a more strident voice of consumer activism. It has pointedly declined to join FOMCA – founded some months after CAP – and has not shied away from commenting on contentious consumer issues, often more vociferously than FOMCA. Despite its geographically regional title and location in Penang, CAP has played a national role. Like FOMCA, CAP is also affiliated to Consumers International.

More than three decades ago CAP organized a major national seminar on health which included a formal declaration and resolutions, subsequently published by CAP (CAP 1987). The declaration highlighted rising costs, questioned their consequences for the equitable provision of services, urged prevention as a priority, and appealed for a holistic approach to health that recognized the impact of housing, water supply, sanitation and nutrition (CAP 1987: 36–7). These themes have continued in CAP's criticisms of the Malaysian health care system. In 2007 CAP called for 'a primary focus on public health measures that are aimed at safeguarding and improving the health of the public', and stressed the need to address 'the determinants of health – be they social, political, environmental or lifestyle' (CAP 2007).

The Declaration also affirmed democratic principles:

> Health is not only the government's business; it should be made the people's. A concept and policy of community health should be developed as health is too serious a matter to be left only to the government or the medical service. The community should ... participate in arriving at better health for all. Meanwhile public concerns should be mobilised in a watchdog role. (CAP 1987: 37)

In certain cases, CAP has vigorously opposed some health care policies, especially the privatization of health services. In a memorandum to the Minister of Health in 1995 it argued that:

> The Government's rationale for privatisation just does not hold water because statistics show that the Government is not spending much on health care. Health is a

basic need … It is therefore the Government's responsibility to provide health care
to its people … We therefore urge the Government to retain the present Government
health services and control the costs of private services. (CAP 1995)

CAP's concept of fairness in financing has led to demands that the policy of
offering public hospital outpatient and clinic services to all citizens at a heavily subsidized price, or for free for those unable to pay, be changed to a means-
tested system. Those able to pay would be charged for a greater proportion of
the cost of their treatment, thereby generating income for the public sector
(S.M. Mohamed Idris 2004).

CAP has also strongly criticized the national medical tourism policy under
which the Ministry of Health has established a number of committees in
collaboration with the Association of Private Hospitals of Malaysia to regulate
and facilitate health services for foreign patients. In CAP's view, this diverts
health care professionals from the public to the private sector and allows
public resources to be used to promote private for-profit activities. CAP has
decried the decision of the Ministry of Health to permit the publicly owned
National Heart Institute to recruit foreign patients under the medical tourism
policy (S.M. Mohamed Idris 2009).

As well as opposing certain health care policies, CAP has supported those
it considers beneficial to consumers. For example, in January 2010 CAP's
president, Haji Mohamed Idris, countered criticisms from the MMA about an
initiative to establish public primary health clinics in urban areas throughout
Malaysia. The MMA president had criticized the policy as hastily conceived
and allowing medical assistants (health auxiliaries), rather than qualified
doctors, to provide primary care (*The Star* 2010). In supporting the policy Idris
claimed that this timely programme would provide an urban equivalent to the
rural clinics that had successfully served the needs of the rural population
since the 1960s. He further predicted that people from lower socio-economic
backgrounds would prefer public clinics (S.M. Mohamed Idris 2010).

The Coalition Against Health Care Privatization

The involvement of CAP and FOMCA in the mobilization of opposition to
government policy on health sector privatization represents a major chapter in
their role in participatory democracy. This opposition was clearly ideological in
that it sought to challenge neo-liberal directions in a policy area characterized
historically by a state commitment to welfare policies and equity. It was also
undisguisedly political, seeking to unify a cross-section of civil society against
articulated government policy on an increasingly electorally sensitive subject.
Both FOMCA and CAP found themselves in a coalition, which included not
only health and welfare interest groups but also opposition political parties.

The coalition was an organizational manifestation of growing concerns about the government's effort to reorientate the health care system towards greater private provision. These concerns had led in 1997 to the formation of the Citizens' Health Initiative (CHI) in the wake of a national conference on privatization and health care financing, conducted under the auspices of CAP, Universiti Sains Malaysia and the MMA. The CHI, in turn, promulgated the 'Citizens' Health Manifesto', advocating the preservation of equity in the face of neo-liberal policy changes. The Manifesto was supported by several civil society organizations. Disturbingly for the government, it was also endorsed by two opposition parties, the Democratic Action Party and *Parti Rakyat Malaysia*. The politicization of health care as a policy issue deeply concerned the government. On the eve of the 1999 general elections it announced that public hospitals and clinics would not be corporatized further and that government funding of public hospitals would be increased (Chee and Barraclough 2007a).

Despite the government's reconsideration of privatization policies, in 2004 it announced the introduction of private wings in public hospitals, allowing government specialists the right to practise privately in government hospitals, and the privatization of hospital pharmacies. It was suggested that a future 'National Health Financing Scheme' would involve compulsory contributions by all Malaysian workers and would permit the use of private hospitals. Moreover, purchase of private health insurance would be encouraged (Chee and Barraclough 2007a).

In response to these proposals, in 2005 the Coalition Against Health Care Privatization was formed, with the backing of 81 NGOs, trade unions and political parties, many of which had been involved with the Citizens' Health Manifesto. The Coalition argued that all Malaysians should have access to comprehensive care irrespective of their financial means. More specifically, it argued that any future financing scheme should not be based on fee for service, and that there should be no more privatization of any public health services. Democratic values were also affirmed through the demand that local health and hospital boards be established to permit local citizen involvement in governance of the system (Chee and Barraclough 2007b).

While not leading the Coalition, both FOMCA and CAP have been active participants. This has given these consumer groups access to a range of individuals and organizations with specific system expertise and has permitted them to articulate wider policy concerns in concert with like-minded bodies.

Social movement theory – especially its 'resource mobilization' variant – focuses on how civil society groups mobilize and deploy resources to achieve movement objectives and goals in conditions where their efforts may be opposed by other groups or by the state. Resources used by social movements include new technology, economic resources, ideologies, symbols and rhetorical efforts to 'frame' the debate in their favour. Success or failure can be crucially affected by the quality of leadership, the existence of pre-existing solidarity or communication networks, timing, and political or professional connections (Scott and Marshall 2009).

Thus the civil society groups that mobilized against neo-liberal policies in health have argued that continued government funding and provision of highly subsidized health care services have helped to promote social solidarity. Civil society activists provided effective leadership while making use of often over-lapping, pre-existing solidarity and communication networks (such as the Penang-based Aliran social justice movement, which offered the Coalition the use of its website). Allies in the form of sympathetic MMA office-holders and opposition political party leaders also contributed to the success of the NGO activists.

MALAYSIAN HEALTH CONSUMER GROUPS: ACHIEVEMENTS AND CHALLENGES

As this chapter has demonstrated, FOMCA and CAP have sought to contribute to health policy through both functional and political roles. In terms of democratic practice these groups have demanded transparency of process, parliamentary scrutiny of policy, and the right of civil society to participate in policymaking. The articulation of such demands is acceptable to the regime and the views of CAP and FOMCA are frequently reported in the regime-controlled mass media. These demands do not destabilize the political system since they do not touch upon officially designated 'sensitive issues' (race, language and religion); rather they give the political system a degree of democratic credibility.

To date, the functional role of consumer organizations has gained greater acceptance by the Ministry of Health and they have gradually gained limited official recognition as stakeholders in the policy process. FOMCA is funded by the government to run a complaints service, which includes health care complaints, and has been included in various official bodies concerned with food and nutrition policy.

The Malaysian Patient Safety Council, established in 2003, is specifically empowered to appoint representatives from consumer organizations, including CAP and FOMCA, alongside the Association of Private Hospitals Malaysia, teaching hospitals and divisions of the Ministry of Health. The Ministry's most recent documentation does not however identify participation by either CAP or FOMCA (Ministry of Health 2008). Ad hoc consultations with stakeholders in the health care system are arranged by the Ministry of Health and both FOMCA and CAP are invited to attend, but there is still an unwarranted degree of secrecy surrounding such interactions.

Despite occasional stakeholder consultations involving consumer groups in policy development, there is still no formal institutional recognition of such groups in the policy process. The National Health Advisory Council has yet to be realized. There is virtually no funding of consumer groups to participate in the policy process, although some funding of health promotion campaigns has occurred. By contrast, the Ministry of Health has set up a number of committees in collaboration with the Association of Private Hospitals Malaysia to further policy on medical tourism and has actively promoted the interests of private hospitals.

In their political roles, both FOMCA and CAP have offered an alternative and challenging discourse to that of neo-liberalism. At times, this counter-discourse is viewed sympathetically by certain civil servants in the Ministry of Health, many of whom are committed to preserving equity and are uncomfortable with a reformist policy agenda promoting privatization.

Through their associations with the Coalition Against Health Care Privatization, these consumer groups have been part of a movement which has transcended ethnic divisions and united various civil society elements in partially restraining public policy favourable to neo-liberal policies and reasserting the value of the public sector. Yet this wider political role poses risks to organizations whose articles of association ostensibly eschew politics. Although it did not eventuate, there was a risk for FOMCA and CAP that the Ministry would come to regard them as 'oppositional', especially as the Coalition was also endorsed by opposition political parties.

According to Alford (1975), the activities of particular US equal health advocacy groups may have improved health care available to the community but did not change the essential and inequitable structures of the system. These observations on the US health system are apposite for Malaysia. Both FOMCA and CAP have been strong advocates of a public system, opposing privatization and upholding equity as an essential value in policy. Yet despite their advocacy and the restraining influence of the Coalition Against Health Care Privatization, public policy has continued to embrace neo-liberal ideas and the private sector in health continues to grow. Consumer groups will need to develop a clearer policy approach to the realities of Malaysia's pluralistic health care system with a vision for how equity can be guaranteed and the interests of consumers of private health care upheld.

From the perspective of social class, the policy role of consumer groups, essentially led by a small group of urban middle-class activists, presents a contradiction. FOMCA and CAP are not mass-based organizations and they participate in what is essentially elite-based policymaking. It has been the growing middle class that has largely fuelled the demand for private facilities and which has benefited from health system pluralism, and yet the consumer groups' commitment to equity and public provision is of greater benefit to lower socio-economic groups. The Malaysian experience is not dissimilar however to that in Western developed countries where sometimes relatively small groups, with narrow membership bases, call upon the expertise of a coterie of supporters in an effort to influence policy.

At a practical level, it must be recognized that both FOMCA and CAP are generic consumer groups with limited specialist expertise in heath care and limited financial resources. While both consumer organizations usually have a full-time officer allocated to deal with health matters, this person's wide brief multiplies consultation invitations but leads to an inability to accept them. There is a need, therefore, for the creation of a specialized health consumer group similar to bodies in some other countries. How to finance such a body is problematic. A government subsidy might risk compromising independence, while funding from a foreign source might cause suspicion of interference in Malaysian internal affairs. Perhaps a consortium of Malaysian civil society bodies could provide expertise and assist in operating a secretariat, as was the case with the Coalition Against Health Care Privatization.

Certainly the nature of Malaysia's political system has placed constraints on the public policy role of Malaysian consumer organizations. Yet it is clear that FOMCA and CAP have succeeded in gaining both official, in-principle recognition of the legitimacy of consumer participation in health care policy and ad hoc access to consultations on policy. It is difficult to assess the influence on policy achieved by these two groups, given the secretive nature of the Malaysian policy process.

The Coalition Against Health Care Privatization, in which these consumer groups played an active role, undoubtedly caused the government to rethink both the extent and pace of its neo-liberal agenda. It is perhaps appropriate to conclude that the consumer voice in Malaysian health care policy is at an early stage of development, with considerable potential for intensification. This was, after all, the situation in many Western nations only three decades ago, when consumer demands for policy participation began to lead to the incorporation of consumer groups into the policy process. Indeed, the experience of such nations may cause Malaysian policymakers to realize that an advanced health care system needs institutionalized consumer participation and that the influence of the medical profession and other powerful interests in the policy process needs to be counterbalanced by representatives of those paying for and receiving health care.

ACKNOWLEDGEMENTS

The authors wish to thank both CAP and FOMCA for supplying documents relating to their activities. They also appreciate Hans Lofgren's and Mick

Leahy's comments on an earlier draft of this chapter. All opinions and any factual errors remain the responsibility of the authors.

REFERENCES

Alford, R. (1975), *Health Care Politics: Ideological and Interest Group Barriers to Reform*, Chicago, IL: The University of Chicago Press.

Barraclough, S. (1984), 'Political participation and its regulation in Malaysia: opposition to the Societies (Amendment) Act 1981', *Pacific Affairs*, **57** (3): 450–61.

Barraclough, S. (1997), 'The growth of corporate private hospitals in Malaysia: contradictions in health system pluralism', *International Journal of Health Services*, **27** (4): 643–59.

Barraclough, S. (1999), 'Constraints on the retreat from a welfare-oriented approach to public health care in Malaysia', *Health Policy*, **47**: 53–67.

Brown, P. and S. Zavestoski (eds) (2005), *Social Movements in Health*, Malden, MA: Blackwell Publishing.

Chee, H.L. and S. Barraclough (2007a), 'Introduction: the transformation of health care in Malaysia', in H.L. Chee and S. Barraclough (eds), *Health Care in Malaysia: The Dynamics of Provision, Financing and Access*, London: Routledge, pp.1–16.

Chee, H.L. and S. Barraclough (2007b), 'Epilogue: civil society and health care policy in Malaysia', in H.L. Chee and S. Barraclough (eds), *Health Care in Malaysia: The Dynamics of Provision, Financing and Access*, London: Routledge, pp. 208–17.

Consumers' Association of Penang (CAP) (1987), *Curing the Sick or the Rich? The Rising Cost of Medical Care in Malaysia*, Penang, Malaysia: Consumers' Association of Penang.

Consumers' Association of Penang (1995), 'Memorandum on privatisation of health services – is it justified?', submitted to Y.B. Dato Lee Kim Sai, Minister of Health, 1 March.

Consumers' Association of Penang (2007), 'National Health policy must focus primarily on public health', 30 August, accessed 28 January 2010 at www.en.cap.org.my/index.php?option=com_content&task=blogcategory&id=0&Itemid=3&limit=13&l imitstart=65.

Crouch, H. (1996), *Government and Society in Malaysia*, St Leonards, NSW: Allen and Unwin.

Department of Statistics Malaysia (2008), 'Population statistics', accessed 23 July 2010 at www.statistics.gov.my/english/frameset_census.php?file=pressdemo.

Federation of Malaysian Consumers Associations (FOMCA) (2007), 'Memorandum for the national budget consultation 2008', 20 April, Kuala Lumpur: FOMCA.

Federation of Malaysian Consumers Associations (2008), *National Budget 2009*, 30 March, Kaula Lumpur: FOMCA.

Federation of Malaysian Consumers Associations (2009a), 'Memorandum for the national budget consultation 2010', 22 May, Kuala Lumpur: FOMCA.

Federation of Malaysian Consumers Associations (2009b), *The Consumer Digest*, **1**: 1.

Merican, I. and Rohaizat bin Yon (2002), 'Health care reform and changes: the Malaysian experience', *Asia Pacific Journal of Public Health*, **14** (1): 17–22.

Ministry of Health (2008), *Malaysia. Strategic Plan 2006–2008*, Kuala Lumpur: Ministry of Health.

National Consumer Complaints Centre (NCCC) (2008), *Annual Report 2008*, Selangor, Malaysia: NCCC.

New Straits Times (2004), 'NGOs are our eyes and ears, says Abdullah', 11 May.

Phua, K.L. (2001), 'Corporatization and privatization of public services: origins and rise of a controversial concept', *Akademika*, **58**: 45–57.

Ramasamy, P. (2004), 'Civil society in Malaysia: an arena of contestation', in L.H. Guan (ed.), *Civil Society in Southeast Asia*, Singapore: Institute of Southeast Asian Studies, pp. 198–216.

Roemer, M.I. (1991), *National Health Systems of the World*, vol.1, New York: Oxford University Press.

Scott, J. and G. Marshall (2009), *Dictionary of Sociology*, revised edn, New York: Oxford University Press.

The Star (2010), accessed 10 January at www.thestar.com.my/news/story.asp?file=/2010/1/10/focus/5439349&sec=focus.

S.M. Mohamed Idris (2009), letter to the editor, *New Straits Times*, 6 November, accessed 29 January 2010, www.nst.com.my/Current_News/NST/articles/18put/Article/.

S.M. Mohamed Idris (2010), 'Gov't on right track with Malaysia clinics', *Malaysiakini*, accessed 8 January at www.malaysiakini.com/letters/121498.

Snodgrass, D.R. (1980), *Inequality and Economic Development in Malaysia*, Kuala Lumpur: Oxford University Press.

12. From activism to state inclusion: health consumer groups in Australia

Hans Löfgren, Michael Leahy and Evelyne de Leeuw

This chapter examines the experiences of Australian consumer groups at the interface with national health policy development. Many community groups concerned with health issues – women's organizations, disease-oriented patient support groups and older citizens' organizations – were formed long before their designation as 'consumer' groups. Members of health groups founded in the 1960s and 1970s understood themselves as activists for social change, not 'consumers' (Short 1998). Influenced by radical and collectivist political ideas, they challenged established models of health care and mobilized to redress inequities of access to care and inequalities of power between the medical profession and the 'lay' population. The major campaign in this period was to establish universal health insurance. Community activists played an important role in the achievement of such a scheme under the Whitlam Labor government (1972–75). Following its dismantling by the Fraser government (1975–83), they played a similar role in its restoration as Medicare in 1984.

The policy influence of the organized consumer movement peaked in the decade from the mid-1980s, when access to the policy table was provided for the first time under Labor governments federally and in several Australian states. Both peak and disease-oriented health consumer groups were increasingly funded by governments and integrated into mainstream policy processes. These gains, however, came at a price: in exchange for their recognition as legitimate policy actors, consumer groups came under mounting pressure to moderate their activist role to exclude systemic critique. Assured access to the policy table, we contend, has weakened the influence of the organized consumer movement by limiting its ability to autonomously mobilize critical patient, carer and community opinion. While it purported to enhance consumer engagement among service providers and policymakers, mainstreaming in fact reduced such engagement to ascertaining the views and experiences of service users, with users conceived of as individual consumers with 'rights to information, access, choice, and redress' (Gregory 2007: 17).

The role of the organized consumer movement was thus rendered only peripheral. Here we sketch the metamorphosis from social movement activism to co-option as marginal actors within the policy mainstream. Three political theories provide particular warrants for the contentions of this chapter.

First, the new public management (NPM) reform programme, based on neo-liberal ideology, was one source of pressure on health policy actors, including consumer groups. By defining health care provision as a market exchange, with 'choice' as the central value, neo-liberal ideology limited the role of consumer groups to protecting consumer interests in that exchange. Rather than questioning the definition itself on the democratic ground that 'the concept of consumer is defined by a philosophical world view that places importance on participation and representation as expressions of citizenship and social connection' (Carter and O'Connor 2003: 24), NPM converted public administration to fit the market paradigm. In so doing, we suggest, it sought to co-opt consumer groups to the limited role of protection of health consumer interests.

Second, Alford's influential model, which explains the health care policy contest in terms of competing 'structural interests' – the professional monopolists, the corporate rationalizers and the community interest – remains useful (Alford 1975; Duckett 1984). Typically, according to Alford, the community interest is repressed, even if it has periods of success, by one or both of the other interests. In essence, the professional monopolists are the medical profession; the corporate rationalizers the bureaucrats and policymakers in the government sector, and in public and private hospital administrations; and the community interest that of consumers. We shall argue that this analysis captures much of what has occurred in the health policy contest in Australia.

Third, Dryzek provides an insightful general perspective on relationships between governments and social movements. Actors based in civil society such as health consumer organizations 'sometimes face a choice between action in the public sphere and action within the state' (Dryzek 2000: 82). Dryzek contends that where the state seeks to exclude social interests, such groups have no choice but to mobilize autonomously outside the state. But where the state takes an inclusive approach and permeates civil society – as in Australia – such groups have a choice between action inside or outside the state. A choice to act inside the state does not, however, necessarily ensure advancement of the aims of a social movement or indeed broader democratic objectives. 'Benign inclusion' through cooperative policymaking mechanisms will further these aims only if two conditions hold: 'a group's defining concern must be capable of assimilation to an established or emerging state imperative [and] civil society's discursive capacities must not be unduly depleted by the group's entry into the state'. State imperatives operate 'irrespective of the desires or preferences of particular public officials' and include domestic order, economic prosperity (capital accumulation) and the legitimacy of the political system (Dryzek 2000: 83). Where a social movement cannot link in with a state imperative, its inclusion into the state is likely to be largely symbolic and ultimately detrimental to the vitality of civil society. We will argue that this reasoning illuminates the Australian experience inasmuch as the objective of radical democratization of the health services system required continuous coincidence with the state's legitimacy imperative but enjoyed it only periodically. Consequently, the quest for radical democratization was largely abandoned, following a brief upsurge of autonomous activism before the inclusion of state-supported peak health consumer groups into the policy mainstream.

Our argument begins with an account of the context that shaped the health consumer movement. We provide a sketch of the changes in the Australian health services system since the 1970s. We then describe the rise of the movement itself in more detail. The third section describes the development of the national medicines policy, an area where consumer groups have made an impact.

THE AUSTRALIAN HEALTH SERVICES SYSTEM

The Australian health services system presents a complex mix of public and private funding and service provision within a federal system of government (Duckett 2007). The Commonwealth (federal) government operates Medicare, a programme of universal health insurance covering health services costs at rates negotiated with stakeholders for five-year periods, and pharmaceutical benefits. Medicare is funded partly from a levy on taxable income but mainly from general taxation. Where doctors charge more than the Commonwealth Schedule Fee for particular services, patients pay the excess 'out of pocket'. Where consumers choose to use more expensive hospital service providers, the excess is paid either out of pocket or by private health insurance or both. The states are responsible for community health services and public hospitals, which are partially funded through Commonwealth grants. Australia is said to be 'unique in having substantial private hospital and private insurance industries operating alongside a universal public program' (Deeble 2000).

As in other domains, the Commonwealth since federation in 1901 has progressively extended its role in health policy. Since the Commonwealth Health Department was established in 1921 there has been often acrimonious contestation over health insurance arrangements between the Australian Labor Party (ALP) and its conservative opponents allied with the Australian Medical Association (AMA; known as the British Medical Association until 1961). This conflict was fiercest in periods of Labor government, notably 1941–49 and 1972–75 (Gray 2004).

Labor governments in the 1940s attempted to introduce a National Health Scheme (NHS) like Britain's but were frustrated by at least three factors. First, there was doubt whether the Commonwealth had the constitutional power to fund a health scheme, a doubt which forced a referendum in 1946. Second, the doctors' monopoly over medical provision frustrated Labor's NHS proposals. The doctors forced the government to include in the referendum proposition an amendment banning the 'civil conscription' of medical practitioners (Hunter 1966). Third, the Liberal opposition's conservative philosophy, seeing citizens as independent, self-reliant individuals participating in public life to contribute to the common good rather than to obtain benefits for any particular class, led it to stoutly resist such schemes (Brett 2003: 63). The opposition argued that health insurance was the responsibility of individuals and families, public provision being only for those unable to insure themselves; that such insurance should be provided by private bodies; and that doctors were the independent and competent authorities in health matters and thus entitled to charge fees for service and to direct most expenditure on hospitals. The Liberals' free-enterprise ideology bolstered the monopoly status of doctors and treated health care as a commodity rather than as the democratic right claimed by the ALP and their community supporters.

The conservative parties' victory in the 1949 national election entrenched the dominance of 'private medicine'. A publicly subsidized private insurance scheme, introduced in consultation with the AMA, lasted until Labor's return to office in 1972. Pensioners received free general practitioner services and pharmaceuticals, but a significant proportion of the population (never below 17 per cent) remained uninsured (Scotton and Macdonald 1993: 13). Over time, dissatisfaction with voluntary private health insurance grew because of its complexity and the inefficiencies of operating hundreds of separate medical and hospital funds, rising contribution rates, social inequities and gaps in coverage. In 1967 the Labor opposition initiated detailed work on a universal national health insurance system (Medibank), financed through general taxation and a hypothecated levy, which was ready for implementation when the Whitlam government was elected in 1972.

This electoral mandate did not result in the smooth establishment of universal health care. The conservative opposition, supported by the AMA, fought a ferocious battle for 3 years, twice blocking legislation in the Senate, before Medibank could finally be introduced in 1975, and then only after a double dissolution and the first and only joint sitting of parliament. Medibank marked a watershed in Australian health policy: 'universality and equity became explicit policy objectives in a way which had not previously been the case' (Scotton and Macdonald 1993: 76). This programme enhanced the power of the Commonwealth relative to the states over health policy and weakened 'the veto power of organised medicine in general, and the AMA in particular, over the structure of the health system' (Scotton and Macdonald 1993: 77) and thus caused some redistribution of power between the contending health policy actors (see also Hunter 1984; Kay 2007). However, the hope that breaking the monopoly power of the medical profession through Medibank would mark an increase in community influence was soon shown to be ill-founded. The conservative Fraser government (1975–83) dismantled Medibank through a series of incremental changes, culminating in the removal of the universal right to free hospital care. The power had shifted significantly instead to the state.

Medibank's successor, Medicare, was introduced by the Hawke Labor government in 1984. Medicare 'promised access to high quality, affordable health care based on clinical need … funded according to ability to pay, combining general revenue with a levy on taxable income' (Cook 2006: 197). Prima facie the reintroduction of universal health insurance appeared to be an expression of social democratic ideology premised on a conception of 'consumers' as citizens. But this was also the period when NPM made powerful inroads into Australian public administration, driving Labor governments to compromise commitments to democratic participation implicit in health and other social policy measures. Indeed, Labor governments in the Commonwealth and the states were the principal drivers of a wave of public sector changes in the 1980s and 1990s underpinned by neo-liberal ideology (Yeatman 1997). The NPM focus on rationality, outcomes, performance measures and customer satisfaction was consistent with a conception of the consumer as a market actor exercising individual choice. The opening up of the health services system to consumer representatives from the mid-1980s was 'predicated on the view that a level of consumer participation is necessary to ensure appropriate services and products are available in the marketplace … and to ensure informed consumer choice as to which services and products best suit the treatment needs experienced by individuals' (Carter and O'Connor 2003: 23). The inclusion of consumer groups as legitimate actors within a more pluralist health policy system can also be seen as diluting the power of the medical profession:

> In the struggle with the medical profession over programmes and schemas which jeopardize its sovereignty, successive administrations [in both the United States and Australia] found it expedient to creatively adapt the health consumer imaginary to resolve some of the novel problems generated by managerialism. Consumer rhetoric created a point for the managerialist discourse to penetrate professional authority. (Irvine 2001: 37)

The health consumer movement, evolving in the late 1980s from a tradition of community activism into a relatively coherent actor in national health policy, never fully embraced the NPM agenda. Yet its newfound acceptance by government and dominant provider interests – in Dryzek's terminology, its inclusion in the state – was premised on consumer groups contributing to the fairness of exchange relations and the quality of services provided. There was less scope for pursuing issues of equity and for questioning whether health care should be regarded as a market transaction at all. The limits imposed on the organized consumer movement through co-option into the state will become clearer in the next section.

THE RISE OF HEALTH CONSUMER GROUPS

In Australia, as elsewhere, health consumer groups first formed around particular illnesses, with a focus on assisting patients and their families. A broader consumer organization, the Australian Consumers' Association (today named CHOICE), which also contributed to the organization of health consumers, was formed in 1959. Self-help activism and critiques of traditional medical authority gained momentum in the 1970s when the 'health consumer' emerged as 'a central organizing principle and figure of speech' (Irvine 2001: 33). In this period, reform groups and activists for the rights of women and the physically and mentally disabled campaigned vigorously to change norms, practices and power relationships (Dwyer 1992). The rise of the new, more radical forms of health activism was intertwined with Labor's democratic reform aspirations and, as emphasized, the ongoing mobilization for universal health insurance.

Active community participation was advanced by the Whitlam Labor government through the creation of the Hospitals and Health Services Commission (Hospitals and Health Services Commission 1973). The adoption of the recommendations of the Commission resulted in the extension of Commonwealth primary care funding to community-managed health centres, community nurses, regional geriatric and rehabilitation teams, day hospitals, community mental health services, women's health centres and Aboriginal medical services. Perhaps peripheral when measured against mainstream health services, the significant result of these reforms was the emergence of a new sector of local and regional institutions supported by politicized health professionals and activists wedded to the ideas and practices of community health. Until the mid-1980s at least there was a close relationship between the community health movement and incipient health consumer organizations (Andersen 1984; DeVoe 2003). In the state of Victoria, health and consumer activists from organizations such as the People's Health Collective, the Health Left and Health Feedback Study Groups, Community Health Action and Information Network, the Medibank Action Coalition, the Workers Health Action Group, Women in Industry, Contraception and Health, Women's

Repetition Injury Support Team, the Women's Health Resource Collective and Workers Health Action came together in the early 1980s in defence of the community health programme and Medibank. In 1984 the Health Issues Centre, which today still operates as the de facto Victorian peak body for health consumer research and advocacy, emerged from this network of activists (Wadsworth 1989).

The relationship between the consumer/community health movement and Labor governments at both Commonwealth and state levels was reciprocal. In the central conflict on universal health insurance, consumer groups were the natural allies of reform advocates like the Australian Consumers' Association, the Australian Council of Social Services and the Doctors' Reform Society. Such organizations formed 'an emergent countervailing force' in support of Medibank and the Labor government's reform programme (Hunter 1984: 33). In turn, the ALP government made the health policy system increasingly accessible to such groups. The Fraser government (1975–83) held back their entry into the mainstream but the process recommenced with Labor's return to federal office in 1983 and around the same time in several of the states. The culmination of this development was the establishment of a peak organization, the Consumers Health Forum of Australia (CHF), in 1987, the first organization 'in the world' of this type (Baldry 1992: 156).

The government's intention was for a consumers' health forum to be established as 'a coalition of community and consumer groups' to provide 'a "community voice" on health issues' to balance the influence of well-organized professional and industry groups (Department of Health 1985: 22). It was to be funded by the Department but to operate as an independent, separate, incorporated body. The CHF's membership today encompasses most health consumer groups of any significance, including peak organizations in each state. With around 15 full-time staff, it is engaged in submission writing, workshops and educational initiatives, policy advocacy and the publication of newsletters and other publications. Importantly, it nominates consumer representatives to more than 150 government, industry, research and professional committees (Consumers' Health Forum of Australia 2009).

The historically blurred lines between the ALP and community activism for universal health insurance, social equity and a more participatory democracy made the 1980s, when Labor formed government federally and in several of the states, a period favourable to the inclusion of consumer groups in health policy. The consolidation of the peak health consumer movement through government funding entailed, however, a degree of domestication of its role. The CHF was established as the voice of the *community* with a particular commitment to preventive and public health and was seen as an influence that could to some extent counter the power of the medical profession (Department of Health 1985). Yet, as a government funded entity, it was in reality from the very outset absorbed into mainstream policy processes, with a focus on activities such as writing submissions and nominating and training consumer representatives on government committees. It has provided 'consumers with a "player" among the other active stakeholders with corporate representation in health' (Bastian 1998: 16) rather than allowing them a more independent and critical role.

The policy influence of the CHF peaked in its first decade, a period of stable Labor governments committed to NPM reforms. In Alford's terms the CHF contributed to the dispersion of power in the health domain, somewhat weakening the influence of the medical profession. The CHF's channelling of government funding to consumer and community organizations for autonomous research formed the 'high water mark in terms of community participation in the health policy process' (Short 1998: 140). Between 1987 and 1992, 75 consumer research projects were funded in this way: 'This research, and research conducted by the Forum, underpinned the Forum's policy advocacy work in Aboriginal health, maternity care, mental health, [and] aged care' (Short 1998: 137). This programme ceased in 1992 when conditions were tightened for peak health and community organizations (House of Representatives Standing Committee on Community Affairs 1991). The government funding the CHF continued to receive was targeted increasingly to closely audited consultative projects directed to the service of government ends, rather than to autonomous community development (Short 1998: 141).

The co-opting of the CHF to voicing consumer preferences as interpreted by officials funded by the government and the downplaying of its role of democratic criticism fits the neo-liberal and managerial reform programme. Despite the statement of a recent high-level government review that 'the health system of the future should be organized around the integral roles of consumer voice and choice, citizen engagement and community participation' (National Health and Hospitals Reform Commission 2009:122), the fact is that 'health policy decisions rarely involve significant levels of consumer engagement' (Gregory 2008: 2). Once having accepted the role of ascertaining and channelling consumer preferences within constraints determined by dominant policy actors, consumer groups can be readily embraced or ignored according to their practical usefulness to those other actors.

The health consumer movement in Australia today presents a relatively cohesive structure through peak bodies at the state level and the national leadership exercised by the CHF. Australia is generally considered a less corporatist polity than countries like Austria, Germany or the Netherlands, but by comparison with these countries (see elsewhere in this volume) the health consumer movement appears remarkably well coordinated. We have only fragmentary knowledge of the dynamics of the several hundred local and state-based groups which make up the greater part of health consumer activities, and the extent to which they exercise influence in health policy. No empirical research comparable to that of Baggott et al. (2005) in the United Kingdom has been undertaken in Australia. But the formal consumer presence within the policy system through well-established organizations such as the CHF does not seem to be sustained by vigorous or resourceful mobilization of large numbers of patients and carers, nor is there a sense of a new generation of activists following on strongly from those of the 1970s and 1980s. There is no sense of consumer organizations contributing a strong and distinct voice in the public debate on health reform. Disease-oriented groups provide much-needed services and support for their particular constituencies, but typically officials and volunteers are preoccupied with issues of funding and organizational survival through government project grants and pharmaceutical industry funding. The type of value-driven autonomous mobilization explored in the social movement literature is not conspicuous today. A recent analysis suggests that consumer groups 'have the capacity to offer high-level, long-term input ... [but] ... provide very low reach in terms of the numbers of consumers engaged' (Gregory 2008: 8).

Yet, while the capacity to mobilize autonomously appears to have been largely drained from the sector, the notion of 'consumer engagement' has evolved into a principal objective in health policy at all levels. Most initiatives that come under this heading are however oriented towards individual service users or towards citizens more broadly, and the role of consumer organizations tends to be peripheral at best. Their contribution is typically to provide representatives on committees and working groups and to advise on government activities, such as the trials of deliberative democracy in health policy planning implemented in Western Australia between 2001 and 2005 (Gregory 2008: 31). To illustrate this trajectory from vigorous social movement activism to inclusion into the state we describe in the next section the role of the CHF in Australian national medicines policy.

EXERCISING INFLUENCE: THE CASE OF MEDICINES POLICY

The health consumer movement is active on many issues, but its most sustained and significant influence has been on medicines policy. Over more than 20 years the CHF and other consumer groups have issued a stream of reports, proposals, policy papers and submissions on matters relating to medicines. These include advertising codes and standards, pharmacy practices and product information for consumers, quality use of medicines, and regulatory, access and affordability issues associated with the Pharmaceutical Benefits Scheme (PBS), Australia's tax-financed medicines insurance programme.

Consumers are represented on most regulatory committees and working groups in the medicines sector, including the Pharmaceutical Benefits Advisory Committee (PBAC) and the Pharmaceutical Benefits Pricing Authority (PBPA). The PBAC, which recommends to the Minister for Health which medicines should be included on the PBS, and the conditions for their listing, is the central node of the regulatory system. The role of the consumer representative on the PBAC is the provision of 'expertise in relation to consumer/community issues and to raise issues that may not be covered in the submissions or evaluations' (Messer 2005). The consumer representatives on the PBAC and the PBPA, which negotiates the prices paid to suppliers, have access to sensitive information and get to rub shoulders with senior figures in industry and the bureaucracy.

Membership of these committees would seem to suggest a degree of real influence in the policy process. Yet, constrained by confidentiality requirements, the consumer representatives are to all intents and purposes co-opted as marginal players into a highly complex regulatory system. Positively, the knowledge gained from participation in regulatory and advisory committees ensures the availability of expertise within the consumer movement, but only a small number of activists are engaged with medicines regulation on an ongoing basis. A mostly passive monitoring role can perhaps serve also as a constraint on more powerful actors. The CHF brings to the table, on key policy issues, their capacity to mobilize public opinion – industry and government are well aware of the political sensitivity of medicines policy. But consumer organizations are excluded from key deliberations between major policy actors, which occur in quasi-secret contexts, such as the Access to Medicines Working Group. Since 2007 this forum has enabled the 'Department of Health and Ageing and Medicines Australia [the 'Big Pharma' groups of companies] to … work together more effectively and to consider issues regarding timely and appropriate access to new medicines for the PBS' (Department of Health and Ageing 2010).

When health consumer activists first made medicines policy a key focus of their activities in the 1980s, they encountered a great deal of suspicion on the part of the medical profession, pharmacy retailers and the pharmaceutical industry. But between 1987 and 1996 aversion gave way to acceptance of a legitimate role for consumer groups in this policy sector. The dominant actors each recognized that participation by consumer groups in the policy process provided opportunities for new alliances within the policy network. The federal Labor government in this period was implementing major regulatory change to foster pharmaceutical industry R&D and investments. In this context, the formation in 1987 of the CHF brought forth a credible voice in support of the government on critical aspects of the reform agenda. In Alford's terms, incorporation of the previously excluded community interest strengthened the position of the corporate rationalizers. In particular, the pursuit of PBS efficiencies, notably the introduction of cost effectiveness as a condition for the government subsidy, was compatible with the social equity and 'rational medicines policy' programme of the consumer movement. For its part, recognizing the potential political significance of the health consumer movement, the Pharmacy Guild, representing retail pharmacists, for the first time acknowledged an interest in forging 'alliances with such key interest groups as they develop' (Bronger 1995). Similarly, there was the beginning of more cooperative relations between consumer groups and the pharmaceutical industry. This relationship was subsequently deepened through, for example, consumer representation on the industry committee which oversees adherence to a code of conduct for the ethical marketing and promotion of prescription pharmaceuticals. Today several pharmaceutical companies, including Pfizer and GlaxoSmithKline, are 'corporate members' of the CHF.

The inclusion of the CHF into a set of 'partnerships', within constraints laid down by the pharmaceutical industry and the government, is most evident in the development of Australia's 'national medicines policy'. Yet the CHF played an influential role in the original development of this concept in the early years after 1987. The notion of a national medicines policy derives from the World Health Assembly and the World Health Organization, in particular its Action Programme on Essential Drugs established in 1981 (Murray et al. 1995). It was envisaged that health policy in all countries should aim to provide the population with access to appropriately prescribed, safe, effective and affordable medicines. For the Australian Labor government, these aims dovetailed with the economic imperative of containing the costs of meeting the popular expectation of access to affordable medicines – and the increasingly important objective of promoting a 'viable' pharmaceutical industry. Given the regulated nature of the system, the pharmaceutical industry had an interest in being seen to be committed to these aims, as well as in securing government support for the industry's research base.

Australia's health ministers in 1988 adopted a series of general health policy targets in a document titled 'Health for all Australians' (Rational Drug Policy Task Force 1989: 1). This was followed by the establishment by the health ministers of the Health Targets and Implementation (Health for All) Committee. The CHF became a co-opted member of this committee, and 'was instrumental' in ensuring the committee recommendation that a comprehensive medicinal drugs policy be adopted (Harvey and Hodge 1995: 264). The inclusion of the consumer movement in this process as a legitimate policy actor was partly in recognition of the intellectual and advocacy work for a national medicines policy undertaken by the CHF. A model had been presented in a 1988 CHF discussion paper, co-authored by academic John Braithwaite. This document was circulated to all relevant interest groups and 'obtained replies supportive of many of the issues raised' (Murray 1995: 175). Indeed, the discussions triggered by the initiatives of the CHF paved the way for the de facto adoption around 1994–95 of a national medicines policy (Rational Drug Policy Task Force 1989; Sylvan and Legge 1989).

The concept of a national medicines policy has since proven a durable de facto policy framework and a reference point for lobbying by all stakeholders. It encompasses four 'arms': timely access to the medicines that Australians need, at a cost that individuals and the community can afford (provided through the PBS); medicines that meet appropriate standards of quality, safety, and efficacy; quality use of medicines; and maintenance of a responsible and viable medicine industry (Department of Health and Ageing 2000). The consumer sector has been a particularly prominent driver of initiatives to meet the third of these objectives, quality use of medicines (QUM). It is now generally accepted 'that consumers [should be] directly involved in all aspects of the QUM process in order to achieve successful behaviour change' (Kirkpatrick et al. 2005: 5 of 7).

The limits on the influence of the consumer movement are also clearly discernible from this analysis. Participation in a wide range of cooperative arrangements has hardly strengthened the capacity and inclination of health consumer groups to mobilize autonomously for radical democratization. The national medicines policy was not achieved principally as a result of CHF lobbying, and much less through the mobilization of its member organizations and supporters. Rather it evolved through the convergence of the interests of the dominant actors in this arena. For the pharmaceutical industry the national medicines policy process, as noted, provided the opportunity to gain acceptance for the objective of a 'viable pharmaceutical industry', with implications for the operation of PBS pricing arrangements. That the initial misgivings of industry about the national medicines policy could be overcome is due also to the convergence of industry and government interests. As noted, in the early 1990s the Labor government was negotiating major changes within this industry sector. In this context, the research-based drug industry sought to advance its interests within a comprehensive approach to health policy which recognized the need for 'a viable medicines industry', or, as others have suggested, for a more profitable pricing system (Löfgren 2009). In short, although the consumer movement has won an established place in this policy arena, the limited influence it has gained does not pose a challenge to the power of dominant actors.

CONCLUSION

In this chapter we have described the role of consumer groups in Australian health policy. While no theory provides an exhaustive explanation of the meta-morphoses of this role, our argument has been that neo-liberal/NPM theory, Alford's 'structural interest' analysis and Dryzek's concept of 'state imperatives' all shed light on them. The influence of community and consumer groups in health policy has varied with the objectives pursued, at different times, by the 'corporate rationalizers', but also with the broader 'state imperatives' of the government of the day. As activist groups born of the wider social movements of the 1960s and 1970s, these organizations have continued to lend vital support to the Labor Party in the perennial political contest in Australia over universal health insurance.

The establishment of Medibank, which finally broke the monopoly power of the medical profession, was a limited measure of their success in mitigating the medical dominance over health policy and practice and in opening the door, to some extent, to democratic participation in health policy. Their accessing of the power of the state, however, exposed consumer groups to the forces driving and constraining that power. When corporate rationalizers in periods of Labor government were concerned with the state's legitimation imperative of popular support for health services reform, the democratizing efforts of activist groups were encouraged and their policy role embraced. But when governments shifted to a focus on efficiency and economic and managerial objectives rather than democracy, community activist groups came under pressure to redefine their role more narrowly in accordance with neo-liberal and managerialist paradigms. Having long accepted their designation as 'consumer groups', they tempered their commitment to radical reform of the health system in favour of participation in the mainstream policy process.

Consumer groups have continued to play a role in preserving an important democratic achievement: universal health insurance. They can also boast significant achievements in representing consumer interests on many other issues, including in relation to the national medicines policy. But we cannot fail to observe the effects on the autonomy and vitality of such groups of having gained entry into the state and a degree of influence, albeit severely constrained, on government policy. Except in circumstances where their own interest in democratizing health policy coincides with the state's legitimation imperative, access to the policy table appears to co-opt such groups to the service of the corporate rationalizers' interests, which are themselves subordinate to the state imperatives of the day. Co-option, while assuring entry to the policy mainstream, marginalizes their capacity for mobilizing health services users, and citizens more broadly.

The health consumer movement has been almost entirely ineffectual in, if not totally absent from, recent political debates over health services reform, such as those that followed the election of the Rudd Labor government in late 2008. In Australian health policy it is clear that the dominant actors have conceded only as much influence as is required to preserve their dominance.

REFERENCES

Alford, R.R. (1975), *Health Care Politics: Ideological and Interest Group Barriers to Reform*, Chicago, IL: University of Chicago Press.

Andersen, N.A. (1984), 'Community health services in action', in R. Walpole (ed.), *Community Health in Australia*, Melbourne, VIC: Penguin Books, pp. 99–106.

Baggott, R., J. Allsop and K. Jones (2005), *Speaking for Patients and Carers: Health Consumer Groups and the Policy Process*, Basingstoke: Palgrave Macmillan.

Baldry, E. (1992), 'The development of the health consumer movement and its effect on value changes and health policy in Australia', PhD thesis, University of New South Wales School of Health Services Management, Sydney, NSW.

Bastian, H. (1998), 'Speaking up for ourselves: the evolution of consumer advocacy in health care', *International Journal of Technology Assessment in Health Care*, **14** (1): 3–23.

Brett, J. (2003), *Australian Liberals and the Moral Middle Class*, Cambridge: Cambridge University Press.

Bronger, J. (1995), 'Influence', *Australian Journal of Pharmacy*, **76**: 1116.

Carter, M. and D. O'Connor (2003), 'Consumers and health policy reform', in P. Liamputtong and H. Gardner (eds), *Health, Social Change and Communities*, Melbourne, VIC: Oxford University Press, pp. 22–37.

Consumers Health Forum of Australia (2009), *Annual Report 2008–2009*, Canberra: Consumers Health Forum of Australia.

Cook, B. (2006), 'Privatising health: the demise of Medicare?', *Australian Journal of Social Issues*, **41** (2): 195–208.

Deeble, J. S. (2000), 'Medicare's maturity: shaping the future from the past', *Medical Journal of Australia*, **173**: 44–7.

Department of Health (1985), *The Review of Community Participation in the Commonwealth Department of Health: Final Report*, Canberra: Department of Health.

Department of Health and Ageing (2000), 'National medicines policy', accessed 3 September 2006 at www.health.gov.au/internet/wcms/publishing.nsf/Content/nmp-objectives-policy.htm.

Department of Health and Ageing (2010), 'Pharmaceutical Benefits Scheme (PBS): access to Medicines Working Group', accessed 18 June at www.health.gov.au/internet/main/publishing.nsf/Content/amwg, .

DeVoe, J. (2003), 'A policy transformed by politics: the case of the 1973 Australian Community Health Program', *Journal of Health Politics, Policy and Law*, **28** (1): 77–108.

Dryzek, J.S. (2000), *Deliberative Democracy and Beyond: Liberals, Critics, Contestations*, Oxford: Oxford University Press.

Duckett, S.J. (1984), 'Structural interests and Australian health policy', *Social Science & Medicine*, **18** (11): 959–66.

Duckett, S.J. (2007), *The Australian Health Care System*, South Melbourne, VIC: Oxford University Press.

Dwyer, J. (1992), 'Women's Health in Australia', in F. Baum, D. Fry and I. Lennie (eds), *Community Health: Policy and Practice in Australia*, Leichhardt, NSW: Pluto Press, pp. 211–25.

Gray, G. (2004), *The Politics of Medicare: Who Gets What, When and How*, Sydney, NSW: University of New South Wales Press.

Gregory, J. (2007), *Conceptualising Consumer Engagement: A Review of the*

Literature, Australian Institute of Health Policy Studies working paper 1 (revised), Melbourne, VIC.

Gregory, J. (2008), *Engaging Consumers in Discussion about Australian Health Policy: Key Themes Emerging from the AIHPS Study*, Melbourne, VIC: Australian Institute of Health Policy Studies.

Harvey, K. and M. Murray Hodge (1995), 'Australian medicinal drug policy', in H. Gardner (ed.), *The Politics of Health: The Australian Experience*, Melbourne, VIC: C. Livingstone, pp. 238–3.

Hospitals and Health Services Commission (1973), *A Community Health Program for Australia: Report of the Interim Committee of the National Hospitals and Health Services Commission*, Canberra: Australian Government Printer.

House of Representatives Standing Committee on Community Affairs (1991), '*You Have Your Moments': A Report on Funding of Peak Health and Community Organisations*, Canberra: Australian Government Publishing Service.

Hunter, S. (1984), 'The politics of national health insurance: "plus ça change"?', in M. Tatchell (ed.), *Perspectives on Health Policy: Proceedings of a Public Affairs Conference held at the Australian National University, Canberra, 27–29 July, 1982*, Canberra: Public Affairs Committee, Australian National University and Health Economic Research Unit, Australian National University, pp. 28–36.

Hunter, T.A. (1966), 'Planning national health policy in Australia, 1941–45', *Public Administration*, **44** (3): 315–32.

Irvine, R. (2001), 'Fabricating "health consumers" in health care politics', in S. Henderson and A. Peterson (eds), *Consuming Health: The Commodification of Health Care*, London: Routledge, pp. 31–46.

Kay, A. (2007), 'Tense layering and synthetic policy paradigms: the politics of health insurance in Australia', *Australian Journal of Political Science*, **42** (4): 579–91.

Kirkpatrick, C.M.J., E.E. Roughead, G.R. Monteith and S.E. Tett (2005), 'Consumer involvement in Quality Use of Medicines (QUM) projects: lessons from Australia', *BMC Health Services Research*, **5**: 75.

Löfgren, H. (2009), 'Regulation and the politics of pharmaceuticals in Australia. Prescribing cultures and pharmaceutical policy in the Asia-Pacific', in K. Eggleston (ed.), *Prescribing Cultures and Pharmaceutical Policy in the Asia-Pacific*, Washington, DC: Walter H. Shorenstein Asia-Pacific Research Center, Stanford University and Brookings Press, pp. 129–44.

Messer, M. (2005), 'Listing and pricing of PBS medicines: profile of a consumer representative', *The Australian Health Consumer* (3): 26–8.

Murray, M. (1995), 'Australian national drug policies: facilitating or fragmenting health?', *Development Dialogue*, **1**: 148–92.

Murray, M., N. Gasman and G. Tomson (1995), 'Health and drug policies: making them the top of the agenda', *Development Studies*, **1**: 5–24.

National Health and Hospitals Reform Commission (2009), *A Healthier Future for All Australians: Final Report*, Canberra: Department of Health and Ageing.

Rational Drug Policy Task Force (1989), *Towards a National Medicinal Drug Policy for Australia*, Canberra: Consumers Health Forum of Australia.

Scotton, R.B. and C.R. Macdonald (1993), *The Making of Medibank*, Kensington, NSW: School of Health Services Management, University of New South Wales.

Short, S. (1998), 'Community activism in the health policy process: the case of the Consumers Health Forum of Australia 1987–96', in A. Yeatman (ed.), *Activism and the Policy Process*, St Leonards, NSW: Allen & Unwin, pp. 122–45.

Sylvan, L. and D. Legge (1989), 'Community participation in health', in M. Miller and

R. Walker (eds), *Health Promotion: The Community Health Approach*, Sydney, NSW: Australian Community Health Association, pp. 58–78.

Wadsworth, Y. (1989), 'Inventing the Health Issues Centre', *Health Issues*, **18**: 40–1.

Yeatman, A. (1997), 'The concept of public management and the Australian state in the 1980s', in M. Considine and M. Painter (eds), *Managerialism: The Great Debate*, Melbourne, VIC: Melbourne University Press, pp. 12–38.

13. Health consumers in Canada: swimming against a neo-liberal tide

John Church and Wendy Armstrong

This chapter examines the significant changes that have occurred to the role of broadly defined consumer groups in Canada's publicly financed health care system, as mediated through ideas, institutions and interests. The development of the Canadian system first took shape around organic processes driven by local interests, including those of consumers. But once national and provincial governments became involved and the system became more complex, consumers' direct role in political and service delivery decision-making was overshadowed by other interests. The constitutional division of responsibilities and taxing power between the federal government and the provinces, the particular set of institutional and professional arrangements that were negotiated between 1945 and 1970, and the more recent emergence of neo-liberal ideas have effectively relegated citizens to a secondary role in decision-making related to health care policy and service delivery. The emergence of neo-liberal thinking in government since the mid-1980s – heavily influenced by new right-wing think tanks, anti-tax groups and the Chicago school of economics – has led to a rethinking of the relationship between the state and its citizens. This reframing has increasingly replaced the language of citizenship with that of market 'consumerism', while historic protections and voices for consumer interests have been eroded or eliminated through delegation, deregulation and programme cuts. The net result has been a shift from an organic to an instrumental view of the role of consumers and consumer organizations in relation to the Canadian state. Related to this shift has been a trend towards centralization of governance in health care away from local communities.

This chapter begins with a discussion of the ideas that shaped the debate around the relationship of the state to its citizens. It then describes the historical context, including the interaction of interests and institutions that shaped the role of consumers in the health care system. This is followed by discussion of emergent patterns of consumer participation and related challenges. The chapter ends with an examination of the implications of these changes for the role of consumers in Canadian health care policy.

IDEAS SHAPING THE CONSUMER ROLE

The role of the state in the lives of Canadians has been shaped by a continuous debate between those who assign a minimal role to government and those who propose a much more robust intervention. The common assumption prior to the 1940s was that the family (and by extension the local community) and private market were responsible for providing relief for those unable to support themselves if faced with some misfortune. State-sponsored agencies were regarded as the last resort for relief and then only on an emergency or temporary basis. This equated well with the allocation of powers and responsibilities through Canada's founding constitutional document, the British North America Act 1867, which assigned primary responsibility for health and social services to the provincial level of government.[1]

The counter assumption – which emerged as a result of the rapid industrialization of Canada at the end of the nineteenth century, the impacts of two world wars and the Great Depression – held that society had an obligation to protect and compensate those who bore the costs of industrial and urban modernization. The emergence of Keynesian economics during the Great Depression provided governments with a theoretical justification to support a growing popular sentiment in favour of government intervention to redress the consequences of industrialization and market failure (Owran 1995).[2] This intervention included developing a vast network of programmes and services during the post-Second-World-War period that collectively became known as the social safety net. A crown jewel in this undertaking was the development of a universal, egalitarian, publicly funded, national health insurance plan for comprehensive hospital and physician services. As will be discussed below, the evolution of health care insurance encompassed three societal bargains. The first, between local communities and the state, centred on the development of hospital services based on direct public funding, and public oversight of the existing system of public and private not-for-profit hospitals including chronic care facilities. This bargain recognized the organic nature of citizenship that prevailed during the early decades of the twentieth century when local health systems began to emerge.

Such a conception of citizenship

> requires certain habits and dispositions, a concern for the whole, an orientation to the common good. They require constant cultivation. Family, neighborhood, religion, trade unions, reform movements, and local governments all offer examples of practices that have at times served to educate people in the exercise of citizenship by cultivating the habits of membership and orienting people to common goods beyond their private ends. (Sandel 1996: 117)

The second bargain centred on a model of private fee-for-service medical practice (reimbursement) that was preferred by organized medicine (Lavis 2002). An implicit third core bargain was the remaining private (for-profit and non-profit) insurance market for products and services provided outside of hospitals, such as pharmaceuticals and ambulance services, and the emergence of extended public health plans to cover such services in many provinces for the otherwise uninsurable, such as the elderly.

These core bargains remained untouched until the 1990s, when most provincial governments dissolved existing hospital boards and created new regional governance structures charged with responsibility for hospitals and a broader continuum of care. As part of this process the hospital sector was downsized dramatically and services were decanted to other settings and service providers – often with terms and conditions of coverage very different from those in hospitals, including income testing and user fees for many services. Preceding this significant development in health care was a more general swing in government thinking during the 1980s towards neo-liberalisms (Lewis 2003). This included opening up traditional hospital services to for-profit service providers (like private surgical clinics) and expanding the role of commercial insurers (and fault-based insurance premi-ums). In a sense this was a rejection of Keynesian economics and a return to the residual ideas of old, although within a very different social, political and economic context. Aside from the retreat of government from an intervention-ist role in many policy sectors, the language accompanying this shift began to reflect a changing view of the relationship between the state and the citizen. As Ignatief notes: 'Most political rhetoric, whether left or right, addresses the electorate not as citizens but as taxpayers or as consumers. It is as if the market were determining the very language of political community' (1995: 71).

The net result of this rethinking was an increased emphasis on market approaches to the delivery of public services, including an increasing central-ization of public decision-making in an effort to maximize efficiency and facilitate contracting-out functions and services to a range of old and new providers. Within this context the role of the consumer and consumer groups has been recast from an organic conception in which citizenship involves 'a mix of rights and responsibilities and mutual support for collective action' to an instrumental conception in which the consumer as citizen is the customer of government and the role of government is to deliver a broad basket of services in the most cost-efficient manner (Fafard et al. 2009: 556). Thus, the organic citizenship reflected in the first core bargain has increasingly given way to a notion of citizenship in which individual empowerment, purchasing power, speed, efficiency, accessibility and customer satisfaction are empha-sized.

As the language of neo-liberalism has been promoted, publicly funded health care has come under attack as inefficient and incapable of providing consumers with sufficiently quick access to, or choice of, health services and products. In the midst of this discussion, democratic notions of empowerment and responsibility have been transformed into economic justifications for increased access to an ever expanding array of public and private health care services within a competitive market (Feldberg and Vipond 1999).

This shift expressed itself in government through the new public management movement and its rejection of traditional bureaucratic values and practices in favour of fostering collective policy action through consultation, cooperation and coordination with industry interests, both within and outside of government.

The business concepts of continuous quality improvement, performance measurement, risk management, outsourcing, competition and 'client' satisfaction began to replace traditional bureaucratic values (Kernaghan 2000). At the same time, Canadian governments began courting investments in private health care companies and commercial research in order to attract foreign investment. As we demonstrate below, direct government support for organized and informed consumer voices in public policy has softened significantly since the 1980s.

EARLY HISTORY

As discussed above, care of the ill and injured or disabled in Canada prior to the Second World War was conceived of primarily as an individual and family responsibility and only secondarily as a local/community/employer/ church responsibility. Stemming from Britain's Elizabethan poor law tradition, major responsibilities for health and social services were assigned to provincial governments, which in turn assigned them to local governments which also had to maintain safe water and sewage systems. But because of the sparseness of population in many regions few municipalities were able to fulfil all of these responsibilities.

Religious orders built hospitals and ministered to the sick with the help of local community fundraising. Other voluntary groups, particularly local women's groups, played an important role in fundraising for health services and creating greater pressure for safer childbirth, health care and public health measures. All of this could be characterized in terms of a 'private market'. Within this context the response of civil society was to develop a variety of cooperatives. The basic principles of these cooperatives were that anyone could join, everyone had an equal right to vote, benefits were distributed according to level of participation, and cooperatives would provide educational activities for their members (*Canadian Encyclopedia*).

While a number of experiments with cooperatives emerged in British North America (Canada) during the early to mid-nineteenth century, farmers were the first group to effectively apply the concept during the latter half of the nineteenth century and into the twentieth century. In eastern Canada, over 1200 cooperatives emerged around the dairy industry. In western Canada cooperatives emerged around the grain industry. Other segments of the agriculture sector (fruit, livestock and tobacco) also organized to protect their collective interests in the marketplace.

In Saskatchewan the provincial government became involved in health care through creating local districts and legislating to enable municipalities to levy money for hiring physicians and building hospitals. A key point to note here was that the provincial government responded to requests from municipalities supported by citizens to enable them to raise taxes to provide basic health services for their citizens. This was especially the case during the Great Depression when an increasing number of municipalities experienced significant financial hardship and were unable to pay the physicians contracted to provide these services. The provincial laws created to support local aspirations for publicly funded health care became the building blocks for the development of other provincial responses, and eventually Canada's national health insurance programme (Taylor 1987: 71).

The role of cooperatives in facilitating this development was important:

> In 1945, the average farmer belonged to four or five cooperatives. Saskatchewan co-operative associations had a combined membership of at least 300,000 and it is likely that 'most ... Saskatchewan families, especially in the rural areas[,] belonged to some form of co-op'. Co-operative institutions permeated rural life and underpinned local rural governments, giving them enormous strength and resiliency. (Ostry 2002: 29)

Much of the activity prior to 1945 fed into discussions taking place between the federal and provincial governments about the role of government in social security. With respect to health care, the Canadian Federation of Agriculture called for a national and universal plan that borrowed from 'the municipal doctor plans of the western provinces which were successful from a preventive and treatment point of view because of total community involvement' (Taylor 1987: 33–4). The combined vision of labour and community interests at the national level supported a universally accessible health care system managed by lay-dominated provincial commissions structured around health regions and community health clinics. The preferred method of payment for physicians was a salary.

However, across the country physicians were wary of third-party intervention in health care:

> In the early 1940s most leaders of Canadian organized medicine still had limited expectations of the voluntary approach to health insurance. Private-sector programs

operating without formal professional sponsorship carried a threat of undue lay influence upon conditions of medical work and remuneration, with negative repercussions for both autonomy and incomes. (Naylor 1986: 101)

But the medical leadership acknowledged that some sort of state-sponsored health insurance was coming. Keeping in mind the sentiments of its membership, the Canadian Medical Association was successful in ensuring that the financial and professional autonomy of physicians would be protected whatever plan emerged. Thus, the counter-proposal from organized medicine called for a provincially administered, universally accessible system, with physicians in dominant decision-making roles and payment based on non-salaried methods. Subsequently the profession bowed to political pressure and softened its position on having total medical control. A major difference between the two visions of the system revolved around the extent to which lay individuals would exert control over physicians.

When the federal and provincial governments failed to reach agreement on a national health insurance scheme in 1945, organized medicine responded over the next decade by developing its own physician-run voluntary health insurance schemes. While this was occurring nationally, Saskatchewan, with a left-of-centre government, chose to move forward on the development of universal hospital insurance (1947) and universal medical care insurance (1962). Both insurance plans served as a model for the federal initiatives in hospital insurance and medical care insurance, in 1957 and 1966 respectively. Saskatchewan became the 'crucible' for health care policy in Canada.

Failure to reach agreement in the federal arena meant that a more comprehensive scheme that included physicians' services was not financially viable. In this political vacuum physician-sponsored insurance schemes that were designed to be more portable began to challenge the municipal doctor schemes, even though many Canadians were unable to afford these plans. As these schemes, conceived largely in urban areas, began to gain in popularity in rural areas, the government was compelled to take action to curb the potential growth in the market share of private plans. Thus, on the cusp of an election in 1961, the government of Saskatchewan passed legislation to create Canada's first universal plan to cover services provided by physicians outside of hospitals. The plan called for universal, compulsory, contributory health insurance for physicians' services outside of hospitals. The reaction from organized medicine was swift and decisive. The majority of doctors across the province closed their offices and went on strike:

What the SCPS [Saskatchewan College of Physicians and Surgeons] feared was a concentration of purchasing power in government hands, that could countervail the profession's own considerable market strength and potentially lead to interference with the doctors' clinical autonomy as well. (Naylor 1986: 200)

In response to the physicians' strike, consumers and sympathetic physicians launched community clinics with lay governance to deliver basic health services. Spearheaded by the Community Health Services Association, a community cooperative, clinics were established in five municipalities. By the end of the strike ten other clinics were under development (Taylor 1987: 326).[3]

In addition to the larger issues relating to medical representation on the provincial commission (which would administer the plan and method of remuneration), the development of community clinics during the strike was viewed as a major threat to the autonomy of doctors because it coincided with the original government plans of 1944 to organize physicians' services as salaried group practices. The clinics were quietly supported by the government, which was actively recruiting physicians from outside the province to staff the clinics. Ironically, the clinics (with salaried physicians and community governance) proved pivotal in effectively limiting the role of consumers in health care decision-making such that one aspect of the eventual settlement between the government and physicians (article 14) included the following:

> There may be places where few or no doctors have enrolled for direct payment by the Medical Care Insurance Commission, so that patients are denied the choice of such doctors. It is not for the Commission to appoint doctors in such places. The remedy is in the hands of the citizens themselves. They can establish premises and invite doctors who wish to enroll for direct payment to rent such premises and set up a practice in them ... The interests of such enrolled doctors must be safeguarded from improper citizen pressure. The role of the citizen group in the provision of insured services must be limited to that of landlord. (Tollefson 1963: 123).

Overall, many aspects of the original legislation that would have assigned a significant role to consumers in health care decision-making were significantly weakened to appease organized medicine. No provision was made for the payment of physician services provided through community clinics other than fee for service. Communities were required to raise their own funding if they chose to pay physicians by alternative means. The Saskatchewan experience produced the blueprint for national Medicare and through this model consumers were effectively excluded as decision-makers in primary care. Arguably the professional and economic interests of organized medicine were given and continue to receive preferential treatment across Canada.

When mediated through national constitutional arrangements, national mechanisms that evolved from these local and provincial experiments left the provinces with responsibility for the provision and regulation of health care and the federal government with responsibility for the safety and marketing of health-related products, like pharmaceuticals and medical devices. It is also a major funder and moral guardian of the patchwork of provincial plans that form the Canadian public health care plan. Provincial and federal governments share responsibilities in the area of public health, health research and economic development, as well as rules governing the private health insurance industry.

FROM HOSPITAL BOARDS TO HEALTH REGIONS

The introduction of publicly financed hospital insurance left the local governance infrastructure largely untouched. Hospital and public health boards continued to be accountable primarily to local communities and to use, to varying degrees, democratic mechanisms in support of this relationship. This changed however during the 1990s when most provincial governments dissolved local health care governance structures, replacing them with regional governance (Church and Barker 1998). Where local governance had previously been divided among several sectors locally (hospitals, long-term care, home care and public health), the new health regions were responsible for governance of hospitals, public health and service delivery for most areas of health care, including services in licensed long-term care facilities (private, for-profit and not-for-profit) which are privately funded but publicly subsidized in most provinces. Thus, the original societal bargain enshrining local governance arrangements most closely tied to an organic notion of citizenship was largely discarded.

For example, from 1994 to 1995 in the province of Alberta, the government eliminated approximately 200 local health boards, replacing them with 17 appointed regional health boards, and in 2003 reduced them to nine. A similar pattern has emerged in most jurisdictions across Canada, although in Ontario and British Columbia existing hospital boards have remained in place, within regional governance structures. As Lomas (1997) notes, in moving from several hundred formal local decision-making structures (per province) to less than two dozen, opportunities for formal consumer input into health care decisions declined dramatically, resulting in a potentially significant loss of social capital. Although some jurisdictions promised at least partial election of regional board members, only Saskatchewan has implemented and sustained this approach. Even here, the democratic effectiveness of this mechanism has been challenged. More tellingly perhaps, a 1997 survey of regional health board decision makers found that in only Prince Edward Island province did regional boards feel 100 per cent accountable to local citizens. In the remaining jurisdictions, less than 50 per cent of respondents felt accountable to local citizens (Brunelle et al. 1998: 31). Other structural factors limiting opportunities for consumer input and influence on health policy have included greater contracting-out of the management and provision of health care services to commercial interests, the gutting of internal policy staff, and increased reliance on global consulting companies for policy advice. All of this has been part of a shift in government practices aimed at 'steering, not rowing' (Osborne and Gaebler 1992). Mechanisms like commercial confidentiality and reliance on new intermediaries to interpret and filter information from consumers and consumer groups have made the activities of both government and providers less transparent.

Since the early 1990s Canadians have also become more reliant on commercial insurance policies (automobile, disability and extended health), provincial workers' compensation funds (for workers injured on the job) and out-of-pocket spending to obtain necessary health care services (Insurance Bureau of Canada 2001; Hurley et al. 2008; Canadian Women's Health Network 2002). The locations and organizations providing both public and privately paid services have also shifted from predominantly small profes-sional group practices and mission-driven, non-profit care organizations (Victorian Order of Nurses, Good Samaritan Society) to regional (and global) companies (Comcare, CML Inc., MDS, LifeMark, Cambie Surgical Centre, Dynacare, The Katz Group, Medysis) with investor and shareholder obliga-tions. Bureaucrats and industry executives move easily and confidently between sectors. Federal and provincial governments now actively court phar-maceutical company investments. The private insurance industry is also lobbying to expand their historically limited market. Governments are doing little to rein in aggressive marketing and problematic practices in these sectors. When compared with many other countries, lack of reliance on corporate suppliers and private insurers in Canada during the latter half of the twentieth century has left this sector woefully underregulated.

EMERGING CONSUMER GROUP STRATEGIES

Faced with decreasing formal opportunities for direct control and influence over health care from the 1960s onwards, consumers turned to other mecha-nisms to influence provincial and national decision-makers. As the historical pattern described so far suggests, these opportunities have developed through both public and private resources. During the 1960s large-scale social movements (human rights, civil rights, women's rights and environ-mental protection), the passage of the Canadian Charter of Rights and Freedoms in 1982 under the second Trudeau government, and the advent of mass television contributed to the mobilization of many new consumer and public interest-oriented groups, as well as specific disease or disability groups (Boscoe et al. 2004). Some of these organizations represented broader consumer and citizen interests while others represented narrower population or member interests. Mandates and activities also differed with the range of foci, including provision of services and social support to individuals and families (Breast Cancer Action), public education (Aids Network), and professional education to improve quality of care; public policy development through promoting expert/consumer views and mobilizing public opinion; mobilization around enhanced drug and product safety, food safety, environmental laws and stronger social programmes; and fundraising for disease-specific research. Many played a crucial role in informing and educating the public about health policy issues. During this period numerous government programmes were created to help fund and facilitate the activities of these groups, in recognition of the need to ensure adequate resources to balance more powerful provider and industry interests – a hallmark of more collectively oriented governments and cultures (Aberbach and Christensen 2005).

A number of these organizations played a critical role in protecting public health care programmes from erosion through changes in government and vested interests. For example the Canadian Health Coalition was created in 1979 in the face of new threats to programmes. The negative effects of the growth of extra billing[4] by physicians and user fees by hospitals exposed in the late 1970s led to a government commission and the Canada Health Act (1984), resulting in prohibitions on these practices.

THEN CAME THE 1990s

Changes in government and government thinking as well as new economic pressures led to significant changes in the structure, funding and nature of consumer and public-interest groups and the way in which they interacted with government and industry during the 1990s (Consumers' Association of Canada [Alberta] 2003). New business and industry strategies, new technologies such as email and the internet together with NPM strategies, including greater reliance on consensus, voluntary initiatives and the use of consulting firms and pollsters or internet surveys to interact with the public, changed the nature of the relationship between consumers and governments.

Aside from the general movement of government towards forging partnerships with industry and industry organizations, together with programme cuts, the 1990s saw a renewed discussion of the role of consumer and public-interest groups. A federal member of parliament pejoratively calling them 'special interest' groups and a government paper entitled 'Federal Government Relations with Interest Groups: A Reconsideration' contributed to the demise of core funding for many, though not all, traditional civil society groups in both the federal and provincial arenas (Finkle et al. 1994).

Federal policies and court decisions relating to interpretation of the national Income Tax Act meant organizations risked losing their charitable status (which attracted donations and provided access to foundation funding) if they spent more than 10 per cent of their funds on 'advocacy' that attempted to influence the policy process (Webb 2000). Consequently many health consumer organizations found it difficult to participate meaningfully in the policy process or even to maintain a significant public presence. Any small grants or funding that remained were largely tied to specific deliverables and contracts – and government agendas. The once influential Consumers' Association of Canada exemplifies this point. The loss of its core government funding and its national magazine (with more than 100 000 subscribers in the mid-1990s) effectively crippled the Association, although some of its provincial affiliates have made important contributions to the health care policy process (Armstrong 2000).

There were numerous efforts to convince policymakers to support the development of informed consumer participation in health policy. Yet in 2002 a national Health*Insider* poll of Canadians following the Royal Commission on the Future of Health Care in Canada (the Romanow Report) found that:

> Canadians feel disenfranchised from the health care debate and policymaking, and feel that, although they would like a greater voice, they are excluded from participating in a significant way. Canadians want an increased role in the future direction of health care and support for increased citizen input is high. Nine out of ten feel that individually they should have greater input on the direction of the health care system; and 94% feel that the Canadian public as a whole should have greater input. (IBM 2002: 1)

As a consequence of many of these changes, consumer organizations became more narrowly focused, often being restricted or influenced by available funding sources rather than taking up the issues raised by their constituencies. Many older groups have also chosen to withdraw from the policy process out of frustration, while others have attempted to influence the public and raise awareness in the media (Consumers' Association of Canada [Alberta] 2003). Governments are turning to online workbooks and surveys with carefully selected background information (deliberative polling) to obtain input from the general public. Overall, there are fewer interactive dialogues or opportunities to put new items on policy agendas.

Perhaps the most interesting development in consumer advocacy in recent years has been the emergence of consumer and patient groups and coalitions funded by corporate interests, especially the pharmaceutical industry. As Batt observes:

> Once passive patient organizations are now outspoken and governments are eager to engage the public in policy decision-making. To advocate effectively, organizations need money for research, training, community consultation and public education. Government policies, which once supported community-based advocacy, have

eliminated or restricted most funding to advocacy groups over the past two decades. Any group involved with advocacy is likely to confront the dilemma of ambitious goals and limited funds, especially for core operations and advocacy. Fundraising and grant writing have become overwhelming requirements for community groups and many, particularly those with a health protection rather than a disease mandate, have ceased to exist ... Government policies encourage charitable groups to form partnerships in the private sector. (2005: 1)

Pharmaceutical companies have responded by devoting increasing resources to partnering, with large and small consumer and disease groups advocating for public funding for the treatment of specific existing or emerging diseases. Often this advocacy involves convincing political decisionmakers of the efficacy of rapid approval of certain new drugs by the federal government and adding them to provincial formularies, as well as extended patent protections. In short, pharmaceutical companies are now an important source of funding for patient and disease-specific groups.[5] A new phenomenon is transient consumer groups or coalitions created by public relations firms working for industry clients and interests (called 'astroturf groups'), which focus on the regulation of health supplements and quicker safety approvals of and access to new pharmaceutical products.

CONCLUSION

The role of consumer groups in Canadian health care has evolved over the past century, reflecting changes in how the relationship between the state and civil society is viewed. After moving from a residual perspective prior to the Second World War, which assigned a minimal role to government in the lives of its citizens and private markets, to an institutional perspective, which assigned a major role to government, the emergence of neo-liberal and NPM thinking during the 1980s caused government to once again rethink its role. The outcome was greater emphasis on market approaches to the delivery of public services, including both increased centralization and the devolution of public-decision making in an effort to maximize efficiency and facilitate delegation and contracting out. As this corporate view of the relationship between the state and society has become embedded, the role of the consumer and organized consumer groups has been recast from an organic conception with a broad collective focus to an instrumental conception with a narrow individual and economic focus.

In this context governments have gradually abandoned the structures that formalized the organic citizenship that produced cooperatives and the local governance structures on which Canada's health care system was built. Elimination of local health care governance and legal limitations placed on collective action by consumer groups have increasingly driven consumer interests into an unholy alliance with private corporate interests. Citizenship is being redefined to emphasize the neo-liberal attributes of individual empowerment, purchasing power, speed, efficiency, accessibility and customer satisfaction. This narrowing of the dimensions of citizenship to its economic elements fails essentially to recognize inherent inequalities and a broader, collective public interest and associated collective action. More fundamentally, this narrow definition is antithetical to sustaining democracy.

If Canada is to achieve a better balance between private and public goods and individual and collective interests, then regaining a greater sense of organic citizenship will be essential. Properly empowered health care consumer groups could play a crucial role in this process.

NOTES

1. Constitutionally, local governments are created at the pleasure of provincial governments.
2. The Leonard Marsh Report of 1943 proposed a number of organized programmes to deal with common risks and contingencies in family life and the economy, such as prolonged family unemployment, sickness, disability and invalidity, widowhood and old age (Marsh 1943 [1975]).
3. The Saskatchewan Community Health Co-operative Federation comprises five cooperative community health centres which service approximately 80 000 people. It advocates for progressive reform in health policy and consumer-sponsored alternatives in the planning, organization, financing and delivery of health services. Features of this model include providing a variety of services in one location, group medical practice and better use of other health professionals. They emphasize prevention and education and promote remuneration of health service professionals by salary rather than fee for service.
4. Extra billing was a practice employed by a minority of physicians, charging patients directly at the point of service an additional amount of money on top of what was paid through publicly funded health insurance. The Canada Health Act 1984 banned this practice along with user fees at hospitals. The practice was an attempt by these physicians to exercise what they saw as their economic right to determine the price of their service and to maintain a direct market relationship with their patients. Note that Canadian physicians are free to bill Canadians for non-insured medical services at whatever price they wish.
5. The problem goes beyond pharmaceutical policy. For example in 2002 the Consumers' Association of Canada National Secretariat was publicly accused by the British Columbia regional affiliate of partnering with government and industry to promote genetically modified food with money from big food biotechnology companies (Perrin and Nunn 2002). The national Canadian Association of Retired Persons also relies heavily on advertising from private health and life insurance companies which market group products to members and subscribers to its magazine to support the organization's work (Armstrong and Deber 2006).

REFERENCES

Aberbach, J.D. and T. Christensen (2005), 'Citizen and consumers: an NPM dilemma', *Public Management Review*, **7** (2): 225–45.
Armstrong, W. (2000), 'The consumer experience with cataract surgery and private

clinics in Alberta: Canada's canary in the mine shaft', accessed 20 May 2010 at
www.albertaconsumers.org/CanaryReportrevised2.pdf.

Armstrong, W. and R. Deber (2006), 'Reading the fine print: focus on long term care
insurance', accessed 20 May 2010 at www.teamgrant.ca/M-THAC%20Greatest%
20Hits/M-THAC%20Projects/Reading%20the%20Fine.html.

Batt, S. (2005), 'Marching to different drummers: health advocacy groups in Canada
and funding from the pharmaceutical industry', Women and Health Protection,
accessed 20 May 2010 at www.whp-apsf.ca/pdf/corpFunding.pdf.

Boscoe M., G. Basen, G. Alleyne, B. Bourrier-Lacroix and S. White (2004), 'The
women's health movement in Canada: looking back and moving forward',
Canadian Women Studies, **24** (1) (Summer): 17, accessed 20 May 2010 at
www.cwhn.ca/resources/cwhn/cwhn-cws04.pdf.

Brunelle, F., P. Leatt and S. Leggat (1998), 'Healthcare governance in transition: from
hospital boards to system boards ... a national survey of chairs of boards', *Hospital
Quarterly* (Winter): 28–34.

Canadian Women's Health Network (2002), 'Health care privatization: women are
paying the price', National Coordinating Group on Health Care Reform and
Women, Women's Health Network, accessed at www.cwhn.ca/node/39564.

Canadian Encyclopedia (undated), 'Cooperative Movement', www.thecanadianency-
clopedia.com/index.cfm?PgNm=TCE&Params=A1ARTA0001903, accessed 22
Feburary 2010.

Consumers' Association of Canada (Alberta) (2003), 'Consumer representatives – linking them to consumer', www.albertaconsumers.org, accessed 22 February 2010.

Church, J. and P. Barker (1998), 'Regionalization of health services in Canada: a critical perspective', *International Journal of Health Services*, **28** (3): 467–86.

Fafard, P., F. Rocher and C. Cote (2009), 'Clients, citizens and federalism: a critical
appraisal of integrated service delivery in Canada', *Canadian Public
Administration*, **52** (4): 549–68.

Feldberg, G. and R. Vipond (1999), 'The virus of consumerism', in D. Drache and T.
Sullivan (eds), *Health Reform: Public Success, Private Failure*, London:
Routledge, pp. 48–62.

Finkle, P., K. Webb, W.T. Stanbury and P. Pross (1994), 'Federal government relations
with interest groups: a reconsideration', paper prepared for the Consumer Policy
Framework Secretariat of Consumer and Corporate Affairs Canada.

Hurley, J., D. Pasic, J. Lavis, A. Culver, C. Mustard and W. Gnam (2008), 'Parallel
payers and preferred access: how Canada's Workers' Compensation Boards expe-
dite care for injured and ill workers ', *HealthcarePapers*, **8** (3), accessed 22
February 2010 at www.longwoods.com/home.php?cat=546.

IBM (2002), 'Canadians and the future of health care in Canada: was Romanow on the
mark?', *IBM* Health*Insider*, (December).

Ignatief, M. (1995), 'The myth of citizenship', in R. Beiner (ed.), *Theorizing
Citizenship*. Albany, NY: State University of New York, pp. 53–78.

Insurance Bureau of Canada (2001), 'Restoring confidence: Insurance Bureau of
Canada submission to the Commission on the Future of Health Care in Canada and
the Standing Committee on Social Affairs, Science and Technology', accessed 22
February 2010 at www.teamgrant.ca/M-THAC%20Greatest%20Hits/Bonus%
20Tracks/CP32-80-3-2001E.pdf.

Kernaghan, K. (2000), 'The post-bureaucratic organization and public service values',
International Review of Administrative Sciences, **66** (1): 91–104.

Lavis, J.N. (2002), 'Political elites and their influence on health-care reform in

Canada', accessed 22 Feburary 2010 at www.dsp-psd.communication.gc.ca/Collection/CP32-79-26-2002E.pdf.

Lewis, T. (2003), *In the Long Run We're All Dead: The Canadian Turn to Fiscal Restraint*, Vancouver, BC: University of British Columbia Press.

Lomas, J. (1997), 'Devolving authority for health care in Canada's provinces: 4 emerging issues and prospects', *Canadian Medical Association Journal*, **156** (6): 817–23.

Marsh, L. (1943) [1975], *Report on Social Security for Canada*, reprinted (1975) Toronto, ON: University of Toronto Press.

Naylor, C.D. (1986), *Private Practice, Public Payment: Canadian Medicine and the Politics of Health Insurance, 1911–1966*, Montreal, QE: McGill-Queen's University Press.

Osborne, D. and T. Gaebler (1992), *Re-inventing Government*, New York: Plume.

Ostry, A. (2002), 'The roots of North America's first comprehensive public health insurance system', *Hygeia Internationalis*, **2** (1): 25–44.

Owran, D. (1995), 'Economic thought in the 1930s: the prelude to Keynesianism', in R.B. Blake and J. Keshen (eds), *Social Welfare Policy in Canada: Historical Readings*, Toronto, ON: Copp Clark, pp. 172–200.

Perrin, J. and J. Nunn (2002), 'Does the Consumers' Association of Canada speak for Canadians', *CBC Market Place*, 6 March, accessed 22 February 2010 at www.healthcoalition.ca/cbc-cac.pdf.

Sandel, M.J. (1996), *Democracy's Discontent: America in Search of Public Philosophy*, Cambridge, MA: Harvard University Press.

Taylor, M.G. (1987), *Health Insurance and Canadian Public Policy: The Seven Decisions that Created the Health Insurance System and their Outcomes*, Montreal, QC: McGill-Queen's University Press.

Tollefson, E.A. (1963), *Bitter Medicine: The Saskatchewan Medical Care Feud*, Saskatoon, SK: Modern Press.

Webb, K. (2000), *Cinderella's Slippers? The Role of Charitable Tax Status in Financing Canadian Interest Groups*, Vancouver, SC: SFU-UBC Centre for the Study of Government and Business.

14. Empowering health care consumers in the United States

Michael H. Fox and Anna Lambertson

In welcoming remarks at a ceremony introducing the Obama administration's new director for health reform in April 2009, representatives of two large consumer-oriented health care organizations likened health care reform to the life cycle of the cicada (Henry J. Kaiser Family Foundation 2009b). Like the homopterous members of the Cicadidae family that emerge from underground every 17 years shrilling loudly, the voices of health care consumerism emerge periodically demanding change.

Indeed, in the United States, the rhythm of health care policymaking is cadenced by the periodic outcry of the major stakeholders – consumers, hospitals, employers, insurance companies and physicians. Since the second term of the Truman presidency in 1948, these cries have emerged every 15 to 20 years, leading to a pattern of incrementalism in US health care policy that Paul Starr aptly referred to as the 'politics of accommodation' (Starr 1982). Crises develop and are defused through health reform that characteristically modifies existing programmes, or creates new ones on the shoulders of others, until fault lines lead to cracks that lead to chasms that lead to crises, when a renewed outcry for health reform goes out, at which point the cycle begins again.

So in the late 1940s crises over access to medical care for the elderly and Second World War veterans led to legislation (known as the Hill-Burton Act) that introduced widespread hospital construction for free medical care to indigent patients, while under parallel legislation (known as the Kerr-Mills Act) state services were provided for poor, elderly residents (Starr 1982). But these actions only met the needs of a portion of those requiring health care. Later, in 1965, using momentum generated in the aftermath of the death of President Kennedy, President Lyndon Johnson took advantage of the climate for political change to improve care for low-income and elderly Americans. With the passage of Medicare and Medicaid, new entitlements created programmes for people over 64 and individuals the states deemed to be 'deserving poor', such as single mothers, infants and people with disabilities unable to work. While meeting the needs of many socially marginalized people these programmes had the unintended consequence of increasing the market value of health insurance products, leading to inflated medical costs associated with the 'usual and customary' fee-for-service payments made to physicians and hospitals. In an unregulated environment, as more people became insured, charges for services rose. Under these early free-market conditions 'usual and customary' became 'usurious and customary', with providers increasingly charging patients whatever they felt insurers would pay. In the mid- to late-1970s, Medicare and Medicaid officials led efforts to redesign the way providers were paid, leading to fixed payments made in advance for certain services, the development of managed care, and more regulated access to services.

In spite of these changes, overall costs continued to rise as managed care limited its reach to healthier segments of the population, making for a very profitable sector. In effect, healthier and wealthier Americans were being cross-subsidized by the rest of the population, including poor and uninsured individuals. In the early 1990s, consumer reaction to the restricted availability of managed care and its failed promise of constraining costs led to futile efforts to overhaul the entire system. The Clinton administration misguidedly used a variation of managed care, so-called 'managed competition', as the centrepiece of their reform efforts. Its spectacular failure (Hacker 1997; Rushefsky and Patel 1998) led to the 'consolation prize' of a joint federal and state health insurance venture known as the State Children's Health Insurance Program, which offered free or inexpensive coverage to poor children not poor enough to qualify for Medicaid. A reduction in the number of uninsured Americans followed, but this was reversed within a few years when a section of the population lost their insurance as a result of reductions in work benefits.

This brings us to the 2009–10 cycle, when Americans again found themselves facing unsustainable cost increases for medical care and insurance, and limited access to many services. Even more shocking, 15 per cent of the population was found to have no insurance cover of any kind over the course of a year (Centers for Disease Control and Prevention 2009). Once again the din of cicadas resounded through Washington, with hope *and* scepticism in no short supply. But has the latest round of changes got it right?

The extent to which there is hope depends upon the success of the consumer voice in health care, perhaps the single most important element significantly lacking in earlier major health policy initiatives. Who is the consumer and why is the consumer voice so important? 'Consumer' is the term of choice in many health policy discussions. In contrast to the 'patient', who is treated by medical providers, the 'consumer' actively accesses the health care system seeking diagnosis and treatment. As key participants in the health care system consumers may reasonably expect that their perspective will be central to health policy discussions. After all, people who use the health care system have a stake in its effectiveness and in part determine whether reforms succeed or fail.

Consumers have already achieved a milestone of sorts in that virtually all major health reform platforms being considered at present claim to speak for people denied something in some way by the current system (Henry J. Kaiser Family Foundation 2009a). From those proposing a single-payer system of only not-for-profit providers to those promoting tax cuts that would allow the purchase of affordable health insurance on the open market, all claim to speak for the consumer.

FRAMING HEALTH CONSUMERISM AND ITS ROLE IN THE US HEALTH CARE SYSTEM

Introducing the *Social Science & Medicine* journal's edition devoted to patient organizations, Kyra Landzelius argues that the consumer voice is a vehicle that extends beyond self-interest and personal suffering, providing opportunities for 'examinations of sociality and morality, nature and culture, freedoms and duties, and for a constellation of inscriptions from human rights to consumer rights to legal rights to citizens rights' (2006: 536). This expression of patienthood becomes a parameter of personhood in ways that could increasingly lead to forms of empowerment.

Brown and Zavestoski (2004) view the empowerment of consumers in the United States as a counterbalance to the inherited authority of the biomedical professions and a challenge to their social, cultural and economic dominance. They describe the 'scientization of decision-making' and the frequent medicalization of social problems as inevitable precursors to technical rather than social solutions, many of which directly remove power from consumers. They hold it is of the greatest value for what they call 'health social movements' 'to reveal the manner in which science and medicine are used as instruments of coercion', citing examples such as the Tuskegee syphilis experiment and the testing of contraceptives on women in Puerto Rico (2004: 683). But like others, Brown and Zavestoski see the future of health consumerism as dependent on building strategic alliances with other social movements, such as those related to environmental justice.

In the next chapter, Christina Nuñez Daw, Denise Truong and Pauline Vaillancourt Rosenau provide an overview of health consumerism in the United States, beginning with an analysis of consumer involvement in the regulation of food and drugs by the US government through the Food and Drug Administration. This involvement is a direct result of the kind of excesses noted by Brown and Zavestoski, though a far cry from the proactive strategic alliances they believe will have to develop for consumer activism to move forward. A relevant parallel to the current health consumer movement is the US disability movement, also described by Daw et al. in this volume. Here, patient and public involvement is neither strictly rights-based nor regulatory, but rather compensatory and opportunistic (Tritter 2009). Paralleling the growth of the disability movement, health consumerism has developed in response to policies and practices that have directly contributed to hardship among certain sections of the population brought about by excesses in the free market. The free market has traditionally failed to provide adequately for the elderly, children, minorities, low-paid workers and the disabled. Policies fuelled by social movements, which have seldom been in complete alignment with their aggrieved populations, have developed as compensation and in that respect have had the disadvantage of often being perceived as reactive in nature.

The opportunistic nature of US health consumerism (most frequently described using Kingdon's (1995) 'window of opportunity' model) has again shaped debate, successfully demonstrating how a far wider proportion of the American middle class than previously thought was experiencing hardship. The election of Barack Obama on a campaign pledge to overhaul the health care system was a tangible expression of this process and echoes the disability movement's achievement in the enactment of the Americans with Disabilities Act (1991).

WHAT DOES HEALTH CONSUMERISM MEAN IN THE UNITED STATES?

In their UK study, Baggott et al. characterize health consumer groups according to three categories: condition-specific (for example, cancer survivors), population-based (for example, the elderly) and formal alliances (for example, business–labour–low-income consortia for health reform) (2005: 21). While these three types of consumer groups can be identified in the United States, such distinctions serve little purpose because whether condition-specific, population-based or associated with specific alliances, US health consumers are motivated less by their association with their peers than by identification with the health care system overall. The situation is highly politicized. On one side there is the view that the United States has 'the best health care system in the world' – moulded by business, specifically the health insurance industry and supporters of the free market. Here the principal role of consumer organizations is seen as protection of the freedom to choose between different health insurance products. Conversely, those who believe the existing system has severe shortcomings conceive of consumer empowerment in ways that align with the European model: that organizational strength will make for progressive social policy.

Given that the profit motive underpins much health care delivery, a clear line is drawn between consumer involvement related to personal or family health issues and consumer involvement that is more closely tied to business and profit generation. Any of the categories of consumer group noted by Baggott et al. (2005) may be underwritten by business interests. While some consumer groups operate in ways that serve the needs of profit in the health sector, others have been established to assist consumers facing unique hardships independent of or caused by the business of health care.

The free market model is clear in so-called consumer-directed health care. Consumer-directed health care has become a pervasive force in recent years, promising the benefits of an unfettered free market and branding almost all governmental interventions as counterproductive to health care consumerism (Herzlinger 2004; Bonney 2005; Goodman 2004). Framing consumerism as a populist type of control over purchasing options in the health care market has allowed it to attain a degree of credibility not otherwise associated with industry-driven campaigns to limit regulatory consumer protections. As related in earlier work by one of the authors of this chapter (Fox 2008), the notion of consumer-directed health care has flourished amid widespread suspicion that while its name suggests empowerment for people at risk it delivers the exact opposite.

We thus find in the United States that both approaches to consumer interaction with the health care system are represented in consumer health organizations. Among groups closely aligned with business while claiming to speak for the health consumer are Consumers for Health Care Choices (www.chcchoices.org) and the National Center for Policy Analysis (www.ncpa.org). Groups whose interests align more closely with those of individuals who use health care services and experience its hardships include Health Care for All (www.hcfama.org) and Families USA (www.familiesusa.org). Consumer-directed health care, a concept which suggests that the interests of health consumers are identical to those of business, is ultimately about health care as a commodity.

Proponents of consumer-directed health care reason that comprehensive health insurance provides an incentive for making frivolous demands for services; that it creates a 'moral hazard' of consumers seeking care that is not really needed because insurers will pay for it regardless (Fox 2008: 673). Their preferred approach is to have consumers divert a pool of money that would otherwise go towards paying for insurance into what are known as 'health savings accounts' or related vehicles, providing banks with investment capital while reserving savings for the purchase of health-related services in what they claim is a free market.

This approach has been subject to intense criticism by analysts (Kuttner 2008; Cross 2003; Marshall et al. 2000; Hibbard et al. 1997; Weissman et al. 2004; Marquis et al. 2006; Fox 2008). The basic challenge to this vision of unfettered consumer control in health care is around the spurious assumption that health care operates in a free market. Few consumers find it possible to overcome the lack of cost transparency, making it virtually impossible for them to shop comparatively for health services. Add to this incentives not to spend their money on the care they need in order to save, and the movement of such 'health savings' from the pockets of employers and insurers into the banks which use this bonus capital to further their own investment strategies, and the concept seems entirely discredited. Perhaps the easiest way to understand this is to see it through the eyes of those who actually use the health care system, in particular the idea that market choice gives people the right and opportunity to negotiate directly with health service providers. It is patently obvious that negotiating with physicians over cost is not something American consumers experience in the present system, nor will they in the near future.

Consumer-driven health care is part of a wider ideology centred on a reduced role for government and putting more money in the hands of individuals to pass along to investors. Many would consider this a straw man that diverts citizens from recognizing the actual voice of those people who play by the rules and still encounter hardships disproportionate to their means, irrespective of their needs.

One such person, disturbingly characteristic of many others in the United States, is described in the report *Playing by the Rules but Losing: How Medical Debt Threatens Kansans' Healthcare Access and Financial Security*:

> Suzanne and her husband live in Americus, Kansas with five children. Both she and her husband are employed full time and everyone in the household is insured. The family has accumulated several thousand dollars of medical debt over the past few years because of insurance deductibles and uncovered services. Initially, the couple's debt resulted from three trips to the emergency room – one when Suzanne's husband was injured in a farm accident and the other two when their second youngest daughter suffered severe asthma attacks. The debt worsened due to the $1500 deductible for care during Suzanne's pregnancy with her youngest child. The hospital was unwilling to work with Suzanne and her husband to develop a reasonable payment plan, so some of the bills were sent to collection agencies and now appear on their credit report.
>
> The family's medical debt makes it difficult for Suzanne and her husband to keep up with other bills. In addition, the medical debt contributed to the accumulation of credit card debt used to deal with other unexpected emergencies. Ongoing health care costs, particularly those related to her daughter's asthma, further complicate the family's financial situation. The family's slim budget forces Suzanne to make hard choices about when to seek care and what procedures, tests, and prescriptions are really necessary. Although Suzanne has health problems of her own, she often delays treatment so she can pay for her children's care. (Pryor and Prottas 2006: 8).

It would be tempting to dismiss this family's dilemma as symptomatic of living on the margins, but this was not the case. Indeed, almost 51 million

Americans do not have health insurance and many who do are denied services because their coverage is inadequate or they are in debt. For many millions of people, the free-market defence of a system that regularly inflicts hardship on them and their family and friends rings hollow.

A gap exists between health consumers' reality and the policy and organizational models that purport to include a consumer perspective. We need to evaluate the model of discourse used to solicit consumer feedback. After all, how can an organization claim to speak for the consumer unless it has reached out to the users of the system in a way that listens to and documents their unique opinions? To truly incorporate the consumer voice into the policymaking process, to amplify and translate situations like Suzanne's into political action to create health policies that improve lives requires a discourse that engages consumers from the vantage point of their own values. This represents a relatively new role for organizations like the Kansas Health Consumer Coalition (www.kshealthconsumer.com) described below, which has developed such a discourse to advocate for consumer legislation at local, state and federal levels.

ENSURING KANSANS ARE HEARD: A CASE STUDY

Tucked away from the hubbub of either coast, Kansas is a state built on Midwestern values of community engagement and solidarity. The rising number of uninsured Kansans threatens to dismantle these values by creating greater disparities between the 'haves' and the 'have-nots'. Kansas's firmly rooted sense of community is being challenged by social disconnectedness as many people struggle to pay for health care.

According to the United States Census Bureau, the number of Kansans without health insurance rose from 10.5 per cent in 2004–5 to 12.5 per cent in 2006–7 (United States Census Bureau 2007). Kansas was one of only ten states in which the uninsured rate increased during this period (Smit et al. 2009). The number of uninsured children increased from 7 per cent in 2005–6 to 9.6 per cent in 2007–8 (Kansas Health Institute 2009).

The uninsured are up to four times more likely to lack a regular source of care, three times more likely to delay seeking care, and are significantly more likely not to have had a physical examination in the past year or been diagnosed with a disease in an advanced state (Wikler and Bailey 2008). Lack of comprehensive health insurance or inadequate insurance coverage jeopardizes families' incomes, leading to medical debt, further affecting credit, housing and potential employment (Pryor and Prottas 2006; Fox and Haas 2006).

The Kansas Health Consumer Coalition is a non-profit organization whose mission is to advocate for affordable, accessible, quality health care.

It puts the consumer face on health care access issues and injects the consumer voice into all health policy conversations, providing consumers with effective, strategic opportunities to maximize their civic engagement and truly make an impact. Kansas's political environment poses unique challenges for consumer engagement. In 2005, the Kansas Health Policy Authority (www.khpa.ks.gov) was created as the state's primary health care agency with the task of developing a comprehensive health policy agenda. The Authority has undertaken several initiatives to respond to consumer needs, including establishing advisory councils and committees whose members represent broad constituencies across Kansas. However ongoing tension, distrust and an ineffective governance structure between legislators, the executive branch (the Governor) and the Authority have made advancing strategic recommendations virtually impossible, despite widespread public support.

For example, prior to the 2009 legislative session in Kansas, the legislature had failed to make any real progress towards passing clean indoor air legislation and increasing the cigarette tax. Yet a poll commissioned by the Sunflower Foundation in 2007 found that an overwhelming majority of registered voters favoured a statewide indoor smoking ban, while a strong majority (64 per cent) supported increasing the tax on a packet of cigarettes (Sunflower Foundation 2007). Despite this level of public support, successful lobbying from tobacco companies and other opposition groups prevented significant change around either issue. While strong grassroots mobilizing around clean indoor air in Kansas led to the eventual passage of clean indoor air legislation by the state Senate in 2009 and both chambers in 2010 (signed into law by Kansas's Governor Mark Parkinson on 12 March 2010), a proposed tobacco tax increase was, once again, not included in the state's final tax package at the conclusion of the 2010 session.

This dissonance between public opinion and policy decisions also reflects how strident voices in Kansas have overtaken more pragmatic ones, a trend seen nationally in many contexts (Ridgeway 2009). In Kansas, town hall meetings about health care in 2009 became, more often than not, shouting matches between supporters of reform and those opposing what they saw to be government intrusion (Garber 2009; Rothschild 2009). One reporter writing in Iola suggested: 'Suggest that the government programs Medicare and Medicaid be abolished, and "a riot" would likely ensue. But propose that a similar health-care program be established for all Americans, and all of a sudden, government has become "too big," "all-controlling," and "inefficient"' (Lynn 2009).

Following media coverage of town hall meetings in Topeka, described as being 'dominated almost entirely by opponents of Democratic plans to reform the health care system' (Rothschild 2009), a reader responded with the following criticism:

Americans don't need or want elected officials to decide what is in our best inter-est. I have faith that the American people are strong enough and intelligent enough to be able to make these kinds of decisions on their own, without any intervention at all from the federal government. So in the future, leave the opinions to the opin-ion page, and present the news as impartial and unbiased. (Schaeffer 2009)

So how can the voices of ordinary health consumers makes themselves heard by policymakers who themselves are being shouted down when discussing health reform? The Kansas Health Consumer Coalition has found success with one major project, Voices for Health Care (www.voicesforhealthcare.org). During this project, staff witnessed consumers engage in civil discussion with fellow citizens in their communities then alter their perspectives about how health care should be reformed.

Voices for Health Care is a public engagement initiative implemented in Kansas by the Coalition in collaboration with California-based Viewpoint Learning and funded by the W.K. Kellogg Foundation. It seeks to engage consumers and policymakers in productive discussions about health care access and quality to reach common ground on key policy issues. Since 2007, this model of deliberation, which prioritizes dialogue over debate, has been seeded in the states of Kansas, Mississippi and Ohio (Voices for Health Care 2007). Policymakers and citizens engage in dialogue, listening to and learning from others and thereby enhancing their own understanding of policy issues. The process is values-based rather than data-driven and emphasizes the process of 'working through' issues by evaluating choices and considering trade-offs. The process of working through issues is critical because it is only by going through this stage that individuals come to make more-balanced and considered judgements (Viewpoint Learning 2008).

In March 2008, randomly selected residents of three small to mid-size Kansas communities participated in day-long citizen dialogue on health reform called Choice Dialogues. Participants were representative of their communities and of the state as a whole. In each dialogue they were presented with scenarios describing how health care could look in Kansas in the future. Using the scenarios as a guide, participants discussed what they were willing to trade off to achieve their preferred system.

They gradually realized that there were no easy solutions, yet participants felt strongly that change needed to occur and that the current system could not just be tweaked but required a major overhaul. Their opinions developed through interaction with other members of their communities who came from all walks of life and socio-economic backgrounds, and were of a variety of political persuasions. The primary outcomes of the Choice Dialogues process follow.

Altered Personal Views

Many participants changed fundamentally their perspectives on how the health care system could and should be reformed. A Viewpoint Learning report (2008) found that participants came to see health care as a right. While participants initially expressed restrained support for covering the uninsured, when the process concluded, 88 per cent said that providing insurance for all Kansans was 'absolutely essential' or 'very important'. In addition, 79 per cent supported switching to a publicly run health insurance programme funded by taxes and 80 per cent voiced a willingness to have their taxes increased to ensure health coverage for every Kansan.

Changed Perceptions of Community Members

While not all participants changed their minds about reforming health care, many whose opinions remained unchanged came away with a different understanding of how other members of their community perceived the issues. Through dialogue, participants re-evaluated their personal views and the assumptions of others. One participant expressed surprise 'at how many people were willing to pay for the health care of others who couldn't afford it'.

Enhanced Understanding of the Value of Dialogue

Many participants were impressed by the civility with which all participants engaged in conversation throughout the discussions. One participant said that the results proved that 'people can be respectful and come to a consensus. They don't have to find a solution right now but they can identify the underlying problem and its triggers.'

Providing a Stepping Stone for Increased Public Engagement

For many participants the Choice Dialogues became a starting point for greater engagement in their communities around health care issues. As one participant put it, the experience served as a 'first step for making [her] voice heard'.

The Voices for Health Care project provided a unique opportunity for increased public engagement in Kansas around health reform. Through it, Kansans had the opportunity to consider thoughtfully the views of others, and in so doing clarified and solidified their own opinions. Since they were asked to reach consensus on a shared health reform vision by the end of the day, participants saw the necessity of compromise; they realized that they might not be able to have everything they wanted in a reform package, but they could develop a vision that worked to satisfy the needs of the group overall. This process emulated the challenges of policymaking and convinced many participants of the necessity for public engagement.

THE ONGOING ROLE OF HEALTH CONSUMERS IN DEVELOPING HEALTH POLICY

Robert Laszewski, a respected US health policy observer, has noted that

> in spite of all of our health care problems, I don't believe we will have a big comprehensive health care reform bill in 2009 or 2010 [because:] 1. There is no consensus in the Congress or the country on what a comprehensive health care bill would look like; 2. Our people don't want health reform badly enough to force the Congress to stand up to the powerful stakeholders and make them do it; and 3. We don't have the money. (Laszewski 2008)

While Mr Laszewski could not have predicted the convoluted path that health reform has taken during the Obama years, the fact that both the House of Representatives and the Senate passed separate versions of the most comprehensive reform bill in over 40 years (Hulse and Pear 2009; Pear 2009) is testament to the power health consumers can exert to ensure their voices are heard over those of powerful stakeholders' strident cries. Massive letter-writing and call campaigns initiated by consumer groups, along with steady and supportive federal leadership, were successful in keeping health reform alive in spite of formidable odds.

To maintain and strengthen this voice, consumer-oriented groups need access to sufficient financial resources to compete against Political Action Committees and other arms of the health care industry. They also need to understand the strength of their personal and professional networks and use them effectively to convey their perspectives to their elected leaders. In turn, political leaders need to make more honest efforts to listen to and understand the perspectives of real consumers, not just those vocal consumers calling their offices. Elected leaders must hold each other accountable for taking the voice of the consumer seriously, and consumers must never give up.

If health consumers come to understand their strength, many of the funding challenges associated with grassroots health consumer organizations may become a distant memory. Philanthropic foundations, the source of most current funding for health consumer organizations, are under increased pressure themselves to justify investments in terms of encouraging stronger consumer involvement. As more health consumers become part of organizations that they feel speak on their behalf, consumer organizations' financial situations will improve: foundations will be assured their money is being spent well and will consider future investments more positively; and increased support from foundations will mean individual donors will be more likely to contribute funds.

To enhance dialogue and civic engagement, policymakers need to improve their understanding of the complexity of the issues faced by all of their constituents instead of focusing on their financially most well-connected contributors. They could perhaps learn from medical practitioners who develop best-practice guidelines based on shared knowledge and measurable outcomes.

Report cards that record not just votes on health policy issues of interest to consumers but also the health outcomes for constituents within a voting juris-diction could prove extremely helpful in making policymakers more account-able to those living within their jurisdiction. If health outcomes in voting district A appear significantly different from voting district B, policymakers would be obliged to work with consumers to address those differences.

Finally, consumers need to remain patient and must not underestimate the importance of their views. We know that historically health reform in the United States has been cyclical, surfacing as part of broader social movements – that have come to characterize different chapters in the nation's develop-ment. Health consumerism as a movement, set apart from institutions support-ing a grossly inefficient health care system, presents a uniquely American approach to effecting change. It offers a stark contrast to a conception of health care founded in the profit motive and its practical consequences. While the cicadas may soon stop chirping following the latest attempts at reform, the challenge to ensure quality, accessibility and affordability of health care for all will be met in the future only if a strong consumer voice continues to develop. With this nascent voice gradually weaving its way into the fabric of American political dialogue, its greatest impact may yet be before it.

REFERENCES

Baggott, R., J. Allsop and K. Jones (2005), *Speaking for Patients and Carers: Health Consumer Groups and the Policy Process*, Basingstoke: Palgrave Macmillan.

Bonney, R. (2005), *Consumer-Directed Healthcare and Its Implications for Providers*, Ann Arbor, MI: Health Administration Press.

Brown, P. and S. Zavestoski (2004), 'Social movements in health: an introduction', *Sociology of Health & Illness*, **26** (6): 679–94.

Centers for Disease Control and Prevention (2009) 'Early release of selected estimates based on data from the 2008 National Health Interview Survey', accessed 13 August at www.cdc.gov/nchs/nhis/released200906.htm.

Consumers for Health Care Choices (n.d.), accessed 13 August 2009 at www.chcchoices.org/about.html.

Cross, M. (2003), 'Consumer-directed health care: too good to be true?', *Managed Care,* **12** (9): 18–25.

Families USA (n.d.), accessed 13 August 2009 at www.familiesusa.org.

Fox, M.H. and T. Haas (2006), 'Being underinsured in Kansas', *Kansas Policy Review*, **28** (2): 14–23.

Fox, M.H. (2008), 'Who speaks for the health consumer?', *Journal of Health Care for the Poor and Underserved*, **19** (3): 671–6.

Garber, K. (2009), 'Behind the rage at healthcare town hall meetings', accessed 21 October at www.usnews.com/articles/news/national/2009/08/18/behind-the-rage-at-healthcare-town-hall-meetings.html.

Goodman, J. (2004), 'Health savings accounts will revolutionize American health care', National Center for Policy Analysis brief analysis no. 464, Washington, DC: NCPA.

Hacker, J. (1997), *The Road to Nowhere: The Genesis of President Clinton's Plan for Health Security*, Princeton, NJ: Princeton University Press.

Health Care for All (n.d.), accessed 21 October 2009 at www.hcfama.org.

Henry J. Kaiser Family Foundation (2009a) 'Side-by-side comparison of major health care reform proposals', accessed 13 August at www.kff.org/healthreform/sideby-side.cfm.

Henry J. Kaiser Family Foundation (2009b), 'Transcripts of health care reform news-maker series: Nancy-Ann DeParle, Director, White House Office of Health Reform', accessed 13 August at www.kff.org/healthreform/upload/041509_kff_deparletranscript.pdf.

Herzlinger, R. (2004), *Consumer-Driven Health Care: Implications for Providers, Payers, and Policy-Makers*, San Francisco, CA: Jossey-Bass.

Hibbard J.H., P. Slovic and J.J. Jewett (1997), 'Informing consumer decisions in health care: implications from decision-making research', *Milbank Quarterly*, **75** (3): 395–414.

Hulse, C. and R. Pear (2009), 'Sweeping health care plan passes House', *New York Times*, 7 November, accessed at www.nytimes.com/2009/11/08/health/policy/08health.html?_r=1.

Kansas Health Consumer Coalition (n.d.), accessed October 2009 at www.kshealth consumer.com.

Kansas Health Institute (2009) 'Fact Sheet', accessed 21 October at www.khi.org/resources/Other/1363NoChangeInKSUninsuredRate.pdf.

Kansas Health Policy Authority (n.d.), www.khpa.ks.gov, accessed 21 October 2009.

Kingdon, J.W. (1995), *Agendas, Alternatives, and Public Policies*, 2nd edn, New York: HarperCollins College Publishers.

Kuttner, R. (2008), 'Market-based failure – a second opinion on US health care costs', *New England Journal of Medicine*, **358** (6): 549–51.

Landzelius, K. (2006), 'Introduction: patient organization movements and new meta-morphoses in patienthood', *Social Science & Medicine*, **62** (3): 529–37.

Laszewski, R. (2008), Health Care Blog, 'Despite Democratic control, major health reform still unlikely', accessed 9 November 2009 at www.thehealthcareblog.com/the_health_care_blog/2008/11/despite-democra.html.

Lynn, S. (2009), '"Hot" conversation cordial', accessed 21 October 2009 at www.iola register.com/Local%20News/Stories/Hot%20conversation%20cordial.html.

Marquis, M.S., M.B. Buntin, J.J. Escarce, K. Kapur, T.A. Louis, and J.M. Yegian (2006), 'Consumer decision making in the individual health insurance market', *Health Affairs*, **25** (3): 226–34.

Marshall, M.N., P.G. Shekelle, S. Leatherman and R.H. Brook (2000), 'The public release of performance data: what do we expect to gain? A review of the evidence', *Journal of the American Medical Association*, **283** (14): 1866–74.

National Center for Policy Analysis (n.d.), accessed 21 October, 2009 at www.ncpa.org.

Pear, R. (2009), 'Senate passes health care overhaul on Party-Line Vote', *New York Times*, 24 December accessed at www.nytimes.com/2009/12/25/health/policy/25health.html.

Pryor, C. and J. Prottas (2006), *Playing by the Rules but Losing: How Medical Debt Threatens Kansans' Healthcare Access and Financial Security*, Boston, MA: The Access Project.

Ridgeway, J. (2009) 'Town Hall meetings and the far right', accessed 21 October at www.motherjones.com/mojo/2009/08/town-hall-meetings-and-far-right.

Rothschild, S. (2009), 'Reform advocates drowned out in uproar', accessed 21 October at www2.ljworld.com/news/2009/aug/16/reform-advocates-drowned-out-uproar.

Rushefsky, M. and K. Patel (1998), *Politics, Power and Policy Making: The Case of Health Care Reform in the 1990s*, Armonk, NY: M.E. Sharpe.

Schaeffer, G. (2009), 'Biased report', accessed 21 October at www2.ljworld.com/news/2009/aug/20/biased-report.

Smit, R., S. Barfield, G. Maree and C. Huang (2009), *Health Insurance and the Uninsured in Kansas, Updates from the March 2008 Current Population Survey*, Topeka, KS: Kansas Health Institute.

Starr, P. (1982), *The Social Transformation of American Medicine*, New York: Basic Books.

Sunflower Foundation (2007), 'Public opinion poll – tobacco and other related issues', accessed 21 October 2009 at www.sunflowerfoundation.org/user/file/Tobacco%20Poll%20Summary%20of%20Findings.doc.

Tritter, J. (2009), 'Revolution or evolution: the challenges of conceptualizing patient and public involvement in a consumerist world', *Health Expectations*, **12** (3): 275–7.

United States Census Bureau (2007), 'Small area income and poverty estimates, state and county data, Kansas', accessed 21 October 2009 at www.census.gov//did/www/saipe/index.html.

Viewpoint Learning, Inc. (2008), *Public Voices for Health Care in Kansas: Topline Findings*, accessed at www.viewpointlearning.com.

Voices for Health Care (n.d.), accessed 21 October 2009 at www.voicesforhealthcare.org.

Weissman, J.S., D. Blumenthal, A.J. Silk, M. Newman, K. Zapert, R. Leitman and S. Feibelmann (2004), 'Physicians report on patient encounters involving direct-to-consumer advertising', *Health Affairs*, **4**: 219–33.

Wikler, B. and K. Bailey (2008) 'Dying for coverage in Kansas', accessed 21 October 2009 at www.familiesusa.org/assets/pdfs/dying-for-coverage/kansas.pdf.

15. Health policy in the United States: consumers and citizens in a market polity

Christina Nuñez Daw, Denise Truong and Pauline Vaillancourt Rosenau

Patients and consumers in many countries attempt to influence health policy directly and indirectly across the domains of government, the private sector and research (Baggott and Forster 2008; Baggott et al. 2005). The United States, however, does not have a robust history of citizen or consumer participation in health care policy or governance at the national level. This contrasts strikingly with the experience of other industrialized countries (Litva et al. 2009; Learnmonth et al. 2009). There are two forms of consumer engagement – through assigned roles within established decision-making bodies and through activist-oriented groups that come together to advance specific agendas affecting patients and families. In this chapter we present a review of salient examples in the United States, broadly canvassing both approaches. In addition, we do not take for granted that patient participation is always genuine empowerment. On occasion it may be merely 'pro forma' (Van de Bovenkamp and Trappenburg 2009a, 2009b).

There is very little systematic research on consumer involvement in US health care policy. But this is no surprise. It has been observed that there is 'little evidence that [citizen] groups have had much effect on health policy' (Weissert and Weissert 1996). In an initial literature search, we identified over 200 peer-reviewed research publications and found 69 articles relating in some way to consumers and health care policy. But the vast majority of these treated the consumer strictly as a user of a product – health care. This perspective typically sees patients as purchasers of health insurance policies choosing among competing health plans in the marketplace and assessing the cost and quality of individual clinicians or hospitals. In this chapter we also cite research located through purling (or 'snowballing') from the references of papers initially located for this review.

Although the United States Constitution calls on the federal government to 'promote the general welfare', government's role in health care is not clear.

Responsibilities not specifically assigned to federal powers are automatically entrusted to the states, according to the Tenth Amendment. A key characteristic of the US system is its lack of 'collective responsibility ... for the health needs of the individual' (Ter Meulen and Jotterand 2008). That is, the principle of solidarity is largely absent, and indeed is contrary to the individualistic tradition in US culture. Personal responsibility and individual choice are the hallmarks of this society's attitude towards welfare and human services (Beauchamp 1988). In the United States there are few systematic, publicly sponsored or endorsed processes or institutions for including consumers in developing health policy. As noted by Tritter and Lutfey (2009), the relative lack of systematic, even everyday avenues for consumer participation in US health care delivery leads to ad-hoc or 'organic' advocacy efforts, such as in the areas of cancer care and mental health. These social movements are developed and 'framed in terms of protest and lobbying' as part of larger political action (Tritter and Lutfey 2009: 222).

To some extent, efforts at consumer engagement in the United States are local, community-specific and generated by foundation, non-profit or academic initiatives. Morone and Kilbreth (2003) note the disparity in local, direct public participation between the health care sector and the education sector, where there are more opportunities for local, direct input and civic debate on school boards and in parent–teacher organizations.

Tomes (2006a) examines the absence of attention to health care consumers as citizen representatives, laying the blame for perceived consumer disadvantage on medical professionalism. From this perspective, physician and patients/consumers are not natural allies; rather, physicians' self-interest sets them apart. As a result, anti-professional views have taken hold in some corners of mental health patient advocacy, though this is controversial (Isaac and Armat 1990; Torrey 1997). Yet, Morone and Kilbreth (2003) argue that with the advent of privately sponsored managed care and 'corporate medicine', both patients *and* professionals (physicians) have ceded their voice to a managerial top layer.

PUBLICLY SPONSORED CONSUMER INVOLVEMENT

Despite the American ethic of personal responsibility, government health programmes such as Medicare and Medicaid were developed in the 1960s to fund medical care for disadvantaged groups – poor families with children, and poor elderly and disabled adults. Though both Medicare and Medicaid have defined benefits (the responsibility for setting benefits for Medicaid lies at the state level while Medicare benefits are defined federally), consumer involvement in the process of defining them is rare. Another government health programme, the Veterans Health Administration (VHA), provides care to those discharged from the armed services. The VHA has no top-level role for consumers but patient representatives do serve in a minor role on local hospital-level councils.

Several states have consumers on newborn screening advisory panels where they participate in decision-making around what conditions should be tested. Individual participants are involved in the oversight of technology and lab procedures. Sometimes they are in a position to recommend policies related to patient consent and refusal, and to the follow-up of positive screens. Consumers are represented on such panels in 26 of 51 state programmes, including in Washington, DC (Hiller et al. 1997). In 17 states, consumers have played a role in determining the tests to be performed on newborns. Another example of a public entity with a consumer advisory role is the national Bioethics Advisory Panels. In recent years, Presidential Bioethics Advisory Panels have written reports about the protection of human subjects, cloning, stem cell research, access to health care, and ageing. However these panels more often address research issues than the delivery of care (President's Council on Bioethics 2009).

Food and Drug Administration

At the federal level, the Food and Drug Administration (FDA) provides the most visible and effective opportunity citizens have to play a strong role on national policymaking. The FDA has a long history of consumer consultation and participation going back to the early twentieth century (Guilford 1993). Congress granted this agency of the US Department of Health and Human Services the authority to protect and promote the health of the nation, fulfilling this mission by regulating and supervising the safety of food, drugs, medical devices, radiation-emitting devices, vaccines, blood products, biologics, animal and veterinary products, cosmetics and tobacco. It has created strong links to consumer groups and patient representatives over the decades and members of Congress have encouraged the FDA to be open and responsive to such groups. The FDA responds to requests of members of Congress to follow up specific patient queries and it maintains a consumer phone line. Consumers and patients often make presentations at FDA advisory committee meetings during open hearing sessions. The FDA's Office of Special Health Issues, designed to serve as a liaison between patients, patient advocates and health professional organizations, aims 'to encourage and support their active participation in the forming of the Food and Drug Administration's regulatory policy' (FDA 2009a). In December of 2008 the FDA formed a partnership with the important health information organization WebMD, the goals being patient and consumer education, and broadening the FDA's reach (WebMD 2009).

WebMD is a publicly held company providing internet-based medical information in articles and through an interactive website.

To maintain transparency and document its responsiveness to consumers and the broader public, the FDA posts and archives a daily public calendar, listing high-level FDA meetings with outside groups. The breadth of consultations is impressive. It includes consumer groups, though meetings with members of the executive branch of the US government are not posted. Neither are meetings with industry representatives. FDA officials believe this is necessary to protect information that is proprietary and/or given in confidence (FDA 2009b).

Consumers and patients participate on most FDA advisory committees. There are 48 committees and panels tasked with providing the FDA with independent expert advice on a variety of scientific, technical and policy matters, including specific recommendations about the approval of medical products. The FDA is not required to follow advisory committee recommendations, though it usually does. Committees are extremely important in the policy-making process. Consumer and patient representatives on these committees are mandated to serve as a 'liaison between the committee and interested consumer associations, coalitions, and consumer organizations' and to 'facilitate dialogue with the advisory committees on scientific issues that affect consumers'. They are required to be proficient in the science and in risk assessment and to be affiliated with consumer or community organizations. The material some consumer representatives receive and evaluate is confidential, and in this case they are subject to government 'conflict of interest rules'. While they never constitute a majority on an advisory committee, nor serve as chairperson, many do have a vote. When differences among other members on an advisory committee are significant, it is theoretically possible that the consumer or patient representatives could influence an outcome (FDA 2009c, 2009d, 2009e).

While policymakers at the FDA encourage consumer and patient group participation, it is difficult to document the exact degree to which such consultations influence the policymaking process. Still, they are clearly an accepted part of the process. But the FDA is not a democracy, and few would argue that it should be. It would be unfair to say that the FDA's consultations with consumers and education outreach are merely efforts at co-optation, or that consumer groups are no longer vital or autonomous organizations because of their participation in the FDA. Consumer groups press the FDA vigorously for specific actions. They have demanded that the FDA be more vigilant in overseeing patient rights in clinical trials carried out overseas; provide greater transparency in the workings of advisory committees; agree to public airing of dissenting opinion within advisory committees; distance itself from the pharmaceutical industry; pull medication off the market at the first sign of unexpected problems; and list all meetings with industry representatives on its public calendar (Favole 2009).

As far as institutionalized channels for consumer input are concerned, FDA advisory committees are exemplary. Yet, the demand that the FDA distance itself from drug developers arose from sharp concern during the 1990s and 2000s about increasing pharmaceutical industry influence; this competing influence may have weakened consumer input in some areas. Some observers argue that pharmaceutical companies' increasing power coincided with chronic underfunding of the FDA, which hampered its regulatory capacity (Rosen 2007).

Health Systems Agencies

One problem with consumer participation in health policymaking in the United States is that even when they are democratically elected, individuals do not always successfully identify and advocate for the specific perspectives they were designated to represent. Health systems agencies (HSAs) are an example. In the 1960s, the United States initiated federal and regional health-planning efforts to target the oversupply of beds and large projects – essentially medical care inflation. In the 1970s, consumer involvement was integrated into the planning process. The National Health Planning and Resources Development Act 1974 created 205 health systems agencies across the nation. HSAs were charged with evaluating applications for the Certificate of Need, a mechanism for approving capital expenditures and significant service expansions. Of the agencies' members, 51 per cent were to be area residents, not medical providers. Other, less direct examples of public accountability were also required: publication of board proceedings, advertisements of meetings and opportunities for public comment at meetings. Marmor and Morone, however, argue 'these requirements might be said to facilitate public accounting, not accountability' (1980: 133).

HSAs and federally sponsored planning processes have been reviewed extensively in the political science literature, and there appears to be widespread agreement that HSAs did not engage citizens to the extent originally intended (Mick and Thompson 1984; Steckler et al. 1981). In one agency studied by Steckler et al. (located in the southern United States), minority groups and rural communities were well represented, but members tended to be middle-class, white-collar residents. Despite consumer participation being on par with that of providers, citizen representatives had less influence than providers on actual decisions. In other parts of the nation several lawsuits were filed against HSAs seeking better representation of target subgroups, such as minority racial groups and people with incomes under $10 000 a year (Marmor and Morone 1980). The resulting legal rulings favoured specific representation from low-income groups and a balance between metropolitan and non-metropolitan residents, while strict 'mirror representation' regarding race and ethnicity was deemed less important.

Despite the effort to have strong citizen representation on agency boards, there was little public enthusiasm or support for HSAs or adequate understanding of their intended role in containing costs, restricting supply of health care resources such as hospital beds, and limiting access to services considered to be in overabundance so that overall access to scarce services could be expanded. Targeted subgroups of consumers were no more likely to rate these goals as worthy than the general population. Indeed, those groups who were most affirmatively sought were least in agreement with key assumptions about the oversupply of hospital beds, and the idea that HSAs were inherently more trustworthy than physicians and hospitals. Marmor and Morone observed a series of flaws in the statute and regulations that hampered HSAs' work, culminating in a serious 'overreach' in their mission. Most importantly, they did not have any way of enforcing their decisions (Marmor and Morone 1980: 156).

Consumer representation has proven difficult to harness effectively in matters with potentially far-reaching economic effects. The expansion of HSAs is a clear-cut example of this. The National Health Planning and Resources Development Act was relatively short-lived. Five years after enactment, Ronald Reagan was elected President, and in 1987 federal funding was repealed, with HSAs no longer mandated to assess Certificate of Need applications. Still, today, in 36 states some type of certificate of need process exists (National Conference of State Legislatures 2009). Consumers sit on these boards, but the focus of many HSAs has changed from specific planning to providing general consultation on broader, community-level public health projects. In short, health planning and the system of regional and local agencies failed to carry out the intended planning activities and have lost their original official mission and cohesiveness.

Federally Qualified Community Health Centers

Federally Qualified Community Health Centers (FQHCs) are another example of efforts to involve consumers from underserved communities in governance and health policymaking. While over the last three decades HSAs sought consumer representation from widely diverse groups, FQHCs have been particularly interested in low- or moderate-income patients, that is, users of the system who are also viewed as underserved and underprivileged. These clinics emerged from the civil rights and community organizing movements of the 1960s which advocated community participation and 'community control over health services' (Geiger 2005: 318). FQHCs provide care in communities designated by the federal government as medically underserved, both in urban and rural areas. Federal funding and favourable Medicare/Medicaid reimbursement allow FQHCs to serve uninsured individuals on a sliding fee scale based on income level. They are considered non-profit agencies rather than government facilities. FQHCs include migrant health centres, clinics serving homeless people and clinics in public housing estates. There is a defined mechanism for consumer participation in FQHCs (US Public Health Services Act), with governance boards required to have active patients of the organization comprising up to 51 per cent of board membership. FQHCs serve over 18 million people, 70 per cent of whom have incomes below the federal poverty threshold. Half of FQHC patients live in rural areas; 39 per cent have no health insurance; and 35 per cent have either a Medicaid or State Children's Health Insurance Plan (for low-income families whose income is too high to qualify for Medicaid) (National Association of Community Health Centers 2009). Because of support in recent administrations, including during the George W. Bush presidency, the number of patients served has grown by 67 per cent (from 10 million to 18 million), and the number of centres receiving federal funds increased from 700 to over 1000. Under the Obama administration, the American Recovery and Reinvestment Act has provided $1.5 billion in funding for FQHC infrastructure needs and $500 million for expanding services to address spikes in the uninsured population (Department of Health and Human Services 2009). In addition, the more recent health care legislation (Patient Protection and Affordable Care Act) adds $11 billion in funding for health centre expansion over 5 years. It is hoped that nearly 20 million new patients can be served (National Association of Community Health Centers 2010).

In contrast to HSAs, FQHCs have not (to our knowledge) been the subject of published research evaluations; there appear to be no empirically based studies of consumer participation on FQHC boards, or of the impact of citizen participation on board performance. The consumer representative role on FQHC boards has evolved over decades. Patient members do not manage medical care but they often have genuine input into clinics' efforts to increase access, acceptability, utilization and community outreach. They often help shape new programmes, offer initiatives and contribute suggestions on patient–provider interaction, including joint goal-setting (Isbell 2009; Buck et al. 2004). In addition, local FQHC consumer advisers are sometimes given opportunities to serve on national health care advisory boards. In general, the role is viewed as a channel of patient empowerment that enhances the cultural competence of clinicians and clinic administrators.

Another example of federally mandated consumer representation involves participation on councils for disabled individuals in legal services agencies called Protection and Advocacy, which were established in legislation, for example the Protection and Advocacy for Mentally Ill Individuals Act (1986).

These laws require Protection and Advocacy agencies to have consumer advisory boards with significant patient representation. The training and support of consumer participants is also viewed as essential to successful integration of the patient point of view (National Disability Rights Network 2009).

In general, with respect to soliciting consumer input, disadvantaged citizens have often been targeted for programmes serving poor communities, such as poverty remediation programmes. These efforts demonstrate affirmative attention for minorities, with an eye to 'buy-in' and 'ownership' of the programmes. The other role for which consumers are solicited is making decisions, often difficult decisions, about allocating restricted resources. It appears the more enduring and successful role has been in oversight of services, such as with FQHCs and on the FDA, with very structured participation.

From Oregon to Massachusetts

In Oregon, in the 1990s, an attempt to rank health care treatments and thus prioritize them for coverage in the state Medicaid programme became a lightening rod for activity. At this time the state of Oregon sought to expand Medicaid eligibility within its boundaries by increasing the income threshold from 67 per cent to 100 per cent of the federal poverty level (Blumstein 1997; Fox and Leichter 1993). However, the state's Medicaid funding level was never likely to be sufficient to provide comprehensive benefits to the newly expanded Medicaid beneficiary population. State officials therefore sought ways to limit benefits, but to change eligibility and other rules they needed approval in the form of a waiver from the federal Department of Health and Human Services. During the development of the waiver application, a telephone survey, sampling Oregon's residents, assessed public opinion about the effects of various diseases on health status and quality of life. The survey employed the Quality of Well-Being Scale, a health-related quality-of-life metric used in health cost-effectiveness evaluations. Essentially, the questionnaire was a tool to elicit a rating of diseases and disorders based on disruption of health quality, thereby indicating which health problems warranted more or less Medicaid coverage. In addition, public meetings were held around the state to further inform policymakers about citizen preferences. But because of federal government concerns that a 'quality-of-life' emphasis conflicted with protections provided by the Americans with Disabilities Act, the final waiver proposal did not use the cost-effectiveness approach. Instead, medical treatments were included or excluded from coverage on the basis of medical effectiveness, that is, prevention of death. An interim approach gave priority to 'returning patients to an asymptomatic state', yet this approach was not acceptable to disability advocates because it interpreted 'asymptomatic' as non-disabled. In the end, consumer consultation was withdrawn as a factor in determining benefits because it did not sufficiently include the *disabled* consumer's perspective (Fox and Leichter 1993).

Oregon's experience demonstrates the importance of consumer input, but also the potential veto power of specific consumer groups. When the general population, including the insured as well as affluent, participates in decisions that directly affect only vulnerable segments of the population (that is, the poor and disabled) the effort appears inequitable. The Oregon Health Commission is still active, and continues to revise its methods for setting priorities. Its prioritization work is still directed largely at Medicaid beneficiaries; the fact that this perceived 'rationing' of care still targets only the poor may continue to marginalize patient/consumer consultation.

In Massachusetts, a statewide universal health care law took effect in 2006. Known as Chapter 58, it mandated health insurance coverage for all. Under the law, subsidies are provided to low- and moderate-income uninsured individuals to purchase health insurance. People 18 and over must enroll in a health plan, as long as 'creditable and affordable' plans are available in their community. If such plans are available, voluntarily uninsured persons lose their personal income tax exemption (an automatic tax deduction applied to individuals but not firms) and are required to pay a penalty of up to half the cost of the lowest available health plan premium; low-income persons are required to pay less. This legislation also imposes modest fines on companies that do not provide health insurance for their employees.

There is only one official avenue of consumer input into the law's implementation – service on the state's Health Quality and Cost Council Advisory Committee, which develops quality measurement and payment methods. However, the Robert Wood Johnson Foundation (a philanthropic fund endowed by the founder of Johnson & Johnson) simultaneously funded a consumer advocacy programme – Massachusetts Health Care for All – to respond as needed to developments as the new law was implemented. Called the Massachusetts Quality Coverage and Quality Care Initiative, it has focused the group's consumer engagement efforts – public testimony, letters, public position statements, meetings with legislators, hotlines – on the implementation of Chapter 58. A key effort has been the development of the Consumer Health Quality Council, which has created a consumer-driven advocacy agenda on issues such as reduction in hospital-acquired infections, public reporting of serious quality failures and provider apologies without legal penalty.

Massachusetts subsequently moved to institutionalize consumer input, not at state level but by mandating hospital-level Patient and Family Advisory Councils. These bodies are charged with collaborating on quality and patient care issues – for instance, medical error prevention, infection control, rapid response teams and notification of actual and potential adverse events. The

Consumer Health Quality Council will coordinate the development of these newly mandated hospital-based advisory groups (Needleman 2009).

CONSUMERS ORGANIZED FOR ADVOCACY: THE DISABILITY COMMUNITY AND OTHERS

The second type of consumer engagement relates not to groups established by public charter but to those which have come together to address specific health care needs and often play key roles in larger social movements. By default, as solidarity is not embedded in the US system, activist organizations from 'outside' the process are frequently the locus of consumer engagement in health care (Epstein 2008). Participation in policy decisions is often only one of several goals these organizations have. Although several examples are considered in this section, the primary focus is on disability groups.

Groups who work to improve health care and other services for disabled people are collectively known as 'the disability community'. If viewed as one large consumer group, it represents roughly one in five Americans (including those with and without chronic diseases) according to the 2000 US Census. A critical issue for this group is not merely the loss of health but the management of emotions that arise because of physical and mental impairment (Scotch 1989). These problems are obstacles to social participation, which explains why disabled individuals are less educated, less employed and more economically disadvantaged than the general population. Public ignorance and policymakers' insensitivity to the vast assortment of disability types are another problem. For example, grouping disabled individuals together into one group without addressing differences in their disabilities is counterproductive when it translates into global policy strategies that while serving some individuals well are ineffective and harmful to others.

The involvement of disabled people in the policy process has been solidified through the work of the disability rights movement. It has sought to eliminate obstacles to disabled individuals making a contribution to society and supported their efforts towards self-determination. The movement has become active in many parts of a complex policy domain (see Milewa in this volume). As with HSAs and FQHCs, it originated in the 1960s and 1970s and was much influenced by the broad social movements of the time that emphasized identity and social roles. The leadership of the disability rights movement emerged from activity on college campuses and successfully applied lessons learned in a disability context (Fleisher and Zames 2001).

'Consumer direction' is a philosophy of involving disabled persons in the design, policy development and implementation of services and tools (Kosciulek 1999). Centers for Independent Living (CILs) are a vehicle for this input. CILs are not-for-profit, non-residential, community-based organizations directed by disabled people that primarily address environmental and attitudinal barriers. The most common use of CIL electronic services is information and referral, for example guides to accessible housing, facilities, transportation routes and assistive technology providers. The second most common use is advocacy. CILs provide more systemic advocacy than self-advocacy. Systemic advocacy includes disability advocacy news tracking and Americans with Disability Act (ADA) accessibility complaint forms for consumers to complete (these forms are reviewed and may be used to take further actions to investigate public buildings possibly not conforming to ADA stipulations). Self-advocacy includes providing information on how to conduct background checks prior to hiring personal assistants and how to protect oneself from theft and abuse (Richie and Blanck 2003).

The progress in the half-century-old goals of the disability rights movement to eliminate obstacles to societal participation and to promote self-determination among disabled people has proceeded in phases, but is difficult to measure owing to lack of quantitative data. Despite major gains, numerous challenges still face disability advocates. One obstacle to attaining their goals is that not all individuals with a disability wish to be associated with the disability community. For example, as most people over 65 have at least one disability, the entire population of over 65-year-olds is commonly associated with the disability community. But this association is not desired by many senior citizens, whether they have disabilities or not. Another major obstacle is opposition to disability rights by some stakeholders. For example, accessibility standards for public buildings are an additional cost to the construction industry. Thus the industry lobbies Congress, state and local legislatures and corporate policymakers, making it difficult for disability rights advocates to attain their goal of eliminating obstacles to participation and self-determination. Finally, progress towards these goals is unclear because the political impact of disability consumer groups is hard to measure.

The mental health community has also activated consumers (often family members rather than patients themselves) in support of mental health parity legislation and services. The Mental Health Association (MHA) was founded in 1909 as the National Committee for Mental Hygiene. Including consumers and professionals, it was instrumental in seeking passage of the National Mental Health Act, which established the National Institute of Mental Health. Other key pieces of legislation in which the MHA has played a role are the Community Mental Health Centers Act, the Protection and Advocacy for Mentally Ill Individuals Act, the 1996 Mental Health Parity Act, and the 2008 Mental Health Parity and Addiction Equity Act. The 2008 legislation requires that employer-sponsored health insurance policies containing mental health and substance abuse benefits pay reimbursement for mental health and substance abuse treatment on par with payments for other medical and surgical health care, thus eliminating separate and more burdensome cost-sharing for these services (Bender 2009).

Another major national advocacy organization for mental health is the National Alliance on Mental Illness (NAMI), which is a broad grassroots consumer/family support and advocacy group. Local chapters focus on supporting family members of mentally ill people and providing community outreach and education about mental illness. Mental health advocacy has focused both on increasing access to treatment and advocating patients' civil rights – at times promoting the patient's right *not* to have treatment. In this respect, civil rights attorneys (which Isaac and Armat [1990] call the 'mental health bar') have promoted self-determination and autonomy among patients while casting doubt on the veracity of mental health diagnoses. This segment of the legal community has argued that psychiatric treatment is oppressive, with a 'radical patient' movement seeking to minimize hospitalization, particularly involuntary commitment, for severe mental illness. There is still some residual tension between patient advocates surrounding involuntary treatment; nevertheless the federal mental health agencies, the National Institute of Mental Health and the Substance Abuse and Mental Health Services Administration, have included consumer involvement in service and treatment design (Tomes 2006b).

While consumers have an established role in decision-making at the FDA (as discussed earlier), consumer activist groups continue to advocate on FDA rulings from outside the agency. While concerns grow about possibly hasty FDA drug and device approvals, there is also pressure from the opposite direction: consumers directly affected by serious illness complain of excessive delays and manoeuvring in getting treatments to the bedside, and have organized campaigns to shorten the time to drug approval. Indeed, some activists for patients are evolving from advocacy to biotech start-up in an effort to get therapies into the hands of seriously ill patients (Herper 2008).

Along with widespread criticism of pharmaceutical firm behaviour there is growing concern that patient advocacy groups are being financed and may be manipulated by drug companies for their own ends. NAMI has also come under criticism; large donations from pharmaceutical developers to this non-profit advocacy organization are viewed as incentives to advance policy that benefits the industry over patient interests (Torrey 2008). Nevertheless, NAMI maintains that financial support from the drug industry has not tainted its public policy positions.

Despite concerns about conflicts of interest in the case of some funders of consumer advocacy groups, these organizations continue to be a strong force in national policy circles. Some view health care consumer activism according to Kingdon's policy framework, which posits that multiple streams – problem recognition, policy development, and political activity – carry ideas from activism to legislation in the process of agenda-setting (Kingdon 1995). Brendtro (1998) has observed that the increased attention to breast cancer over several years, from the work of vocal patient groups to legislation and increased research funding, is an example of Kingdon's multi-stream idea. Interest groups like the National Breast Cancer Coalition engaged the public through letter-writing campaigns and adopted a symbol of support, the pink ribbon, modelled after the AIDS red ribbon icon. Key policy actors responded with hearings, attention was drawn to the need for additional research funding, more women were elected, and breast cancer became a prominent focus of the scientific agenda.

CONCLUSION

In the United States, we observe uneven success in establishing effective consumer involvement channels. Some consumer-based efforts, such as FQHCs and HSAs, are the result of earlier efforts to strengthen civil rights. In this policymaking pathway, especially publicly sponsored participation, the goal is often to ensure representation of specific population subgroups, for instance, low income, young, elderly, ethnic minority, or otherwise under-served groups. The FDA has arguably the strongest and most enduring official programme of consumer participation, and is focused broadly on involving people affected by its decisions regarding medications and devices. As 'labora-tories' of health policy, states may offer useful models of consumer involve-ment. While Oregon's experience showed that public involvement in health benefits distribution can dissolve into arguments over rationing, Massachusetts is building a consumer voice (with philanthropic help) through health quality committees and complaint hotlines. The efforts of the disability community have stretched beyond health care to seeking independence in all facets of living, such as employment and housing. Yet fundamental access to health care, arguably the ultimate prize for consumer advocacy, is still piecemeal and elusive. For example, disabled people may be able to find work, only to lose their Medicaid eligibility because of the programme's work and income restric-tions. Although recent health care legislation will increase access, most provi-sions will not be implemented until 2014. Compared with other industrialized nations, the United States has had special need of consumer advocacy for basic coverage, as well as for developing new cures and improving service delivery.

While consumer participation in health care policymaking continues along various pathways, it has taken a back seat in recent health care services and policy literature to the concept of the consumer as an economic actor. This approach puts responsibility on individuals to discern good quality and to judge fair and appropriate pricing. We observe this approach in the growth and encouragement of 'consumer-driven health plans', which involve increased patient cost-sharing and are expected to foster cost-conscious health care behaviour. Indeed, the label of consumer-driven health care has led one noted reformer physician to observe that consumers are indeed driven, 'just like cattle' (Woolhandler 2009). Yet, behavioural scientists observe that individual consumers are not well equipped to undertake such responsibility. Consumer-directed health plans, with their high out-of-pocket costs for patients, lead to reduced use of both high- and low-priority services (Hibbard et al. 2008). Although consumers are reported to be interested in finding high-quality providers, report cards and similar quality comparison literature tend to place cognitive burdens on patients (Hibbard 2008). This emphasis drives the focus of consumer engagement further away from solidarity towards individualism. As noted by Tritter, the results of the focus on individual patient choice 'in terms of shifting responsibility, inequality and opportunity cost are significant' (2009: 285). As pointed out by Fox and Lambertson in this volume, the US experiences recurrent cycles of attempts at reform. Although we are witnessing a watershed in health reform activity following the inauguration of a new President, democratization of health care will most likely continue to be fragmented and relatively specialized.

REFERENCES

Baggott, R. and R. Forster (2008), 'Health consumer and patients' organizations in Europe: towards a comparative analysis', *Health Expectations* **11** (1): 85–94.

Baggott, R., J. Allsop and K. Jones (2005), *Speaking for Patients and Carers: Health Consumer Groups and the Policy Process*, Basingstoke: Palgrave Macmillan.

Beauchamp, D.E. (1988), *The Health of the Republic: Epidemics, Medicine, and Moralism as Challenges to Democracy*, Philadelphia, PA: Temple University Press.

Bender, E. (2009), 'MH advocacy group celebrates century of achievement', *Psychiatric News*, **44** (6): 14.

Blumstein, J.F. (1997), 'The Oregon experiment: the role of cost-benefit analysis in the allocation of Medicaid funds', *Social Science & Medicine*, **45** (4): 545–54.

Brendtro, M.J. (1998), 'Breast cancer: agenda setting through activism', *Advanced Practice Nursing Quarterly*, **4** (1): 54–63.

Buck, D.S., D. Rochon, H. Davidson and S. McCurdy, for Members of the CHANGE Committee (2004), 'Involving homeless persons in the leadership of a health-care organization', *Qualitative Health Research*, **14**: 513–25.

Department of Health and Human Services (2009), 'Recovery act: community health centers', accessed September at www.hhs.gov/recovery/hrsa/healthcenter grants.html.

Epstein, S. (2008), 'Patient groups and health movements', in E.J. Hackett, O. Amsterdamska, M.E. Lynch and J. Wajcman (eds), *The Handbook of Science and Technology Studies*, 3rd edn, Cambridge, MA: MIT Press, pp. 499–539.

Favole, J. (2009), 'FDA pressed for transparency', *Wall Street Journal*, 24 June, accessed August at www.wsj.com/article/SB124588492308150255.html.

Food and Drug Administration (FDA) (2009a), 'About FDA: Office of Special Health Issues, mission statement', accessed August at www.fda.gov/AboutFDA/CentersOffices/OC/OfficeofExternalAffairs/OfficeofSpecialHealthIssues/default.htm.

FDA (2009b), 'Public calendars: past meetings with FDA officials', accessed August at www.fda.gov/NewsEvents/MeetingsConferencesWorkshops/PastMeetingsWithFDAOfficials/default.htm.

FDA (2009c), 'FDA advisory committees: membership types', accessed August at www.fda.gov/AdvisoryCommittees/AboutAdvisoryCommittees/CommitteeMembership/MembershipTypes/default.htm.

FDA (2009d), 'Patient representatives to FDA advisory committees', accessed August at www.fda.gov/ForConsumers/ByAudience/ForPatientAdvocates/PatientInvolvement/ucm123861.htm.

FDA (2009e), 'Patient representative program', accessed August at www.fda.gov/ForConsumers/ByAudience/ForPatientAdvocates/PatientInvolvement/ucm123858.htm.

Fleisher, D.Z. and Zames F. (2001), *The Disability Movement: From Charity to Confrontation*, Philadelphia, PA: Temple University Press.

Fox, D.M. and H.M. Leichter (1993), 'The ups and downs of Oregon's rationing plan', *Health Affairs*, **12** (2): 66–70.

Geiger, H.J. (2005), 'The first community health centers', *Journal of Ambulatory Care Management*, **28** (4), 313–20.

Guilford, C.T. (1993), 'Involving consumers in food control in the United States', Food and Agriculture Organization of the United States (FAO), *Food, Nutrition and Agriculture Review*, 08/09.

Herper, M. (2008), 'Patient Power', accessed 15 September 2009 at www.forbes.com/forbes/2008/0915/070.html.

Hibbard, J.H. (2008), 'What can we say about the impact of public reporting? Inconsistent execution yields variable results' (editorial), *Annals of Internal Medicine*, **148** (2): 160–1.

Hibbard, J.H., J. Greene and M. Tusler (2008), 'Does enrollment in a CDHP stimulate cost-effective utilization?', *Medical Care Research and Review*, **65** (4): 437–49.

Hiller, E.H., G. Landenburger and M.R. Natowicz (1997), 'Public participation in medical policy-making and the status of consumer autonomy: the example of newborn-screening programs in the United States', *American Journal of Public Health*, **87** (8): 1280–88.

Isaac, J. and V.C. Armat (1990), *Madness in the Streets: How Psychiatry and the Law Abandoned the Mentally Ill*, New York: Free Press.

Isbell, F. (2009), personal interview at Health Care for the Homeless, Houston, TX.

Kingdon, J.W. (1995), *Agendas, Alternatives, and Public Policies*, 2nd edn, New York: HarperCollins College Publishers.

Kosciulek, J.F. (1999), 'Consumer direction in disability policy formulation and rehabilitation service delivery', *Journal of Rehabilitation*, **65** (2): 4–9.

Learnmonth M., G.P. Martin and P. Warwick (2009), 'Ordinary and effective: the Catch-22 in managing the public voice in health care?', *Health Expectations*, **12** (1): 106–15.

Litva, A., K. Canvin, M. Shepherd, A. Jacoby and M. Gabbay (2009), 'Lay perceptions of the desired role and type of user involvement in clinical governance', *Health Expectations*, **12** (1): 81–91.

Marmor, T.R. and J.A. Morone (1980), 'Representing consumer interests: imbalanced markets, health planning, and the HSAs', *The Milbank Memorial Fund Quarterly:Health and Society*, **58** (1): 125–65.

Mick, S.S. and J.D. Thompson (1984), 'Public attitudes towards health planning under the health systems agencies', *Journal of Health Politics, Policy and Law*, **8** (4): 782–800.

Morone, J.A and E.H. Kilbreth (2003), 'Power to the people? Restoring citizen participation', *Journal of Health Politics, Policy and Law*, **28** (2–3): 271–88.

National Association of Community Health Centers (2009), *America's Health Centers*, accessed 6 September at www.nachc.org/client/documents/America's_Health_Centers_updated_3.09.pdf.

National Association of Community Health Centers (2010), 'Community health centers and health reform', accessed 19 May at www.nachc.org/client/Summary%20of%20Final%20Health%20Reform%20Package.pdf.

National Conference of State Legislatures (2009), 'Certificate of need: state health laws and programs, updated April 30, 2009', accessed 16 September at www.ncsl.org/default.aspx?tabid=14373.

National Disability Rights Network (2009), accessed at www.napas.org/aboutus/PA_CAP.htm.

Needleman, C. (2009), 'Second year evaluation of ensuring the consumer voice in coverage and quality in Massachusetts', July, Robert Wood Johnson Foundation, accessed at www.rwjf.org/files/research/3419.33719massreformrpt.pdf.

President's Council on Bioethics (2009), council reports, accessed September at www.bioethics.gov/reports.

Richie, H. and P. Blanck (2003), 'The promise of the internet for disability: a study of on-line services and web site accessibility at Centers for Independent Living', *Behavioral Sciences and the Law*, **21**: 5–26.

Rosen, C.J. (2007). 'The Rosiglitazone story – lessons from an FDA advisory committee meeting', *New England Journal of Medicine*, **357** (9): 844–6.

Scotch, R.K. (1989), 'Politics and policy in the history of the disability rights movement', *The Milbank Quarterly*, **67** (suppl. 2, pt 2): 380–99.

Steckler, A., L. Dawson, N. Dellinger and A. Williams (1981), 'Consumer participation and influence in a Health Systems Agency', *Journal of Community Health*, **6** (3): 181–93.

Ter Meulen, R.T. and F. Jotterand (2008), 'Individual Responsibility and Solidarity in European Health Care', *Journal of Medicine and Philosophy*, **33** (3): 191–7.

Tomes, N. (2006a), 'Patients or health-care consumers? Why the history of contested terms matters', in R.A. Stevens, C.E. Rosenberg and L.R. Burns (eds), *History and Health Policy in the United States: Putting the Past Back In*, New Brunswick, NJ: Rutgers University Press.

Tomes, N. (2006b), 'The patient as a policy factor: a historical case study of the consumer/survivor movement in mental health', *Health Affairs*, **25** (3): 720–29.

Torrey E.F. (1997), *Out of the Shadows: Confronting America's Mental Illness Crisis*, New York: John Wiley & Sons.

Torrey, E.F. (2008), letter to editor, 'Question of disclosure', *Psychiatric Services*, **59** (8): 935.

Tritter, J. (2009), 'Revolution or evolution: the challenges of conceptualizing patient and public involvement in a consumerist world', *Health Expectations*, **12**: 275–87.

Tritter, J. and K. Lutfey (2009), editorial, 'Bridging divides: patient and public involvement on both sides of the Atlantic', *Health Expectations*, **12** (3): 221–5.

Van de Bovenkamp, H.M. and M.J. Trappenburg (2009a), 'Patient participation in collective health care decision making: the Dutch model', *Health Expectations*, forthcoming; doi: 10.1111/j.1369-7625.2009.00567.x.

Van de Bovenkamp, H.M. and M.J. Trappenburg (2009b), 'Reconsidering patient participation in guideline development', *Health Care Analysis*, **17** (3): 198–216.

WebMD (2009), 'WebMD teams with FDA for new online consumer health information: new partnership to inform and educate tens of millions of Americans', accessed August 2009 at www.investor.shareholder.com/wbmd/releasedetail.cfm?ReleaseID=351973 .

Weissert, C.S. and W.G. Weissert (1996), *Governing Health: The Politics of Health Policy*, Baltimore. MD: Johns Hopkins University Press.

Woolhandler, S. (2009), comments to Annual Meeting of Physicians for a National Health Program, October, Cambridge, MA, October.

16. Health consumer groups and the pharmaceutical industry: is transparency the answer?

Agnes Vitry and Hans Löfgren

It is a commonplace for organizations with different interests to work cooperatively for shared but limited objectives. Yet large power asymmetries present particular hazards for the weaker party. Most health consumer groups operate on small budgets and rely on volunteers. They typically provide mutual support and self-help, information and advice, services, advocacy and efforts to generate public awareness of particular disease conditions, fundraising for research, and participation in the policy process. Small amounts of corporate funding can make a significant difference to their capacity to support members and their families. In contrast, large pharmaceutical corporations develop, produce and sell medicinal products, with the ultimate aim of maximizing returns to shareholders.

It is increasingly acknowledged by both corporations and consumer groups that their interactions must be consistent with ethical standards. For example the Consumers Health Forum of Australia (CHF) jointly with the Big Pharma association Medicines Australia have developed guidelines 'to assist both parties to work together appropriately in a transparent and accountable way' (CHF and Medicines Australia 2008: 2). The guidelines note that '[h]ealth consumer organizations and pharmaceutical companies have collaborated for many years to address the needs of health consumers' (CHF and Medicines Australia 2008: 2). Such relationships have given rise to a vigorous international debate, to which this chapter seeks to make a contribution (Herxheimer 2003; Kent 2007; Mintzes 2007).

Industry–consumer group relations usually entail an exchange of product or corporate visibility for funding and other resources. For companies, consumer groups offer opportunities of reaching consumers directly. This can be through joint 'disease awareness' campaigns with the hidden, or not-so-hidden, message that drugs are available (on prescription) to address the disease in question. Consumer groups also provide opportunities for building pre-launch awareness of new drugs, and they may share with pharmaceutical companies an interest in lobbying for licensing and pricing arrangements that maximize access to particular medicines. The downside of such interaction is that the integrity of decision-making on medicines policy and public health may be jeopardized (Gauvin et al. 2010; Deloitte 2009). We also identify in this chapter an emerging trend towards inclusion of consumer groups into the research and development (R&D) process. Charities and foundations with an origin in patient activism have in some instances themselves become influential drivers of R&D, and in this capacity engage closely with the pharmaceutical industry.

We argue the case for caution on the part of consumer organizations. As these organizations gain influence in the health policy arena they are increasingly viewed as the preferred target for pharmaceutical industry marketing. By accepting corporate donations patient organizations expose themselves to the charge of contributing to industry efforts to 'sell more pills' (Mintzes 2007). Full public disclosure of financial and other ties would be a step forward, but transparency is not a sufficient response to this dilemma.

CORPORATE SPONSORSHIP OF HEALTH CONSUMER GROUPS

From the few studies undertaken (cited in this chapter) it would seem that between a third and two-thirds of health consumer groups in developed countries receive corporate support in some form. Firms 'clearly have much to gain by filtering their marketing messages through such organizations, which tend to engender more trust than do multinational companies' (Marshall and Aldhous 2006: 18). Companies rarely acknowledge this marketing objective explicitly. Instead formulations such as the following are typical, taken from the Novo Nordisk website (which also reports that in 2009 diabetes products accounted for 73 per cent of company sales):

> Novo Nordisk interacts with a wide variety of patient organisations as part of a shared goal of informing and supporting patients about their healthcare needs. We work with patient groups, often on a long-term basis, to raise disease awareness, including the importance of early diagnosis and appropriate treatment. These interactions provide Novo Nordisk with valuable insights about how living with diabetes or other conditions affects patients' lives. (Novo Nordisk 2010)

Of 55 Finnish patient organizations surveyed in 2003, 71 per cent reported funding from pharmaceutical companies. Half of these (55 per cent) considered cooperation with the drug industry important or very important and 33 per cent reported increased industry cooperation in the previous 5 years. Support received included medicines information and expert opinions, advertising in organization magazines and newsletters, participation in seminars, assistance with printing costs, participation in projects, and money donations. All of the 20 top largest drug firms in Finland confirmed that they gave support to patient organizations (Hemminki et al. 2010).

A 2004 survey of 112 Irish 'health advocacy organizations' showed that almost half (47 per cent) accepted funding and/or support in kind from the pharmaceutical industry. Detailed information on pharmaceutical industry funding was generally not provided in the organizations' publications or on their websites (O'Donovan 2007). In 2006 an international survey of 69 websites of patient organizations representing chronic conditions showed that 45 per cent of such groups declared pharmaceutical funding. However, annual reports named more industry donors than did the websites. None of the annual reports provided sufficient information to determine the proportion of organizations' total budgets funded by industry (Ball et al. 2006).

In 2007, 40 per cent of the Association of British Pharmaceutical Industry's 74 full members reported providing financial and in-kind support to consumer groups on their websites (Jones 2008). Each firm supported only one or a few consumer organizations; most consumer groups reported support from only one company while a quarter of groups reported support from two or three companies. Presumably firms were focused on organizations that are active in the disease areas for which they supply medicines. Only four companies revealed the exact funding provided. A cross-check of consumer group websites showed that they were less likely than companies to acknowledge this relationship; only 26 per cent of groups known to receive industry support reported this on their websites (Jones 2008).

In 2006 the *New Scientist* investigated the funding of large US patient groups by pharmaceutical and medical device industries (Marshall and Aldhous 2006). From a database listing, 20 organizations with revenues of more than US$100 000, plus five with revenues in excess of US$10 million, were chosen at random. Also included were four groups with revenues of more than US$100 000 working in areas where the industry has been criticized for 'disease-mongering'. Of these groups, seven received more than 20 per cent of their funding from the industry; the Depression and Bipolar Support Alliance and the Colorectal Cancer Coalition received more than half of their revenue from corporate sources. The report noted that groups not receiving industry funding seemed to be working in disease areas where drug therapies were not available. There was a clear correlation between the commercial interests of a company and donations provided to consumer groups working in that same disease area (Marshall and Aldhous 2006). In an accompanying editorial the *New Scientist* noted that 'the groups most heavily funded by industry are more likely to be those focusing on conditions where the industry has been accused of "disease-mongering" – encouraging relatively healthy people to seek treatment' (Anonymous 2006: 5).

PatientView, an organization with apparent links to the pharmaceutical industry, has reported a survey of 384 patient groups from 49 countries. A third of respondent groups derived some portion of their income from pharmaceutical companies, while 57 per cent received no corporate funding. In total, 58 per cent had regular or occasional contact with pharmaceutical companies and 29 per cent reported no contact (PatientView 2008; PatientView 2009).

The Irish survey showed that the form of engagement with pharmaceutical firms varied from confrontation to close collaboration. Yet a tendency was identified among consumer groups and medical research charities for them to frame the pharmaceutical industry as a partner (O'Donovan 2007). A 2005 Canadian study showed a similar pattern of consumer organizations' attitudes towards the pharmaceutical industry, ranging from gratitude to caution to alarm. Typically, groups opposed to pharmaceutical funding supported a strong government role in drug regulation and opposed direct-to-consumer advertising of prescription medicines. Industry-funded groups contested the assumption that strict government regulations necessarily favoured the public interest, emphasized the need for rapid drug approvals and in some instances supported direct-to-consumer advertising (Batt 2005).

In the PatientView survey only a minority of respondent groups considered pharmaceutical companies 'good' or 'better than good' in terms of trustworthiness (37 per cent), or at managing conflicts of interest (24 per cent) or adverse news about their products (39 per cent). Groups receiving funding from the drug industry had greater confidence in pharmaceutical companies, but not in their management of adverse news. Fewer than half (44 per cent) thought that pharmaceutical companies were good or better than good at innovation to meet patients' needs. Respondents blamed a lack of innovation on the profit motive; in particular they held the view that commercial considerations make innovation to address rare conditions unattractive. Only one-third felt that pharmaceutical companies were good or better than good at being transparent about their relationships with patient groups.

In 2007 conflicting views on partnerships with the pharmaceutical industry were presented in a debate in the *British Medical Journal*. According to Alastair Kent, director of the Genetic Interest Group (the UK alliance of charities and support groups for people affected by genetic disorders), 'if financial support is out in the open and any attached strings are clear and appropriate (for example, restricted to a specific project or publication) then industry money is as good as that from any other source' (Kent 2007). The view of Barbara Mintzes of Health Action International was that patient groups, seen in the pharmaceutical marketing literature as 'allies to help advance brand objectives', 'cannot provide impartial information if they are funded by companies that sell products to treat those illnesses'(Mintzes 2007).

THE INFLUENCE OF THE PHARMACEUTICAL INDUSTRY

The influence of the pharmaceutical industry on prescribers is well documented (Moynihan 2003), as is its capacity to influence regulatory arrangements (Abraham 2008). Industry-sponsored research is more likely to report drug benefits than non-sponsored trials or meta-analyses (Lexchin et al. 2003; Yank et al. 2007) and less likely to report adverse effects (Nieto et al. 2007). But there is very limited research examining whether and how patient organizations are influenced by corporate sponsors. Batt (2005) argues that such influence can result in the gradual and instinctive accommodation of such organizations to the sponsor. Subtle and improper influence is difficult to identify and may not translate into public endorsement of commercial claims for specific products, but may affect the views of consumer organizations on issues such as conditions of access to new medications. Industry support also conceivably contributes to a 'techno-consumption' mindset of excessive trust in new and expensive medicines even should they be less safe or effective than older treatments or lifestyle changes (Deyo and Patrick 2005).

There are numerous case reports of improper corporate influence on consumer groups (Herxheimer 2003; Mintzes 2007). For example Forest Laboratories, charged by the US Justice Department with defrauding the government through illegal marketing of the antidepressants Celexa and Lexapro for unapproved uses in children and teenagers, was a sponsor of several US health consumer organizations in the mental health sector, where their aim was 'to disseminate important brand information to their members' and 'to assist mutual efforts at the state policy level' (Forest Laboratories 2003).

There are also instances of companies or their public relations agents creating their 'own' patient organizations to promote a product or a perspective on particular regulatory issues (Herxheimer 2003; Batt 2005). Such groups are referred to as 'astroturf' organizations because of their false claims to genuine, grass-roots consumer status (O'Donovan 2005). For example the International Alliance of Patients' Organizations (IAPO) founded by Pharmaceutical Partners for Better Healthcare, a consortium of about 30 major companies, to all intents and purposes presents the industry's perspective on medicines issues. Together with other industry-related organizations, IAPO lobbied the European Commission to allow direct-to-consumer information about prescription medicines (Herxheimer 2003). In the United States several seniors organizations have been funded by pharmaceutical companies to lobby against proposed drug policy changes (Batt 2005). In some instances groups with genuine origins as consumer organizations have become virtually indistinguishable from astroturf groups through a process of 'mission drift' (Batt

2005). For example, after collaborating with pharmaceutical companies on developing hormone replacement therapy (HRT), the Society for Women's Health Research (SWHR), established in 1990, reacted negatively when a large, independent clinical trial demonstrated the harmful effects of HRT for menopausal women (Mundy 2003).

In the United Kingdom a House of Commons inquiry recommended that measures be taken to limit the influence of the industry on patient groups (House of Commons Health Committee 2005). A particular concern was that groups lobbying the National Institute for Health and Clinical Excellence (NICE) for approval of specific drugs are often supported by pharmaceutical companies (Ferner and McDowell 2006). A more recent example of such lobbying relates to the Alzheimer's Society. In receipt of substantial funding from manufacturers of dementia products, in 2006 it led a patient campaign against a NICE ruling that the dementia drugs Aricept, Reminyl and Exelon should not be subsidized from public funds (Mintzes 2007).

REGULATING RELATIONS BETWEEN THE PHARMACEUTICAL INDUSTRY AND HEALTH CONSUMER ORGANIZATIONS

Corporate support for health consumer organizations creates conflicts of interest that should be recognized and addressed. A conflict of interest does not necessarily mean that one's judgement has been or will be compromised but refers to a potential for undue influence and the creation of an impression of bias that may undermine public confidence in consumer organizations. The legitimacy of their participation in public policy processes risks being weakened. Participation typically takes the form of representation on committees such as those involved in decisions on public subsidization of new medicines, an area where both consumer organizations and pharmaceutical companies have a strong interest. In response to these concerns consumer organizations, pharmaceutical companies and governmental institutions have developed policies to govern relationships between stakeholders.

Policies Developed by Consumer Organizations

The UK Association of Medical Research Charities has developed guidelines for industry partnership which cover areas such as medical research, sponsorships, policy and advocacy (Association of British Pharmaceutical Industry 2008). The guidelines recommend that members work, where possible, with several industry partners when producing educational material, that they retain editorial control, and do not endorse specific treatments. They recommend a written agreement where a charity is involved in a collaborative lobbying campaign. As already noted, the CHF, the national peak body for Australian health consumers, has, together with Medicines Australia, adopted guidelines for relationships between health consumer organizations and pharmaceutical companies which emphasize principles such as honesty, integrity, trust and respect. The guidelines are non-prescriptive and do not require explicit disclosure of industry support on an organization's website or in its annual reports. The benefits of collaborative relationships are highlighted without reference to possible drawbacks (CHF and Medicines Australia 2008).

In June 2009 several European patient organizations adopted a code of practice for relations with the health care industry (European Cancer Patient Coalition 2009). The principles expressed in this code, such as openness, honesty and transparency, are similar to those of the CHF, but the code is more prescriptive, recommending that funding should be diversified and received on an unconditional basis. Amounts and sources of industry funding should be disclosed and sponsors' logo size and space on websites should be modest to avoid being perceived as advertisements. This code also provides a list of sponsorship activities considered promotional and potentially illegal, such as consumer organizations appearing in promotional materials for particular products or being quoted in industry press releases. This concern is also explicit in a policy adopted by the Australian organization Arthritis Victoria, which notes that the association of some consumer organizations with particular products may contravene the spirit of laws prohibiting direct-to-consumer advertising of prescription products in most countries. Notably, it states that all relationships should be documented in signed memoranda of understanding and that the recipient organization should seek an independent review of information supplied by any pharmaceutical company prior to publication (Arthritis Victoria 2010). At the opposite end of the spectrum, IAPO, which derived more than 95 per cent of its 2009 budget from industry funding, is asking industry partners to provide financial support under four headings: gold (US$50 000 per year), silver (US$25 000 per year), bronze (US$10 000 per year), and standard (US$5000 per year) (IAPO 2008).

Policies Developed by the Pharmaceutical Industry

The European Federation of Pharmaceutical Industries and Associations (EFPIA) has adopted a code of practice for relationships between the pharmaceutical industry and patient organizations (EFPIA 2007). This code requires pharmaceutical companies to have a written agreement in place when providing financial support or significant non-financial support to patient organizations, and companies must make publicly available a list of supported patient organizations, updated annually, with a short description of the nature of each sponsorship. The Code of Practice of the Association of British Pharmaceutical Industry (ABPI) contains similar provisions (Association of British Pharmaceutical Industry 2008). Anything with a value of £500 or more is considered significant support and should be declared. In 2010 the 16th edition of Medicines Australia's code of conduct for marketing by its member firms added a section on relationships with health consumer organizations. Companies must list on their websites those health consumer organizations to which they give financial or significant direct or indirect non-financial support, but the code of conduct does not require disclosure of the amount of funding (Medicines Australia 2010). There seems to have been no systematic assessment of how or to what extent such industry codes have been implemented in practice.

Policies Developed by Governments

Government institutions in several countries have developed or are in the processes of developing detailed frameworks for the participation of consumers in decision-making concerning the licensing and use of pharmaceuticals. Draft guidelines developed by the Canadian Agency for Drugs and Technologies in Health (CADTH) for patient group input into assessment of new medicines propose conflict of interest declarations for corporate members and situations of joint work/sponsorship or funding, and for individuals who play a significant role in compiling submissions (CADTH 2009). In its response to this draft, the Best Medicines Coalition, a Canadian national alliance of patient organizations, expressed concern that it did not explain how conflicts of interest would be taken account of in the review process and that such declarations should not compromise the value of legitimate patient input (Best Medicines Coalition 2010).

The criteria to be fulfilled by consumer organizations involved in European Medicines Agency (EMA) activities require transparency as far as possible in disclosing sources of funding, including individual financial contributions (European Medicines Agency 2005). In August 2009, 23 consumer organizations were eligible to work with the EMA. Of these, 15 received corporate funding, seven did not, and no information was found for one organization (Perehudoff and Alves 2010). Corporate funding for the years 2006 to 2008 ranged from 0.19 per cent to 99.1 per cent of organizations' annual budgets, the average being 45.4 per cent. Individuals nominated by their organization to participate as representatives or as experts have to adhere to the EMA policy on conflicts of interest (European Medicines Agency 2005). However a recent survey found that conflicts of interest statements may be misleading (Corporate Europe Observatory 2010). For example statements by the two consumer representatives on the powerful EMA Management Board failed to mention that the organizations they represented – the European Federation of Neurological Associations and the European Patients' Forum – were funded mainly by pharmaceutical companies. There is no information on how these conflicts of interest are managed in practice at the EMA (Lexchin and O'Donovan 2010). It appears, however, that representatives of consumer organizations funded mainly by drug companies are not restricted in any way from participating in EMA activities.

CONSUMER PARTICIPATION IN BIOMEDICAL R&D

In the early years of the modern pharmaceutical industry, interactions with consumers were mediated by doctors, particularly medical specialists. In that period a business model of dependence on a small number of chemically derived, big-selling 'blockbuster' drugs was established (Galambos and Sturchio 1997). Today multinational companies with familiar names like Pfizer and GlaxoSmithKline depend for new drugs on innovation networks linking many actors. In particular, collaborations between large companies, universities and public sector research institutes, and smaller biotechnology companies, are critical to biomedical innovation.

At the same time the Big Pharma model has come under pressure for a lack of new breakthrough drugs, price constraints imposed through the application of market power by public and private insurers, and more demanding regulatory requirements. The upshot is an environment where external organizations, and public and consumer opinion, must increasingly be taken account of in technical–scientific, regulatory and commercial decisions and strategies. An industry analyst notes that 'the end of the blockbuster generation … [requires] … a new model of commercialization [that] recognize[s] the patient as a key stakeholder and include[s] the direct communication of value messages' (Featherstone 2009). Epstein's (2008) survey of studies of 'patient groups and health movements' in the biomedical field details an important aspect of this trend. He pays particular attention to the 1980s activist mobilization to gain access to HIV/AIDS drugs, which was followed by the formation of other 'disease constituencies' seeking to influence the funding and direction of R&D. For example a high-profile campaign has been waged in many countries by groups advocating for women afflicted by breast cancer (Fricker 2007). Such campaigns have built a momentum for the entry of consumer groups into systems of funding and regulation of research, which often takes the form of representation on advisory committees assessing research proposals or ethical issues.

Participation of this type is increasingly seen as appropriate for moral and ethical reasons that centre 'on concepts of rights, citizenship and democracy specifically related to publicly funded research, whereby the word "consumer" is seen as a synonym for "taxpayer"' (Ward et al. 2010: 64). In the United Kingdom, for example, there is 'a clear policy directive to involve patients and the public in the National Health Service's (NHS) research and development process' (Boote et al. 2002). A related area of active consumer participation is that of technology assessment undertaken by agencies like the National Institute for Health and Clinical Excellence (NICE) in the United Kingdom, and the Pharmaceutical Benefits Advisory Committee in Australia (Fattal and Lehoux 2008). As already noted, at the European level consumer groups have had a significant presence in the consultations and working groups of the European Medicines Agency, ever since its establishment in 1995 (Kermani 2010).

Consumer groups are not likely to exercise major influence on the direction of research, but their participation in this area adds to other reasons for companies to take them seriously (Smits and Boon 2008):

- Consumer organizations and other NGOs have lobbied with some success for governments and corporations to address the need for R&D focused on rare disorders and the 'neglected diseases' of the developing world. For example the National Organization for Rare Disorders (NORD) in the United States and the European Organization for Rare Disorders (EURORDIS) bring together large numbers of advocacy groups (Kermani 2009).
- Corporate innovation can benefit from experiential knowledge of sickness and medicinal products channelled by consumer groups (Caron-Flinterman et al. 2005).
- Consumer organizations in some cases mobilize substantial financial resources for research. Clinical trial participants can be recruited through consumer organizations.
- Norms and attitudes are important for the social acceptance and commercial success of new drugs.

Some disease-specific consumer groups with a focus on rare genetic diseases have become biomedical research organizations in their own right. Terry et al. (2007: 159) list 21 US 'research advocacy foundations', and examples can be found also in other countries, such as the Netherlands (Boon and Broekgaarden 2010) and France (Dalgalarrondo 2004; Franrenet 2007). The Hereditary Disease Foundation, reported to be the first consumer organization of this type, established a research consortium 'which in 1983 led to the identification of a genetic marker for Huntington's disease' (Terry et al. 2007: 158). The Cystic Fibrosis Foundation and similar organizations were established as conventional patient support organizations decades before turning to fundraising 'to accelerate the pathway from basic science to treatments and technologies' (Mackta and Weiss 1994; Terry et al. 2007: 158). In 2009 the revenues of the Cystic Fibrosis Foundation were in excess of US$200 million; at its annual medical conference in that year 'more than 3500 scientists and researchers around the globe' reported on research in this field (Cystic Fibrosis Foundation 2009: 1). While retaining a large network of volunteers, the Foundation provides funding for and works closely with pharmaceutical and biotechnology companies, and reports having more than 30 potential drugs in its 'therapeutics development pipeline' (Cystic Fibrosis Foundation 2009: 5). Gilead Sciences, a major biotech company, is one of the firms receiving funding from the Cystic Fibrosis Foundation. Its chief scientific officer affirms that 'the foundation's stamp of approval gives companies more credibility with investors. "If they have looked at it, and they have funded it, it must be something worthwhile" ' (Herper 2008). This is one of a number of 'patient groups with an entrepreneurial bent [that] have become the drug industry's new power brokers ... By becoming a one-stop source for expertise and research about their disease, these patient groups can use as little as a few million dollars in funding to shift the priorities of the industry' (Herper 2008). US organizations in this category include the Leukemia and Lymphoma Society, the Multiple Myeloma Research Foundation, the Juvenile Diabetes Research Foundation, the Myelin Repair Foundation for Multiple Sclerosis, and the Multiple Myeloma Research Foundation. The National Organization for Rare Disorders in the United States and the European Organisation for Rare Disorders (EURORDIS) have lobbied successfully for the introduction of orphan drug legislation aimed at providing incentives for pharmaceutical companies to develop and market drugs to treat rare diseases. EURORDIS, which reports 434 member organizations in 43 countries, vigorously promotes rare diseases as a priority in EU research policy and funding schemes. In France, the Association Française contre les Myopathies (AFM, French Muscular Dystrophy Organisation) is extensively involved in medical research through direct funding of around 400 projects a year (Franrenet 2007).

Such activities as these point to an intriguing coming-together of patient activism with the pharmaceutical industry. If genuinely responsive to their membership and attuned to broader citizen needs, the organizations involved in this meeting of interests could be a force for the opening up of the biomedical research field to public deliberation and democratization. But the embeddedness of most such groups within the United States or a US-inspired 'culture of innovation' suggests that research-oriented patient activism runs the risk of mutation into commercial entrepreneurialism and a research agenda shaped by corporate partners (Sunder Rajan 2006: 188; Herper 2008).

DOES TRANSPARENCY EQUAL PROBITY?

The role of consumer organizations in many health policy areas has come to be recognized and valued by governments, pharmaceutical companies and the public. Governmental institutions, health care providers and research bodies seek input from consumer groups and provide guidelines and policies to encourage best practice for such participation. But in the same way that health professionals are criticized for close relationships with drug companies, the legitimacy of consumer organizations as genuine representatives of their constituencies may be damaged if relations with the pharmaceutical industry generate perceptions of bias. Policies and codes of practice, and the public disclosure of information about such relations, represent a limited and insufficient response to these concerns. Disclosure is important and may reinforce openness by facilitating further demands for information. But disclosure of information may also make conflicts of interest appear acceptable and may not be an adequate basis for assessments of the risk of bias. Moreover in contrast to conflicts of interest declared by health professionals, which relate to personal involvement with the pharmaceutical industry in research, educational or marketing activities, conflicts of interest are in this context likely to reflect organizational engagements. This is not adequately taken account of in the current EMA criteria for conflicts of interest. Can it be considered appropriate that a representative of IAPO, one of the 25 organizations included in the EMA registry, and more than 95 per cent funded by the drug industry, be allowed to engage in EMA's activities as legitimately representing consumers?

On the basis of Canadian experiences Batt (2005) argues for stricter controls on relations between corporations and consumer groups, including regulation of informational and educational material produced by consumer organizations on the same basis as controls on corporate marketing. That nearly half of Finnish patient organizations are estimated to receive drug information from the pharmaceutical industry raises concerns about the reliability of patient information supplied by consumer organizations. Public participation in drug policy development requires constraints on consumer organizations' dependence on corporate funding, and Batt (2005: 21) for this reason proposes a federal Canadian 'arm's length health advocacy funding agency (or agencies)'. There is at least one international precedent for a broad-based system of non-corporate funding of consumer organizations; Geissler in this volume explains that German health insurers have been required since 2000 to spend 0.56 a year per insured individual in support of consumer groups undertaking self-help activities. Finnish researchers also highlight the need for a sustainable funding model guaranteeing independence of consumer organizations (Hemminki et al. 2010). This concern is shared by European consumer organizations; the European Cancer Patient Coalition notes that very few sources of non-commercial funding are available to patients groups at a European level (European Cancer Patient Coalition 2009).

The role of consumer organizations in health policy is only likely to grow further and the issues around partnerships with the pharmaceutical industry will become increasingly central. While transparency and codes of conduct represent a first response to these concerns, the drawbacks of industry partnerships require new initiatives for independent funding of consumer organizations and clear rules for managing conflicts of interest in governmental, research and health services institutions.

ACKNOWLEDGEMENTS

The authors wish to acknowledge valuable comments on an earlier draft by Barbara Mintzes.

REFERENCES

Abraham, J. (2008), 'Bias and science in knowledge production: implications for the politics of drug regulation', in O. O'Donovan and K. Glavanis-Grantham (eds), *Power, Politics and Pharmaceuticals*, Cork, Ireland: Cork University Press, pp. 43–57.

Anonymous (2006), 'A special relationship: does it matter when patient groups get cosy with drug companies?', *New Scientist*, **192** (2575): 5.

Arthritis Victoria (2010), 'Relationships with pharmaceutical companies', accessed 15 August at www.arthritisvic.org.au/pages.asp?d=5A4C5A717251477C7008060 B0E0800.

Association of British Pharmaceutical Industry (2008), 'Code of Practice for the pharmaceutical industry', accessed 15 August 2010 at www.pmcpa.org.uk/.

Ball, D.E., K. Tisocki and A. Herxheimer (2006), 'Advertising and disclosure of funding on patient organisation web sites: a cross-sectional survey', *BMC Public Health*, **6**: 201.

Batt, S. (2005), 'Marching to different drummers: health advocacy groups in Canada and funding from the pharmaceutical industry, women and health protection', accessed 15 August 2010 at www.whp-apsf.ca/pdf/corpFunding.pdf.

Best Medicines Coalition (2010), 'Submission: CADTH consultation on patient input into CDR review assessments', accessed 15 August 2010 at www.bestmedicines.ca/ node/140 .

Boon, W. and R. Broekgaarden (2010), 'The role of patient advocacy organisations in neuromuscular disease R&D: the case of the Dutch neuromuscular disease association VSN', *Neuromuscular Disorders*, **20** (2): 148–51.

Boote, J., R. Telford and C. Cooper (2002), 'Consumer involvement in health research: a review and research agenda', *Health Policy*, **61** (2): 213–36.

Canadian Agency for Drugs and Technologies in Health (CADTH) (2009), 'Guidance for submitting patient group input to the common drug review and participating drug plans', accessed 15 August 2010 at www.cadth.ca/index.php/en/cdr/cdr-update/cdr-update-issue-63.

Caron-Flinterman, J.F., J.E.W. Broerse and J.F.G. Bunders (2005), 'The experiential knowledge of patients: a new resource for biomedical research?', *Social Science & Medicine*, **60** (11): 2575–84.

Consumers Health Forum of Australia (CHF) and Medicines Australia (2008), *Working Together: A Guide to Relationships Between Health Consumer Organisations and Pharmaceutical Companies*, Canberra: CHF/Medicines Australia.

Corporate Europe Observatory (2010), 'Patient groups need a strong dose of transparency: how a lax conflicts of interest policy allows patient groups to hide pharma-industry funding', accessed 15 August at www.corporateeurope.org/lobbycracy/content/2010/04/patient-groups-need-dose-transparency.

Cystic Fibrosis Foundation (2009), *Annual Report*, Bethesda, MD: CF Foundation.

Deloitte (2009), 'Enhancing consumer involvement in medicines health technology assessment', accessed 15 August 2010 at www.deloitte.com/view/en_AU/au/industries/Lifesciencesandhealth/da8692c1e7495210VgnVCM100000ba42f00a RCRD.htm.

Dalgalarrondo, S. (2004), 'Recherche clinique et innovation médicamenteuse: quelle place pour les patients et leurs représentants? Une comparaison sida, cancer et maladies rares', Maison de la Recherche, Toulouse, France: Université de Toulouse le Mirail.

Deyo, R. and D.L. Patrick (2005), *Hope or Hype: The Obsession with Medical Advances and the High Cost of False Promises*, New York: AMACOM.

Epstein, S. (2008), 'Patient groups and health movements', in E.J. Hackett, O. Amsterdamska, M. Lynch and J. Wajcman (eds), *The Handbook of Science and Technology Studies*, 3rd edn, Cambridge, MA.: MIT Press, pp. 499–540.

European Cancer Patient Coalition (2009), 'Code of practice working with the industry', accessed 15 August 2010 at www.ecpc-online.org/advocacy-toolbox/code-of-practice.html.

European Federation of Pharmaceutical Industries and Associations (EFPIA) (2007), 'EFPIA code of practice on relationships between the pharmaceutical Industry and patient organisations', accessed 15 August 2010 at www.efpia.org/content/default.asp?PagcID=615.

European Medicines Agency (2005), 'Criteria to be fulfilled by patients and consumers' organisations involved in EMEA activities', accessed 15 August 2010 at www.emea.europa.eu/ docs/en_GB/document_library/Regulatory_and_procedural_guideline/2009/12/WC500018099.pdf.

Fattal, J. and P. Lehoux (2008), 'Health technology assessment use and dissemination by patient and consumer groups: why and how?', *International Journal of Technology Assessment in Health Care*, **24** (4): 473–80.

Featherstone, J. (2009), 'Pharma's new commercialization model', PharmExec.com, accessed 15 August 2010 at http://pharmexec.findpharma.com/pharmexec/Europe/Pharmas-New-Commercialization-Model/ArticleStandard/Article/detail/648932?ref=25.

Ferner, R.E. and S.E. McDowell (2006), 'How NICE may be outflanked', *British Medical Journal*, **332** (7552): 1268–71.

Forest Laboratories (2003) 'Lexapro FY 2004 marketing plan', accessed 15 August 2010 at http://dida.library.ucsf.edu/pdf/zwc37b10.

Franrenet, S. (2007), 'Le rôle des associations de patients dans les organismes de recherché', *Etudes et Synthèses*, 10, accessed 15 August 2010 at www.ethique.inserm.fr/inserm/ethique.nsf/f812af09a0a47338c1257153004fa70e/b a7afdbb3233126ac125736b004c2993?OpenDocument.

Fricker, J. (2007), 'Patient advocacy groups: empowering patients in their fight against cancer', *Molecular Oncology*, **1** (3): 252–4.

Galambos, L. and J.L. Sturchio (1997), 'The transformation of the pharmaceutical industry in the twentieth century', in J. Krige and D. Pestre (eds), *Science in the Twentieth Century*, Amsterdam, Netherlands: Harwood Academic Publishers, pp. 227–52.

Gauvin, F.P., J. Abelson, M. Giacomini, J. Eyles, and J.N. Lavis (2010), '"It all depends": conceptualizing public involvement in the context of health technology assessment agencies', *Social Science & Medicine*, **70** (10): 1518–26.

Hemminki, E., H.K. Toiviainen, and L. Vuorenkoski (2010), 'Co-operation between patient organisations and the drug industry in Finland', *Social Science & Medicine*, **70** (8): 1171–5.

Herper, M. (2008) 'Patient power', Forbes.com, accessed 15 August 2010 at www.forbes.com/forbes/2008/0915/070.html.

Herxheimer, A. (2003), 'Relationships between the pharmaceutical industry and patients' organisations', *British Medical Journal*, **326** (7400): 1208–10.

House of Commons Health Committee (2005), *The Influence of the Pharmaceutical Industry. Fourth Report of Session 2004–2005*, London: The Stationery Office.

International Alliance of Patients' Organizations (IAPO) (2008), 'Healthcare industry partners framework', accessed 15 August 2010 at www.patientsorganizations.org/ showarticle.pl?id=222;n=122.

Jones, K. (2008), 'In whose interest? Relationships between health consumer groups and the pharmaceutical industry in the UK', *Sociology of Health & Illness*, **30** (6): 929–43.

Kent, A. (2007), 'Should patient groups accept money from drug companies? Yes', *British Medical Journal*, **334** (7600): 934.

Kermani, F. (2009), 'EU and US unite against rare diseases', PharmTech.com, accessed 15 August 2010 at http://pharmtech.findpharma. com/pharmtech/Spotlight/EU-and-US-unite-against-rare-diseases/ArticleStandard/ Article/detail/605697.

Kermani, F. (2010), 'The changing face of European regulatory affairs', PharmExec.Com, accessed 15 August 2010 at http://pharmexec.findpharma. com/pharmexec/Europe/The-Changing-Face-of-European-Regulatory-Affairs/ ArticleStandard/Article/detail/663632.

Lexchin, J. and O. O'Donovan (2010), 'Prohibiting or "managing" conflict of interest? A review of policies and procedures in three European drug regulation agencies', *Social Science & Medicine*, **70** (5): 643–7.

Lexchin, J., L.A. Bero, B. Djulbegovic and O. Clark (2003), 'Pharmaceutical industry sponsorship and research outcome and quality: systematic review', *British Medical Journal*, **326** (7400): 1167–70.

Mackta, J. and J.O. Weiss (1994), 'The role of genetic support groups', *Journal of Obstetric, Gynecologic, & Neonatal Nursing*, **23** (6): 519–23.

Marshall, J. and P. Aldhous (2006), 'Swallowing the best advice? Does funding from industry influence US groups that are supposed to represent patients' interests?', *New Scientist*, **192** (2575): 18–22.

Medicines Australia (2010) 'Code of Conduct, Edition 16', accessed 15 August 2010. at www.medicinesaustralia.com.au/pages/page251.asp.

Mintzes, B. (2007), 'Should patient groups accept money from drug companies? No', *British Medical Journal*, **334** (7600): 935.

Moynihan, R. (2003), 'Who pays for the pizza? Redefining the relationships between doctors and drug companies 1: entanglement', *British Medical Journal*, **326** (7400): 1189–92.

Mundy, A. (2003), 'Hot flash, cold cash', *The Washington Monthly*, **35** (1): 35–9.

Nieto, A., A. Mazon, R. Pamies, J.J. Linana, A. Lanuza, F.O. Jiménez, A. Medina-Hernandez and F.J. Nieto (2007), 'Adverse effects of inhaled corticosteroids in funded and nonfunded studies', *Archives of Internal Medicine*, **167** (19): 2047–53.

Novo Nordisk (2010) 'Public affairs', accessed 15 August 2010 at http://annual report2009.novonordisk.com/social/public-affairs.aspx.

O'Donovan, O. (2005), 'Time to weed out the Astroturf from the grassroots? Conceptualizing the implications of pharmaceutical industry funding of health advocacy organizations', paper presented at 'Concepts of the Third Sector: The European Debate', ISTR/EMES Conference, Paris, 27–29 April.

O'Donovan, O. (2007), 'Corporate colonization of health activism? Irish health advocacy organizations' modes of engagement with pharmaceutical corporations', *International Journal of Health Services*, **37** (4): 711–33.

PatientView (2008), 'The pharmaceutical industry: a global survey of patient groups – part 1', *Health and Social Campaigners' News International*, **46**: 6–42.

PatientView (2009), 'The pharmaceutical industry: a global survey of patient groups – part 2', *Health and Social Campaigners' News International*, **47**: 4–41.

Perehudoff, S.K. and T.L. Alves (2010), 'Patient and consumer organisations at the European Medicines Agency: financial disclosure and transparency', Health Action International (HAI) Europe, accessed 15 August at www.haieurope.org.

Smits, R.E.H.M. and W.P.C. Boon (2008), 'The role of users in innovation in the pharmaceutical industry', *Drug Discovery Today*, **13** (7–8): 353–9.

Sunder Rajan, K. (2006), *Biocapital: The Constitution of Postgenomic Life*, Durham, NC: Duke University Press.

Terry, S.F., P.F. Terry, K.A. Rauen, J. Uitto and L. Bercovitch (2007), 'Advocacy groups as research organizations: the PXE international example', *Nature Reviews Genetics*, **8** (2): 157–64.

Ward, P.R., J. Thompson, R. Barber, C.J. Armitage, J.D. Boote, C.L. Cooper and G.L. Jones (2010), 'Critical perspectives on "consumer involvement" in health research: epistemology dissonance and the know-do gap'. *Journal of Sociology*, **46** (1): 63–82.

Yank. V., D. Rennie and L.A. Bero (2007), 'Financial ties and concordance between results and conclusions in meta-analyses: retrospective cohort study', *British Medical Journal*, **335** (7631): 1202–5.

Index